Cellular and Cytokine Networks in Tissue Immunity

PROGRESS IN LEUKOCYTE BIOLOGY

TITLES IN THE SERIES

Volume 1: **Viral Mechanisms of Immunosuppression,** Norbert Gilmore and Mark A. Wainberg, Editors

Volume 2: **The Physiologic, Metabolic, and Immunologic Actions of Interkeukin-1,** Matthew J. Kluger, Joost J. Oppenheim, and Michael C.Powanda, *Editors*

Volume 3: **Genetic Control of Host Resistance to Infection and Malignancy,** Emil Skamene, *Editor*

Volume 4: **Macrophage Biology,** Sherwood Reichard and Mizu Kojima, *Editors*

Volume 5: **Leukocytes and Host Defense,** Joost J. Oppenheim and Diane M. Jacobs, *Editors*

Volume 6: **Immunopharmacology of Infectious Diseases: Vaccine Adjuvants and Modulators of Non-Specific Resistance,** Jeannine A. Majde, *Editor*

Volume 7: **Antigen Presenting Cells: Diversity, Differentiation, and Regulation,** Lawrence B. Schook and John G. Tew, *Editors*

Volume 8: **Monokines and Other Non-Lymphocytic Cytokines,** Michael C. Powanda, Joost J. Oppenheim, Matthew J. Kluger, and Charles A. Dinarello, *Editors*

Volume 9: **Cellular Basis of Immune Modulation,** J. Gordin Kaplan, Douglas R. Green, and R. Chris Bleackley, *Editors*

Volume 10A: **Molecular and Cellular Biology of Cytokines,** Joost J. Oppenheim, Michael C. Powanda, Matthew J. Kluger, and Charles A. Dinarello, *Editors*

Volume 10B: **The Physiological and Pathological Effects of Cytokines,** Charles A. Dinarello, Matthew J. Kluger, Michael C. Powanda, and Joost J. Oppenheim, *Editors*

Volume 11: **Cellular and Cytokine Networks in Tissue Immunity,** Monte S. Meltzer and Alberto Mantovani, *Editors*

Cellular and Cytokine Networks in Tissue Immunity

Proceedings of the 12th International RES Congress and the 27th Annual Meeting of the Society for Leukocyte Biology, Held in Heraklion, Crete, Greece, October 14–18, 1990

Editors

Monte S. Meltzer
Department of Cellular Immunology
Walter Reed Institute of Research
Rockville, Maryland

Alberto Mantovani
Laboratory of Immunology
Institute of Pharmacological Research "Mario Negri"
Milan, Italy

WILEY-LISS

A JOHN WILEY & SONS, INC., PUBLICATION
NEW YORK • CHICHESTER • BRISBANE • TORONTO • SINGAPORE

Address all Inquiries to the Publisher
Wiley-Liss, Inc., 605 Third Avenue, New York, NY 10158-0012

Printed in United States of America

Library of Congress Cataloging-in-Publication Data

International Union of Reticuloendothelial Societies. International Congress (12th : 1990 : Hērakleion, Greece)
Cellular and cytokine networks in tissue immunity : proceedings of the 12th International RES Congress and the 27th Annual Meeting of the Society for Leukocyte Biology, held in Hērakleion, Crete, Greece, October 14-18, 1990 / editors, Monte Meltzer, Alberto Mantovani.
p. cm. -- (Progress in leutocyte biology ; v. 11)
Includes bibliographical references.
Includes index.
ISBN 0-471-56097-9
1. Cytokines--Congresses. 2. Second messengers (Biochemistry)--Congresses. 3. Inflammation--Mediators--Congresses. 4. Cellular immunity--Congresses. I. Meltzer, Monte. II. Mantovani, Alberto. III. Society for Leukocyte Biology. Meeting (27th : 1990 : Hērakleion, Greece) IV. Title. V. Series.
[DNLM: 1. Cytokines--congresses. 2. Immune System--congresses. 3. Immunity, Cellular--congresses. W1 PR6703 v. 11 / QW 700 I618c 1990]
QR185.8.C95I575 1990
616.07'9--dc20
DNLM/DLC
for Library of Congress 91-7464
CIP

Contents

Contributors

James P. Allison, Cancer Research Laboratory, Department of Molecular and Cellular Biology, University of California, Berkeley, Berkeley CA 94720 [37]

J. Andrew Alspaugh, Department of Medicine, Duke University School of Medicine, Durham NC 27710 [241]

Tommy Andersson, Department of Cell Biology, Faculty of Health Sciences, University of Linköping, S-58185 Linköping, Sweden [265]

Barbara A. Araneo, Department of Pathology, University of Utah School of Medicine, Salt Lake City UT 84132 [77]

Meir Aridor, Department of Clinical Immunology, The Weizmann Institute of Science, Rehovot 76100, Israel [169]

Lisa M. Baca, Department of Cellular Immunology, Walter Reed Army Institute of Research, Rockville MD 20850 [205]

Andrea Baiocchini, Section of Pathological Anatomy, Department of Human Biopathology, University of Rome, "La Sapienza," I-00161 Rome, Italy [289]

Eddy G. Balentien, Departments of Cell Biology and Medicine, Vanderbilt University, Nashville TN 37221 [111]

Carlo D. Baroni, Section of Pathological Anatomy, Department of Human Biopathology, University of Rome, "La Sapienza," I-00161 Rome, Italy [289]

Gianfranco Bazzoni, Laboratory of Vascular Biology, Istituto di Ricerche Farmacologiche "Mario Negri," I-20157 Milan, Italy [195]

Robert M. Bell, Department of Biochemistry, Duke University Medical Center, Durham NC 27710 [157]

Edward Bernton, Neuropharmacology Branch, Department of Medical Neuroscience, Division of Neuropsychiatry, Walter Reed Army Institute of Research, Washington DC 20307 [69]

Riccardo Bertini, Istituto di Ricerche Farmacologiche "Mario Negri," I-20157 Milano, Italy [131]

Alfons Billiau, Laboratory of Immunobiology, Rega Institute for Medical Research, University of Leuven, B-3000 Leuven, Belgium [131]

Diana Boraschi, Laboratory of Immunopharmacology, Sclavo Research Center, I-53100 Siena, Italy [283]

Manfred Brockhaus, Central Research Units, Hoffmann-LaRoche, Ltd., CH-4002 Basel, Switzerland [325]

Hal E. Broxmeyer, Departments of Medicine and Microbiology/Immunology, Walther Oncology Center, Indiana University School of Medicine, Indianapolis IN 46202 [31]

Miriam L. Cameron, Department of Medicine, Duke University School of Medicine, Durham NC 27710 [241]

The numbers in brackets are the opening page numbers of the contributors' articles.

Debra Chester Kalter, Department of Cellular Immunology, WRAIR and H.M. Jackson Foundation, Walter Reed Army Institute of Research, Rockville MD 20850 **[205, 213]**

Matthias Clauss, Department of Physiology, College of Physicians and Surgeons, Columbia University, New York NY 10032 **[177]**

René Conings, Laboratory of Immunobiology, Rega Institute for Medical Research, University of Leuven, B-3000 Leuven, Belgium **[131]**

George W. Cox, Laboratory of Molecular Immunoregulation, Biological Response Modifiers Program, National Cancer Institute, Frederick Cancer Research and Development Center, Frederick MD 21702-1201 **[301]**

Robert M. Crawford, Department of Cellular Immunology, Walter Reed Army Institute of Research, Rockville MD 20850 **[235]**

Jitendra Dave, Neuropharmacology Branch, Department of Medical Neuroscience, Division of Neuropsychiatry, Walter Reed Army Institute of Research, Washington DC 20307 **[69]**

Raymond A. Daynes, Department of Pathology, University of Utah School of Medicine, Salt Lake City UT 84132 **[77]**

Benny Decock, Laboratory of Immunobiology, Rega Institute for Medical Research, University of Leuven, B-3000 Leuven, Belgium **[131]**

Elisabetta Dejana, Laboratory of Vascular Biology, Istituto di Ricerche Farmacologiche "Mario Negri," I-20157 Milan, Italy **[195]**

Zlatko Dembic, Central Research Units, Hoffmann-LaRoche, Ltd., CH-4002 Basel, Switzerland **[325]**

John Didsbury, Department of Medicine, Duke University Medical Center, Durham NC 27710 **[137]**

Carl Dieffenbach, Department of Pathology, Uniformed Services University of Health Sciences, Bethesda MD 20814 **[205]**

Ian Dransfield, Macrophage Laboratory, Imperial Cancer Research Fund, London WC2A 3PX, England **[253]**

Jean-Claude Drapier, Unite 196 INSERM "Interferons et Cytokines," Section de Biologie, Institut Curie, 75005 Paris, France **[229]**

David F. Eierman, Department of Obstetrics and Gynecology, University of North Carolina, Chapel Hill NC 27599 **[259]**

Igor Espinoza-Delgado, Laboratory of Molecular Immunoregulation, Biological Response Modifiers Program, National Cancer Institute, Frederick Cancer Research and Development Center, Frederick MD 21702-1201 **[301]**

Michael A. Farrar, Department of Pathology, Washington University School of Medicine, St. Louis MO 63105 **[337]**

Jose Fernandez-Luna, Department of Pathology, Washington University School of Medicine, St. Louis MO 63105; present address:, Seccion de Immunologia Hospital, "Marques de Valdecilla," E-39008 Santander, Spain **[337]**

Adriano Fontana, Section of Clinical Immunology, Department of Neurosurgery, University Hospital, CH-8044 Zurich, Switzerland **[91]**

Anne H. Fortier, Department of Cellular Immunology, Walter Reed Army Institute of Research, Rockville MD 20850, **[235,277]**

Karl Frei, Section of Clinical Immunology, Department of Neurosurgery, University Hospital, CH-8044 Zurich, Switzerland **[91]**

Robert M. Friedman, Department of Pathology, Uniformed Services University of Health Sciences, Bethesda MD 20814 **[205]**

Hernando Garcia, Departments of Medicine and Microbiology/Immunology, University of Miami School of Medicine, Miami FL 33101 **[63]**

Howard E. Gendelman, Department of Cellular Immunology, WRAIR and H.M. Jackson Foundation, Walter Reed Army Institute of Research, Rockville MD 20850 **[205,213]**

Reiner Gentz, Central Research Units, Hoffmann-LaRoche, Ltd., CH-4002 Basel, Switzerland **[325]**

Alan M. Gewirtz, Departments of Pathology and Internal Medicine, University of Pennsylvania School of Medicine, Philadelphia PA 19104 **[7]**

Paolo Ghiara, Laboratory of Immunopharmacology, Sclavo Research Center, I-53100 Siena, Italy **[283]**

Donald L. Granger, Division of Infectious Diseases, Department of Medicine, Duke University School of Medicine, Durham NC 27710 **[221,241]**

Patrick W. Gray, ICOS Corporation, Bothell WA 98021 **[337]**

Shawn J. Green, Department of Cellular Immunology, Walter Reed Army Institute of Research, Rockville MD 20850 **[235,271]**

Sergio Grinstein, Department of Cell Biology, Hospital for Sick Children Research Institute, Toronto, Ontario, Canada M5G 1X8 **[151,163]**

Ueli Gubler, Roche Research Center, Hoffmann-LaRoche, Inc., Nutley NJ 07110 **[325]**

Judy Guffee, Departments of Medicine and Microbiology/Immunology, University of Miami School of Medicine, Miami FL 33101 **[63]**

Yusuf A. Hannun, Department of Medicine, Duke University Medical Center, Durham NC 27710 **[157]**

Stephen Haskill, Departments of Obstetrics and Gynecology, and Microbiology and Immunology, Lineberger Comprehensive Cancer Center, University of North Carolina, Chapel Hill NC 27599 **[259]**

Wendy L. Havran, Cancer Research Laboratory, Department of Molecular and Cellular Biology, University of California, Berkeley, Berkeley CA 94720 **[37]**

Yann Henry, Unite 219 INSERM "Biophysique Moleculaire," Section de Biologie, Institut Curie, Batiment Universitaire, 91405 Orsay, France **[229]**

John B. Hibbs, Jr., Division of Infectious Diseases, Department of Medicine, Veterans Affairs Medical Center, University of Utah School of Medicine, Salt Lake City UT 84132 **[221,241]**

Nancy Hogg, Macrophage Laboratory, Imperial Cancer Research Fund, London WC2A 3PX, England **[253]**

Maureen Howard, DNAX Research Institute, Palo Alto CA 94304, **[331]**

Christopher C.W. Hughes, Department of Pathology, Brigham and Women's Hospital, Harvard Medical School, Boston MA 02115 **[183]**

Dominique Kaiserlian, Hôpital E. Herriot, 69437 Lyon, cedex 03, France **[55]**

Irene R. Katz, Department of Pathology, Kaplan Cancer Center, New York University Medical Center, New York NY 10016 **[117]**

Gurjit Khurana Hershey, Department of Pathology, Washington University School of Medicine, St. Louis MO 63105 **[337]**

Michael E. Kleinberg, Division of Infectious Diseases, University of Maryland School of Medicine, Baltimore MD 21201 **[247]**

Andreas Köck, LBI-DVS, Laboratory of Cellbiology, Department of Dermatology II, University of Vienna, A-1090 Vienna, Austria **[105]**

Elizabeth J. Kovacs, Department of Cell Biology, Neurobiology and Anatomy, Molecular Biology Program, Loyola University Stritch School of Medicine, Maywood IL 60153 **[307]**

Hans-Werner Lahm, Central Research Units, Hoffmann-LaRoche, Ltd., CH-4002 Basel, Switzerland **[325]**

James W. Larrick, Exploratory Research Department, Genelabs, Inc., Redwood City CA 94063 **[319]**

David A. Leiby, Department of Cellular Immunology, Walter Reed Army Institute of Research, Rockville MD 20850 **[277]**

Jean-Pierre Lenaerts, Laboratory of Immunobiology, Rega Institute for Medical Research, University of Leuven B-3000, Leuven, Belgium **[131]**

Werner Lesslauer, Central Research Units, Hoffmann-LaRoche, Ltd., CH-4002 Basel, Switzerland **[325]**

Thomas L. Leto, Bacterial Diseases Section, Laboratory of Clinical Investigation, National Institute of Allergy and Infectious Diseases, National Institutes of Health, Bethesda MD 20892 **[247]**

Daniel P. Lew, Division of Infectious Diseases, University Hospital of Geneva, CH-1211 Geneva, Switzerland **[143]**

Peter Libby, Department of Medicine, Brigham and Women's Hospital, Harvard Medical School, Boston MA 02115 **[183]**

Hansruedi Loetscher, Central Research Units, Hoffmann-LaRoche, Ltd., CH-4002 Basel, Switzerland **[325]**

Dan L. Longo, Biological Response Modifiers Program, National Cancer Institute, Frederick Cancer Research and Development Center, Frederick, MD 21702-1201 **[301]**

Thomas A. Luger, Department of Dermatology, University Munster, D-4400 Munster, Germany **[105]**

Gergely L. Lukacs, Department of Cell Biology, Hospital for Sick Children Research Institute, Toronto, Ontario, Canada M5G 1X8 **[151,163]**

Ian A. MacNeil, DNAX Research Institute, Palo Alto CA 94304 **[331]**

Harry L. Malech, Bacterial Diseases Section, Laboratory of Clinical Investigation, National Institute of Allergy and Infectious Diseases, National Institutes of Health, Bethesda MD 20892 **[247]**

Alberto Mantovani, Laboratory of Immunology, Istituto di Ricerche Farmacologiche "Mario Negri," I-20157 Milan, Italy **[131,195]**

Inés Martìn-Padura, Laboratory of Vascular Biology, Istituto di Ricerche Farmacologiche "Mario Negri," I-20157 Milan, Italy **[195]**

Anda I. Meierovics, Department of Cellular Immunology, Walter Reed Army Institute of Research, Rockville MD 20850 **[271]**

Monte S. Meltzer, Department of Cellular Immunology, Walter Reed Army Institute of Research, Rockville MD 20850 **[205,213,235]**

Jean E. Merrill, Department of Neurology, Reed Neurological Research Center, University of California, Los Angeles, School of Medicine, Los Angeles CA 90024 **[99]**

Kevin W. Moore, DNAX Research Institute, Palo Alto CA 94304 **[331]**

John G. Morgan, Exploratory Research Department, Genelabs, Inc., Redwood City CA 94063 **[319]**

Timothy R. Mosmann, Department of Immunology, University of Alberta, Edmonton, Alberta, Canada T6G 2H7 **[331]**

Carol A. Nacy, Department of Cellular Immunology, Walter Reed Army Institute of Research, Rockville MD 20850 **[235,271,277]**

David Nadal, Division of Infectious Diseases and Immunology, University Children's Hospital, CH-8032 Zurich, Switzerland **[91]**

Barbara J. Nelson, Department of Cellular Immunology, Walter Reed Army Institute of Research, Rockville MD 20850 **[271]**

Judith E. Neuman, Department of Cell Biology, Neurobiology and Anatomy, Molecular Biology Program, Loyola University Stritch School of Medicine, Maywood IL 60153 **[307]**

Janet Ng-Sikorski, Department of Cell Biology, Faculty of Health Sciences, University of Linköping, S-58185 Linköping, Sweden **[265]**

Shigeyuki Nozaki, Department of Dermatology, Showa University, Tokyo 142, Japan **[49]**

Satoshi Ogawa, Department of Physiology, College of Physicians and Surgeons, Columbia University, New York NY 10032 **[177]**

Toshiro Okazaki, Department of Biochemistry, Duke University Medical Center, Durham NC 27710 **[157]**

Inge Olsson, Department of Medicine, University Hospital, S-22185 Lund, Sweden **[265]**

Yu-Ching E. Pan, Roche Research Center, Hoffmann-LaRoche, Inc., Nutley NJ 07110 **[325]**

Catherine Pellat, Unite 196 INSERM "Interferons et Cytokines,"., Section de Biologie, Institut Curie, 75005 Paris, France **[229]**

H. Anne Pereira, Department of Microbiology and Immunology, Emory University School of Medicine, Atlanta GA 30322 **[319]**

Laura Pirami, Center of Cytopharmacology, Department of Cytopharmacology, Università degli Studi di Milano, I-20129 Milano, Italy **[313]**

Alberto Pisacane, Section of Pathological Anatomy, Department of Human Biopathology, University of Rome, "La Sapienza", I-00161 Rome, Italy **[289]**

Didier Pittet, Division of Infectious Diseases, University Hospital of Geneva, CH-1211 Geneva, Switzerland **[143]**

Jordan S. Pober, Department of Pathology, Brigham and Women's Hospital, Harvard Medical School, Boston MA 02115 **[183]**

Donatella Pomponi, Section of Pathological Anatomy, Department of Human Biopathology, University of Rome, "La Sapienza," I-00161 Rome, Italy **[289]**

Peter Ralph, Department of Cell Biology, Cetus Corporation, Emeryville CA 94608 **[15,91]**

Paola Ricciardi-Castagnoli, Center of Cytopharmacology, Department of Cytopharmacology, Università degli Studi di Milano, I-20129 Milano, Italy **[313]**

David W.H. Riches, Division of Basic Sciences, Department of Pediatrics, National Jewish Center for Immunology and Respiratory Medicine, Denver CO 80206 **[295]**

Ann Richmond, Departments of Cell Biology and Medicine, Vanderbilt University, Nashville TN 37221 **[111]**

Johan Richter, Department of Medicine, University Hospital, S-22185 Lund, Sweden **[265]**

Marco Righi, Center of Cytopharmacology, Department of Cytopharmacology, Università degli Studi di Milano, I-20129 Milano, Italy **[313]**

Daniel Rotrosen, Bacterial Diseases Section, Laboratory of Clinical Investigation, National Institute of Allergy and Infectious Diseases, National Institutes of Health, Bethesda MD 20892 **[241]**

Ori D. Rotstein, Department of Surgery, Toronto General Hospital, Institute of Medical Research, University of Toronto, Toronto, Ontario, Canada M5G 2C4 **[151,163]**

Luigi P. Ruco, Section of Pathological Anatomy, Department of Human Biopathology, University of Rome, "La Sapienza," I-00161 Rome, Italy **[289]**

Ronit Sagi-Eisenberg, Department of Clinical Immunology, The Weizmann Institute of Science, Rehovot 76100, Israel **[169]**

Luisa Salter-Cid, Departments of Medicine and Microbiology/Immunology, University of Miami School of Medicine, Miami FL 33101 **[63]**

Marica Sassano, Center of Cytopharmacology, Department of Cytopharmacology, Università degli Studi di Milano, I-20129 Milano, Italy **[313]**

Daniel N. Sauder, Department of Dermatology, Sunnybrook Health Science Center, University of Toronto, Toronto, Ontario, Canada M4N 3M5 **[49]**

Caroline O.S. Savage, Department of Pathology, Brigham and Women's Hospital, Harvard Medical School, Boston MA 02115; present address: Vascular Biology Section, Clinical Research Centre, Middlesex HA1 3UJ, England **[183]**

Elisabeth Schauer, LBI-DVS, Laboratory of Cellbiology, Department of Dermatology II, University of Vienna, A-1090 Vienna, Austria **[105]**

Frederick J. Schoen, Department of Pathology, Brigham and Women's Hospital, Harvard Medical School, Boston MA 02115 **[183]**

Robert D. Schreiber, Department of Pathology, Washington University School of Medicine, St. Louis MO 63110 **[277,337]**

Jens-M. Schröder, Department of Dermatology, University of Kiel, D-2300 Kiel, Germany [125]

Thomas Schwarz, Department of Dermatology, Hospital Vienna-Lainz, A-1130 Vienna, Austria [105]

Rebecca L. Shattuck, Departments of Cell Biology and Medicine, Vanderbilt University, Nashville TN 37221 [111]

Ralph Snyderman, Department of Medicine, Duke University Medical Center, Durham NC 27710 [137]

John K. Spitznagel, Department of Microbiology and Immunology, Emory University School of Medicine, Atlanta GA 30322 [319]

Ron H. Stead, Department of Pathology, McMaster University, Hamilton, Ontario, Canada L8N 3Z5 [83]

Joan Stein-Streilein, Departments of Medicine and Microbiology/Immunology, University of Miami School of Medicine, Miami FL 33101 [63]

David Stern, Department of Physiology, College of Physicians and Surgeons, Columbia University, New York NY 10032 [177]

Brigitta Stockinger, Basel Institute for Immunology, CH-4002 Basel, Switerland [313]

Antonella Stoppacciaro, Section of Pathological Anatomy, Department of Human Biopathology, University of Rome, "La Sapienza," I-00161 Rome, Italy [289]

J. Wayne Streilein, Department of Microbiology and Immunology, University of Miami School of Medicine, Miami FL 33101 [43]

Takashi Suda, DNAX Research Institute, Palo Alto CA 94304 [331]

Teresa Sukiennieckі, Exploratory Research Department, Genelabs, Inc., Redwood City CA 94063 [319]

Carol J. Swallow, Department of Surgery, Toronto General Hospital, University of Toronto, Toronto, Ontario, Canada M5G 2C4 [163]

Hisahiro Tabuchi, Central Research Units, Hoffmann-LaRoche, Ltd., CH-4002 Basel, Switzerland [325]

Aldo Tagliabue, Dompe' S.p.A., I-20122 Milano, Italy [283]

LuAnn Thompson-Snipes, DNAX Research Institute, Palo Alto CA 94304 [331]

G. Jeanette Thorbecke, Department of Pathology, Kaplan Cancer Center, New York University Medical Center, New York NY 10016 [117]

Jim A. Turpin, Department of Cellular Immunology, Walter Reed Army Institute of Research, Rockville MD 20850 [205]

Jo Van Damme, Laboratory of Immunobiology, Rega Institute for Medical Research, University of Leuven, B-3000 Leuven, Belgium [131]

Christian Van Delden, Division of Infectious Diseases, University Hospital of Geneva, CH-1211 Geneva, Switzerland [143]

Luigi Varesio, Laboratory of Molecular Immunoregulation, Biological Response Modifiers Program, National Cancer Institute, Frederick Cancer Research and Development Center, Frederick MD 21702-1201 [301]

Malcolm L. Watson, Department of Applied Pharmacology, National Heart and Lung Institute, London SW3 6LY, England [189]

Timothy J. Williams, Department of Applied Pharmacology, National Heart and Lung Institute, London SW3 6LY, England **[189]**

Yu-Chung Yang, Departments of Medicine and Biochemistry/ Molecular Biology, Walther Oncology Center, Indiana University School of Medicine, Indianapolis IN 46202 **[1]**

Albert Zlotnik, DNAX Research Institute, Palo Alto CA 94304 **[331]**

Marjorie B. Zucker, Department of Pathology, Kaplan Cancer Center, New York University Medical Center, New York NY 10016 **[117]**

Cellular and Cytokine Networks in Tissue Immunity, pages 1-6

Molecular Cloning and Characterization of Two Newly Isolated Cytokines, Human Interleukin-9 and Interleukin-11

Yu-Chung Yang

Departments of Medicine and Biochemistry/Molecular Biology and Walther Oncology Center, Indiana University School of Medicine, Indianapolis, IN 46202

INTRODUCTION

Hematopoietic growth factors are a group of hormones responsible for the proliferation and differentiation of blood cells. These regulatory molecules include colony stimulating factors (CSFs), interleukins (ILs), interferons, tumor necrosis factors and various tumor growth factors. The availability of purifed recombinant hematopoietic growth factors, molecular probes for their genes, antibodies and biological assays for these proteins in recent years has not only facilitated our understanding of the role of these cytokines in hematopoiesis but also allowed us to discover other novel growth factors. The discussion here will focus on the identification and characterization of two recently isolated cytokines, namely human IL-9 and IL-11.

IDENTIFICATION AND CLONING OF HUMAN IL-9 AND IL-11

Human IL-9 was first identified based on the ability of this cytokine to stimulate the proliferation of a human megakaryocytic leukemic cell line, MO7E. This cell line was derived from the peripheral blood of an infant with acute megakaryoblastic leukemia and displays several early markers for erythromegakaryoblastic hematopoietic precursors (1). Because of the phenotype of these cells, it was particularly interesting to determine whether they could respond to known or new growth factors and the role of these gorwth factors in regulating erythroid or megakaryocytic differentiation. MO7E cells were found to be highly responsive to granulocyte/macrophage colony-stimulating factor (GM-CSF) and

IL-3. Analysis of the conditioned medium from a human T-cell leukemia virus type I (HTLV-I) transformed T cell line, C5MJ2 (9), indicated that these cells produce an MO7E-growth promoting factor activity distinct from the known cytokines. The cDNA encoding this novel cytokine has been isolated (20) using the functional expression cloning in mammalian cells (21) and was found to have striking similarity to the newly identified murine T cell growth factor, P40 (18). Mouse P40 and this newly isolated human homologue are now designated as IL-9.

The cDNA encoding human IL-11 was isolated from a IL-1 induced human fetal lung fibroblast cell line, MRC-5, by hybridization with a primate IL-11 cDNA probe (15). The primate IL-11 cDNA was originally isolated from a IL-1 induced primate bone marrow-derived stromal cell line, PU-34 (16), by expression cloning method based on the ability of this cytokine to stimulate the proliferation of a IL-6-dependent mouse plasmacytoma cell line (14). PU-34 cell line has been shown to be capable of supporting long-term hemopoiesis as measured by in vitro progenitor assays (16).

MOLECULAR AND BIOLOGICAL CHARACTERIZATION OF HUMAN IL-9 AND IL-11

The nucleotide sequences of human IL-9 and IL-11 cDNAs have been determined and they contain open reading frames of 432 and 597 nucleotides, respectively (15,20). Interestingly, all of the cysteine residues present in human IL-9 aligned with those present in mouse homologue indicating the conservation of tertiary structure of these two proteins. IL-11, on the other hand, encodes no cysteine residue.

Although mouse IL-9, P40, was originally identified based on its ability to support the growth of certain mouse helper T cell clones (18) and can stimulate the mast cell growth elicited by IL-3 or IL-4 (6, 12), these activities have not been successfully demonstrated in the human system. The biological activities of human IL-11 examined so far indicated that IL-11 acts very similarly to another cytokine, IL-6. It is possible that these two cytokines may use similar signal transduction pathway or they may even share common receptor(s).

Table I. Molecular and Biological Characteristics of Human IL-9.

Properties	References
Isolation: cDNA encoding human IL-9 was isolated from a HTLV-I- transformed human T cell line by expression cloning.	20
Sources: Activated human Peripheral Blood Lymphocytes (PBLs); HTLV-I or II-transformed human T cell lines	20
Gene: Location: 5q31-32	7
Structure: Five exons and four introns	
Size: 4.6 kb	
mRNA: Size: 0.8 kb	20
Expression: Constitutive expression in HTLV-I or II-transformed human T cell lines; induced expression in activated PBLs (TPA/PHA) and induced HTLV-transformed T cells (TPA).	7,20
Protein: Size: 20-30 kD	20
pI: 10.0	
Glycosylation: Highly	
Disulfide bond: Many	
Biological activities:	
(1) Stimulates the proliferation of a human megakaryocytic leukemic cell line, Mo7E.	20
(2) Supports erythroid colony formation in vitro.	4,5, 10,19
(3) T cell growth factor activity?	18
(4) Mast cell enhancing activity? Human IL-9.	6,12

Other molecular and biological properties of these two cytokines are summarized in Table I and II.

DISCUSSION

The cloning of human IL-9 and IL-11 will now allow us to produce large quantities of these hematopoietins to study their in vitro activities and evaluate their biological effects in vivo. The availability of their respective genes will also allow us to study the control of gene expression in different cell types. Studies like these should help us understand the role of these growth factors in the complicated cytokine network.

Table II. Molecular and Biological Characteristics of Human IL-11

Properties		References
Isolation: cDNA encoding human IL-11 was isolated from a IL-1 induced human fetal lung fibroblast cell line using primate IL-11 cDNA as the probe; cDNA encoding primate IL-11 was isolated from a IL-1 induced primate bone marrow-derived stromal cell line by expression cloning.		15
Sources: Human fetal lung fibroblast cell line, MRC-5; human trophoblast cell line, TPA 30-1; primate bone marrow-derived stromal cell line, PU-34.		15
Gene:	Location: 19q13 Structure: Five exons and four introns Size: 7.5 kb	11
mRNA:	Size: 2.5 and 1.5 kb Expression: (1) Constitutive expression in TPA 30-1 (only 2.5 kb); (2) Induced expression in MRC-5 (IL-1/TPA induced) and PU-34 (IL-1 induced)	15
Protein:	Size: 23 kD pI: 11.5 Glycosylation: None Disulfide bond: None	
Biological activities:		
	(1) Stimulates the proliferation of a IL-6-dependent mouse plasmacytoma cell line, T1165.	15
	(2) Synergizes with IL-3 in supporting megakaryocyte colony formation in vitro.	3,8 15
	(3) Stimulates the T-cell dependent-development of immunoglobulin-producing B cells.	2,15
	(4) Acts synergistically with IL-3 to shorten the Go period of early progenitors.	13

ACKNOWLEDGEMENT

We thank Becki Rohling for preparing the manuscript.

REFERENCES

1. Avanzi GC, Lista P, Giovinazzo B, Miniero R, Saglio G, Benetton G, Coda R, Cattoretti G, Pegoraro L (1988). Selective growth response to IL-3 of a human leukemic cell line with megakaryoblastic features. Br J Haematol 69: 359-366.

2. Barut B, Morimoto C, Paul S, Williams D, Anderson K (1990). Interleukin 11 augments immunoglobulin secretion through selective stimulation of the T cell helper inducer (CD4+CD45RA-) subset. Blood 76: 201a.

3. Briddell RA, Bruno E, Cooper RJ, Yang YC, Clark SC, Hoffman R (1990). The effect of interleukin-11 on in vitro human megakaryocytopoiesis. Blood 76: 448a.

4. Donahue RE, Yang YC, Clark SC (1990). Human P40 T-cell growth factor (interleukin-9) supports erythroid colony formation. Blood 75: 2271-2275.

5. Holbrook ST, Ohls RK, Schibler KR, Yang YC, Christensen RD (1991). Effects of interleukin-9 on clonogenic maturation and cell-cycle status of fetal and adult hematopoietic progenitors. Blood, in press.

6. Hultner L, Druez C, Moeller J, Schmitt E, Uyttenhove C, Rude E, Dormer P, Van Snick J (1990). Mast cell growth enhancing activity (MEA) is structurally related and functionally identical to the novel mouse T cell growth factor P40/TCGFIII. Eur J Immunol, in press.

7. Kelleher K, Bean K, Clark SC, Leung WY, Yang-Feng TL, Chen JW, Lin PF, Luo W, Yang YC (1991). Human IL-9: Genomic sequence, chromosomal location and sequences essential for its expression in HTLV-I-transformed human T cells. Blood, in press.

8. Larson D, Leary A, Hahn-Cordes L, Fitagerald M, Giannoti J, Sibley B, Bennett F, Calvetti J, Turner K, Clark SC (1990). Interleukin-11 (IL-11) synergizes with IL-3 in promoting human and murine megakaryocyte colony formation in vitro. Blood 76: 464a.

9. Leary AG, Ogawa M (1987). Blast cell colony assay for umbilical cord blood and adult bone marrow progenitors. Blood 69: 953-956.

10. Lu L, Leemhuis T, Srour EF, Yang YC (1991). Effect of human interleukin-9 on highly enriched erythroid progenitors in normal human bone marrow under serum-containing and serum-depleted culture conditions. J Immunol, submitted.

11. McKinley D, Wu Q, Yang-Feng TL, Yang YC (1991). Genomic sequence and chromosomal localization of human IL-11. In preparation.

12. Moeller J, Hultner L, Schmit E, Breuer M, Dormer P (1990). Purification of MEA, a mast cell growth-enhancing activity, to apparent homogeneity and its partial amino acid

sequence. J Immunol 144: 4231-4234.
13. Musashi M, Yang YC, Paul SR, Clark SC, Sudo T, Ogawa M (1991). Direct and synergistic effects of interleukin-11 on murine hemopoiesis in culture. Proc Natl Acad Sci USA, in press.
14. Nordan RP, Potter M (1986). A machrophage-derived factor required by plasmacytomas for survival and proliferation in vitro. Science 233: 566-569.
15. Paul SR, Bennett F, Calvetti JA, Kelleher K, Wood CR, O'Hara RM, Leary AC, Sibley B, Clark SC, Williams DA, Yang YC (1990). Molecular cloning of a cDNA encoding interleukin 11, a stromal cell-derived lymphopoietic and hematopoietic cytokine. Proc Natl Acad Sci USA 87: 7512-7516.
16. Paul SR, Yang YC, Donahue RE, Goldring S, Williams DA (1991). Stromal cell associated hematopoiesis: Immortalization and characterization of primate bone marrow-derived stromal cell lines. Blood, in press.
17. Uyttenhove C, Simpson RJ, Van Snick J (1988). Functional and structural characterization of P40, a mouse glycoprotein with T-cell growth factor activity. Proc Natl Acad Sci USA 85: 6934-6938.
18. Van Snick J, Goethals A, Renauld JC, Van Roost E, Uyttenhove C, Rubira MR, Moritz RL, Simpson RJ (1989). Cloning and characterization of a cDNA for a new mouse T cell growth factor (P40). J Exp Med 169: 363-368.
19. Williams DE, Morrissey PJ, Mochizuki DY, de Vries P, Anderson D, Cosman D, Boswell HS, Cooper S, Grabstein KH, Broxmeyer HE (1990). T-cell growth factor P40 promotes the proliferation of myeloid cell lines and enhances erythroid burst formation by normal murine bone marrow cells in vitro. Blood 76: 906-911.
20. Yang YC, Ricciardi S, Ciarletta A, Calvetti J, Kelleher K, Clark SC (1989). Expression cloning of a cDNA encoding a novel human hematopoietic growth factor: Human homologue of murine T-cell growth factor P40. Blood 74: 1880-1884.
21. Yang YC, Ciarletta AB, Temple PA, Chung MP, Kovacic S, Witek-Giannoti JS, Leary AC, Kriz R, Donahue RE, Wong GG, Clark SC (1986). Human IL-3 (multi-CSF): Identification by expression cloning of a novel hematopoietic growth factor related to murine IL-3. Cell 47: 3-10.

Cellular and Cytokine Networks in
Tissue Immunity, pages 7-13

Antisense Oligodeoxynucleotides as Probes for Studying the Molecular Regulation of Hematopoietic Cell Proliferation

Alan M. Gewirtz

Depts. of Pathology and Medicine, University of Pennsylvania School of Medicine, Philadelphia, PA 19104

INTRODUCTION

The study of hematopoiesis has been greatly facilitated by the advent of in vitro systems for culturing stem/progenitor cells, and by the increasing availability of a large number of molecularly cloned hematopoietic growth factors (Nicola, 1989). With these tools, the factors and events which regulate the developmental flow of hematopoietic stem cells into mature blood cells has begun to be better defined (Leary et al, 1989). Nevertheless, the factor(s) which stimulate stem cells to enter the cell cycle, or undergo lineage committment are essentially unknown, as are their mechanism(s) of action. Accordingly, it would be of great interest to study the effect of recombinant growth factors and other cytokines on the expression of cell cycle and cell proliferation related genes during the course of hematopoietic cell development.

Such studies have heretofore been impossible on normal hematopoietic progenitor cells because of their rarity, and difficulties in purification. However, the advent of several recent technologic advances, including the use of antisense oligodeoxynucleotides to study the role of specific genes in regulating cell proliferation (reviewed in van der Krol et al, 1988) now make such studies possible. Below I summarize a few illustrative examples of how I and my collaborator at the Temple University School of Medicine in Philadelphia, Dr. Bruno Calabretta, have utilized this technique to study the molecular regulation of normal human hematopoietic progenitor cell proliferation.

METHODS

Cells. Light density mononuclear cells (MNC) were obtained from consenting normal donors by Ficoll-Hypaque density gradient centrifugation and enriched for hematopoietic progenitors as previously described (Carraciolo et al, 1990).

Human leukemia cell lines, HL-60, ML-3, KG-1, and KG-1a were obtained from the American Type Culture Collection or as described (Anfossi et al, 1989).

Hematopoietic colony assays. Hematopoietic cell colonies were cloned in plasma clot culture (Gewirtz and Calabretta, 1988), or in methylcellulose (Carraciolo et al, 1990). Colonies were scored after 14-16 d of culture in a humidified 5% CO_2 incubator. CFU-E and G-CSF-stimulated granulocytic colonies were scored at 7-9 d of culture. To determine colony size, 30 consecutive individual colonies from each plate were plucked from methylcellulose, dispersed in tissue culture medium, and then counted in a hemocytometer. Cells in smaller colonies were counted directly in the plates.

Oligodeoxynucleotides. Unmodified, 18-base oligodeoxynucleotides were made on a DNA synthesizer (model 380B, Applied Biosystems Inc., Foster City, CA) by means of β-cyanoethyl-phosphorymidite chemistry. Oligodeoxynucleotides were purified by ethanol precipitation and multiple washes in 70% ethanol. They were subsequently lyophilized to dryness andredissolved in culture medium at a concentration of 1 mg/ml. The sequences of the *c-myb* and *c-abl* antisense oligomers employed for these studies are published (Gewirtz and Calabretta, 1988; Carraciolo et al, 1989).

Oligomer treatment of cells. MNC or leukemia cells from were incubated in tissue culture medium in polypropylene tubes (Falcon Plastics, Cockeysville, MD) in the presence of optimal concentrations of the relevant hematopoietic growth factor (Gewirtz and Calabretta, 1988; Anfossi et al, 1989; Carraciolo et al, 1989). Some cultures were also supplemented with either sense or antisense oligomers for 18 h at final concentrations up to ~ 17.5 μM. Cells placed into semi-solid medium were not washed before plating. Control cultures were left untreated.

Detection of c-myb and c-abl mRNA in bone marrow cells by reverse transcriptase-polymerase chain reaction (RT-PCR) analysis. Expression of *c-myb* and c-abl mRNA in oligomer treated and control cells was performed as published (Gewirtz et al, 1989; Carraciolo et al, 1989). In brief, cells were collected at the end of the required time of culture and total RNA was extracted in the presence of 20 μg of *Escherichia coli* ribosomal RNA. RNA was then reverse-transcribed and the resulting cDNA fragments were amplified with 7.5 U of *Thermus aquaticus* (Taq) polymerase in the presence of *c-myb* or cabl mRNA sequence-specific synthetic primers. 10 μl of the 50-μl polymerase chain reaction was separated in a 4% Nusieve agarose gel and transferred to a nitrocellulose filter. The resulting blot was hybridized with a synthetic [^{32}P]γ-ATP end-labeled oligomer complementary to the amplified *c-myb* or *c-abl* DNA.

Detection of myb and abl protein. Expression of myb and abl protein was assessed by indirect immunofluorescence as described (Gewirtz et al, 1989; Carraciolo et al, 1989). A sheep anti-human myb serum (Cambridge Research Biochemicals, Valley Stream, NY) was utilized at a 1:40 dilution. R. Arlinghaus generously provided antiserum to a c-*abl* peptide.

RESULTS

Role of c-myb encoded protein in normal human hematopoiesis: Exposure of MNC to c-myb antisense oligomers resulted in the generation of small colonies with a statistically significant decrease in total numbers of colonies formed (Gewirtz and Calabretta, 1989). The decrease in granulocyte-macrophage colony forming units (CFU-GM) in four studies was 86% (p=.018), 70% (p=.040), 43% (p=.001), and 74% (p=.001) respectively. Similar data were generated when the effect of c-myb antisense oligomers on erythroid and megakaryocyte progenitor cell growth was examined. In contrast, the c myb sense oligomer had no consistent effect on the formation of hematopoietic colonies of any lineage when compared to growth in control cultures.

We also determined if inhibition of colony formation correlated with oligomer concentration utilized. After progenitor cells were exposed to 0.3, 1.4, 7, and 14 μM of c-myb sense and anti-sense oligodeoxynucleotides, erythroid and megakaryocytic colony formation was examined. The c-myb sense oligodeoxynucleotide had no significant effect on colony formation. In contrast, there was a direct correlation between amounts of the c-myb anti-sense oligonucleotide utilized and the degree of colony inhibition. Exposure to c-myb anti-sense oligomers at the above concentrations led respectively to the formation of 21 $\pm$ 3, 17 $\pm$ 1,10 $\pm$ 2, and 4 $\pm$ 2 megakaryocyte colonies; exposure to 1.4, 7, and 14 μM concentrations of the anti-sense oligodeoxynucleotide led to the formation of 775 $\pm$ 127, 515 $\pm$ 9, and 244 $\pm$ 25 myeloid colonies.

The work just described suggests that c-myb protooncogene encodes a nuclear protein which plays a fundamental role in the development of human hematopoietic cells of the myeloid, megakaryocytic, and erythroid lineages. Since lymphocyte c-myb mRNA levels increase in response to interleukin-2, and remain high during exponential growth phase, c-myb is likely important role in regulating lymphocyte proliferation as well. We tested this hypothesis by determining if blockade of lymphocyte c-myb gene function inhibits the proliferative response to either phytohemagglutinin (PHA) or HL-A non-identical lymphocytes. Normal peripheral blood mononuclear cells

(MNC) were exposed to 18bp (codons 2-7) c-myb sense or anti-sense oligodeoxynucleotides (final concentration7μM) at 6 hrs prior to, and 24 + 48 hrs after PHA stimulation; or while culturing in presence of non-HL-A identical, mitomycin C treated MNC in a one way mixed lymphocyte reaction. Using a semi-quantitative indirect

immunofluorescence assay (see above) it was determined that the c-myb anti-sense oligomer inhibited synthesis of c-myb protein by ~90% (c-myb fluorescense intensity in untreated MNC--~10%; in PHA stimulated MNC-48±2%; in c-myb sense + PHA treated MNC-52±3%; and in c-myb anti-sense + PHA treated MNC- 16±1%). The c-myb anti-sense oligomer also reduced T lymphocyte proliferation (~90%) in response to either stimulus (Fig 1). Exposing MNC to the c-myb sense oligomer had no effect on either parameter.

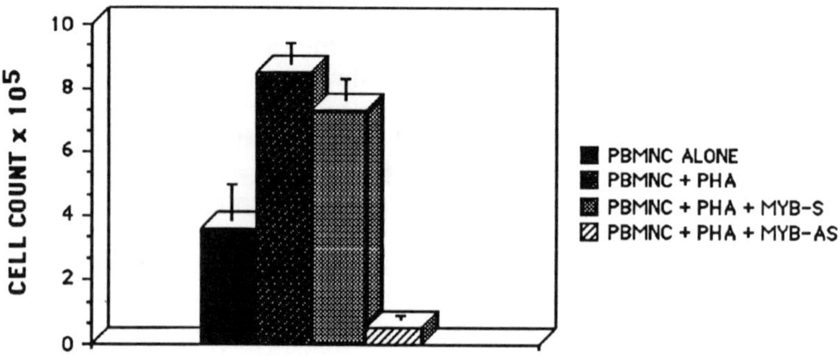

Fig. 1: Effect of c-myb oligomers on PHA stimulated lymphocyte proliferation. Cell count were determined after five days of culture under the condtions indicated in the figure key.

Flow cytometric analysis of MNC labeled with monoclonal antibodies to either the interleukin-2 or transferrin receptor revealed that neither the anti-sense nor sense oligomers affected the expression of either activation marker in PHA stimulated cells. These results suggested that initial cell activation events were unperturbed. However, in situ hybridization studies of anti-sense treated lymphocytes demonstrated a marked decrease in histone H3 mRNA expression , and analysis of DNA content revealed that while c-myb sense treated cells doubled their DNA content after PHA stimulation, the c-myb anti-sense oligomer prevented this occurrence. We conclude that c-myb plays a direct role in regulating normal human T lymphocyte proliferation, and suggest that it is most important in late G1 or early S phase of the cell cycle since inhbition of c-myb protein synthesis appears to prevent subsequent progression through the S/G2 phase of the cell cycle.

c-myb and Megakaryocyte Polyploidization

Since c-myb is expressed in a cell cycle dependent manner and is active in cells that are undergoing DNA synthesis, we have also sought to determine if the myb gene plays an important role in the process of endoreduplication. To address this question normal mature human

megakaryocytes were isolated from bone marrow aspirates by centrifugal elutriation. Cells were then incubated for 24 to 36 hours alone, in the presence of IL-3 (100 U/ml) and IL-6 (300 ng/ml), or the two growth factors plus c-myb sense or antisense oligomers. After incubation, cells were harvested and DNA content measured in arbitrary fluorescence intensity (AFI) units as described (Anfossi et al, 1989). Analysis of >250 cells obtained from a total of three separate bone marrow samples revealed a mean fluorescence intensity of 51 ± 1.4 units. In the presence of the growth factors the expected rightward ploidy shift occurred so that the mean DNA content increased to ~58 ± 1.5 AFI units (n=286; p=.002). Addition of c-myb sense oligomers did not prevent the growth factor mediated shift in ploidy and in fact appeared to augment it slightly. Measurement of cells exposed to the myb sense oligomers during the course of the three experiments revealed a DNA content of 63 ±1.7 AFI units. In contrast to these results, the presence of the c-myb antisense oligomers completely blocked the growth factor induced increase in ploidy so that the mean DNA content of megakaryocytes in this groups was 51 ± 1.3 AFI units (compared to myb sense- p<.001; compared to control- p=.946).

Leukemic cell proliferation and c-myb function

To determine whether the treatment with c-myb anti-sense modified cell cycle distribution of HL-60 cells, we measured the DNA content in exponentially growing cells exposed to either either sense or antisense myb oligomers (Anfossi et al, 1989). Control cells, and cells treated with c-myb sense had essentially equivalent DNA content values which were approximately twice those observed in HL-60 cells treated with anti-sense oligomers. The majority of these cells appeared to reside either in the the G1 compartment, or were blocked at the G1/S boundary.

It has been reported that an oligomer complementary to the first five codons fo c-myc mRNA inhibits proliferation of HL-60 cells and induces differentiation. We therefore compared the effect of two 18nt oligomers complementary to the same region (codons 2-7) in HL-60, KG-1, and KG-1a cells (Anfossi et al, 1989). In each case, c-myb anti-sense inhibited cell proliferation to a much greater extent than the c-myc anti-sense oligomer. For example, untreated HL-60 cells had a cell doubling time of 20-21 hours, c-myc antisense treated cells had a doubling time of 30-31 hours, while the c-myb anti-sense treated cells had a doubling time of 50-52 hours. Of note, the c-myc antisense effect we noted is similar to that observed by other investigators.

These findings indicate that reduction of the c-myb protein level in a number of leukemic cell types is accompanied by a substantial inhibition in their growth rate. HL-60 appeared to be most sensitive to the c-myb antisense effect suggesting that the growth advantage conferred on these cells by c-myc amplification, and by activation of N-ras, is not enough to maintain increased cell proliferation in the absence of c-myb protein.

DISCUSSION

Events which regulate normal human hematopoietic cell proliferation at the molecular level are not well defined. This lack of knowledge is ascribable to the rarity of hematopoietic progenitor cells, and the inability to apply standard molecular analytic techniques to very small numbers of cells. The recent development of molecular "micro-methodologies" such as reverse transcription PCR, the cloning of human hematopoietic growth factors, and refined techniques for growing normal hematopoietic cells in culture now make such studies possible.

We believe that the antisense approach as briefly described in this article will also assist in an important way in examining the functional significance of various genes in regulating hematopoietic and other cell type proliferation. Accordingly, further studies of the type outlined are highly likely to contribute to our understanding of the cell cycle and how the trafficing of cells through this still mysterious circular pathway occurs.

ACKNOWLEDGEMENTS: This work was supported in part by grants from the U.S. Public Health Service (CA36896, and CA01324), and a grant from the WW Smith Charitable Trust. Dr. Gewirtz is the recipient of a Research Career Development Award from the National Cancer Institute.

REFERENCES

Anfossi G, Gewirtz AM, and Calabretta B. (1989). An oligomer complementary to c-myb encoded mRNA inhibits proliferation of human myeloid leukemia cell lines. Proc. Natl. Acad. Sci. USA 86:3379-3383.

Caracciolo D, Valtieri M, Venturelli D, Peschle C, Gewirtz AM, and Calabretta B. (1989). Lineage specific requirement of c-abl function in normal hematopoiesis. Science (Wash. DC) 245:1107-1109.

Caracciolo D, Venturelli D, Valtieri M, Peachle C, Gewirtz AM and Calabretta B. (1990). Stage-related proliferative activity determines c-myb functional requirements during normal human hematopolesis. J. Clin. Invest. 85:55-61.

Gewirtz AM, and Calabretta B. (1988). A c-myb anti-sense oligodeoxynucleotide inhibits normal human hematopoiesis in vitro. Science 242:1303-1306.

Gewirtz AM, Anfossi G, Venturelli D, Valpreda D, Sims R, and Calabretta B. (1989). G1/S transition in normal human T-lymphocytes requires the nuclear protein encoded by c-myb. Science 245:180-183.

Leary AG, Hirai Y, Kishimoto T, Clark SC, and Ogawa M (1989). Survival of hemopoietic progenitors in the Go period of the cell cycle does not require early hemopoiesis regulators. Proc Natl Acad Sci USA 86:4535-4538.

Nicola N (1989). Hematopoietic cell growth factors and their receptors. Ann Rev Biochem 58:45-77.

van der Krol AR, Mol JNM, Stutije AR (1988). Modulation of gene expression by complementary RNA or DNA sequences. Biotechniques 6:958-976.

Cellular and Cytokine Networks in Tissue Immunity, pages 15-29

NEGATIVE REGULATION OF CYTOKINES - INHIBITION OF THE PRODUCTION OF IL1 AND TNF, AND A NEW FORM OF THE IL1 RECEPTOR ANTAGONIST

Peter Ralph

Department of Cell Biology, Cetus Corporation, 1400 Fifty-Third Street, Emeryville, CA 94608

INTRODUCTION

One of the most notable successes in the area of mammalian cell biology in the past decade is the identification of protein factors that regulate cellular function. Many cytokines have been cloned based on stimulatory biologic assays, mainly promotion of cell growth or DNA synthesis. These factors have taken on broader functions than originally envisaged, and methods with increased sensitivity of detection are frequently showing unusual patterns of production of factors. Further, many cells make their own stimulatory cytokines, leading to potentially autocatylic catastrophes. What limits these positive signals? Will autoregulation at the level of a tissue and even of a single cell be recognized as a common method of physiologic control?

Many cloned cytokines and other natural molecules of defined structure are now known to have down-modulatory as well as stimulatory effects. Examples are shown for inhibition of cytokine production (Table 1), cytokine-induced cellular proliferation (Table 2), and other cellular functions (Table 3). This paper will discuss two aspects of negative regulation - the inhibition of cytokine production and inhibition of cytokine activity. The experimental systems are the production of IL1 and TNF, and antagonism of IL1 effects by a recombinant protein coded by a newly discovered gene segment.

INHIBITION OF HUMAN MONOCYTE PRODUCTION OF IL1 AND TNF

We have studied several systems for induction of human IL1 and TNF production. The human monocyte-related THP-1 cell line derived from an acute monocytic leukemia patient has no background production and makes reproducibly large

TABLE 1. Identified Endogenous Inhibitors of Cytokine Production

Inhibitor	Cytokine	Event	Target Cell	Reference
Corticosteroid (CS)	Most, Ig	Production	Various	10,17,42
PGE	Most	Production	Various	7,16,43
IL4 (IL6)	IL1, TNF	Production	Mononuclear phagocyte (MNP)	5,18,23
PP14	IL2	Production	T	27
IFNγ	IL4	Induction of IgE	T	44
TGFβ	IL1	Production	MNP	24
CSIF/IL10	IFNγ, IL2	Production	MNP	45
Acidic Ferritin (FE), LF	CSFs, IL1	Production	MNP	46,47
Vitamin D3	IL2, IFNγ	Production	T	48
IFNγ	IL1	IL1 induced	MNC	49

PP14 = Placental protein 14, LF = lactoferrin

TABLE 2. Identified Endogenous Inhibitors of Cytokine-Induced Proliferation

Inhibitor	Cytokine	Target Cell	Reference
Tetra, Pentapeptide	CSFs	Myeloid progenitor	50,51
TGFβ, IFN, TNF, PGE Acidic Fe, CS	CSFs	Myeloid progenitor	47,52-54
IL1ra, sIL1-R	IL1	B, T, Th	55-57
sTNF-R	TNF	Various	58,59
sIL4-R	IL4	B, T	57,60
PF4	CSFs	CFU-Meg	61
PF4	ECGF	EC	62
IL4	IL2, BCGF, IL1, CSFs	B, T, Th, Myeloid progenitor	63-68
TGFβ	BCGF, IL1, IL2	B, Th, T	69-71
Complement Ba	BCGF	B	72
α-fetoprotein	IL2, etc.	T	73

Fe = ferritin, PF4 = platelet factor 4, CSF = myeloid colony-stimulating factor, Th = thymocyte, CFU-Meg = megakaryocyte precursor, CS = corticosteroid

TABLE 3. Identified Endogenous Inhibitors of Cytokine Action

Inhibitor	Cytokine	Event	Target Cell	Reference
IL1ra, sIL1-R	IL1	Various	B, T, fib, EC, chond.	31-34,55-57
sTNF-R	TNF	Various	Various	58,59
Calcitonin, CGRP	IFNγ	PMA-H_2O_2 Ag present	MNP	74
Epi, Ins, Somatostatin	IFNγ	TNF-R, kill M. avium	Monocytes	75
IL3, IL4	IFNγ, TNF	Cytotoxicity, FcR, H_2O_2	MNP	76-79
GM-CSF	C5a, fMLP	Chemotaxis	Neutrophil	80
IL8	IL1	PMN adhesion	EC	81
IL4, TGFβ	IL2	LAK, CTL	MNC, T	82-85
IL4	IFN	Resistance to virus	fib	86
TGFβ	TNF	EC adhesion	Neutrophil	87
TGFβ	IFN, IL4	FcεR	Myeloid	88
Thrombospondin	bFGF	Chemotaxis	EC	89

sIL1-R = soluble IL1 receptor, CGRP = calcitonin gene-related peptide, Epi = epinephrin, Ins = insulin, LAK = lymphokine-activated killer cell, CTL = cytotoxic T lymphocyte, EC = endothelial cell, fib = fibroblast, MNP = mononuclear phagocyte, MNC = blood or spleen mononuclear cells

amounts of each cytokine after dose-dependent induction with LPS (1-4). In comparison, we found that HL-60 and U937 lines did not make significant amounts of these cytokines in similar induction protocols. IFNγ and GM-CSF could enhance the productions induced by low concentrations of LPS, but generally did not induce in the absence of LPS.

Comparable levels of IL-1 and TNF are produced by human blood mononuclear cells and adherence-purified monocytes under similar inducing conditions. The blood cells have some "constitutive" production and are more variable depending on the donor (1). Previous studies have shown stimulation of TNF production in human blood mononuclear cells or monocytes by LPS, GM-CSF, IFNγ, IL-2, PMA, silica and anti-Ig (e.g., 5-10), and by LPS in total blood cells in their own plasma (heparinized whole blood) (11). There are also many studies on induction of IL1 secretion in blood cells by LPS, GM-CSF, IFNγ, IL2 and silica (e.g. 5-9,12-15). Table 4 shows the conditions we use with THP-1 or blood cells in order to screen for natural inhibitors of cytokine production. Much higher levels of IL1 and TNF can be produced with stronger inducing signals (1). IFNγ is included as a coinducer of TNF to avoid high LPS levels and to provide for a more physiological induction.

We used the THP-1 and blood cell systems to test a number of agents for modulating cytokine production. The corticosteroids and prostaglandin E are known to inhibit expression of cytokines by human mononuclear phagocytes (7,10,16-18). Dexamethasone and PGE2 strongly block the induction of IL1 and TNF production in THP-1 and blood cells (1).

IL4 (18-23) and TGFβ (24) are reported to inhibit human blood cell expression of IL1 and TNF. However, some studies find that IL4 does not block expression of IL1 transcripts (20) and TGFβ does not affect secretion of IL1 bioactivity by LPS-induced monocytes provided that TGFβ protein is removed from the monocyte supernatant before assay (25). TGFβ stimulates IL1 mRNA expression and some IL1-like bioactivities in certain conditions of monocyte culture (26). We find that IL4 and TGFβ at 10 ng/ml or less show weak or no inhibition of the secretion of IL1 and TNF by THP-1 and mononuclear cells when added at the same time as the inducer. With a 4-h preincubation, TGFβ and IL4 have moderate inhibitory effects (1). There may be several reasons for the differences between our results and the above quoted papers. a) We studied mononuclear cells whereas all the papers showing negative regulation used purified monocytes except Chantry et al. (24). b) We used low levels of inducers, less than 1 ng/ml LPS for IL1 and 10 ng/ml for TNF production by blood cells. We chose these conditions of weak factor production to enhance the sensitivity of seeing inhibitor activity. In contrast, most of the quoted papers use 100 ng/ml to 10 μg/ml LPS or other strong inducer. c) Most of

TABLE 4. Induction of Human IL1 and TNF Production

Cell	IL1 (pg/ml)		TNF (ng/ml)	
	Background	Induced	Background	Induced
		1 ng/ml LPS		20 ng/ml LPS + 100 U/ml IFNγ
THP-1	<25	45-250	<0.2	0.5-2.5
		0.5 ng/ml LPS		10 ng/ml LPS + 100 U/ml IFNγ
Blood MNC	<20-1100	65-1500	<0.2	0.8-5.5

0.2 ml THP-1 cells at 4×10^5/ml RPMI 1640 + 10% fetal bovine serum + LPS (List Biochemicals) or IFNγ (Amgen Corp., Thousand Oaks, CA) for 2 days. Donor blood mononuclear cells (MNC), 0.5-1×10^6 per 0.2 ml as for THP-1, for 1 day. Supernatant assayed for IL1β (Cistron Corp., Pine Brook, NJ) and TNF (Cetus) by Elisa (1).

the quoted papers measure the cytokines by bioactivity which could be influenced by other factors. TGFβ is reported to inhibit the readout of the mouse thymocyte coproliferation assay for IL1 (25), and TGFβ or IL4 may induce other molecules that interact in the bioassays.

IFNγ and GM-CSF, and IL1 for TNF production, enhance somewhat the output of the two cytokines above levels induced by our standard culture conditions of LPS induction. IL2, IL6, M-CSF, IL3, PDGF, and melanocyte stimulating hormone (αMSH) have little effect on IL1 and TNF production (1). IL6 is reported to have a moderate inhibitory effect on LPS-induced TNF production by U937 and monocytes (5). The presence of indomethacin to block LPS-induced PGE production enhances factor production moderately (1), as described by others for IL1, TNF (6,7,16) and M-CSF and GM-CSF expression by blood cells (16).

Other physiological molecules can inhibit IL1 or TNF production (Table 1), including placental protein 14 (PP14) (27), serum lipoproteins that act via neutralizing LPS (28), α-globulins (29), and deoxycholic acid and other bile acids by a direct action on monocytes (30).

We find that inhibitors of IL1 and TNF can be found in a number of human sources (Table 5). In the case of dialyzed febrile urine from burn or cancer patients, pleural fluids, and extracts of placentas and platelets, inhibitory activity

TABLE 5. Human Sources of Inhibitors of IL1 and TNF Production

Source	Condition	Possible Identification
Urine	febrile	?
Pleural fluid	cancer	?
Placental extract	normal	?
Platelet extract	normal	?
Cell Line		
Fibroblast		
DE551, Hs275f		PGE
Melanoma		
LD-1, Hs294T		PGE
Lung Ca		
A375		PGE
Epidermoid		
KB-1		?
Other		IL10

does not fractionate as a simple, single protein. With the supernatants of many cell lines, inhibitors are resistant to boiling, pass through a dialysis membrane, and are absent from indomethacin-treated cell. These properties suggest an eicosenoid inhibitor such as prostaglandin E2 (PGE2) (Table 5). An inhibitor in other cell lines is associated with IL10 (unpublished).

DIFFERENTIAL EFFECTS OF PGE ON MONOCYTE CYTOKINE EXPRESSION

No M-CSF gene expression is detected in freshly harvested monocytes (as in Ficoll-Hypaque purified blood mononuclear cells) or Percoll purified monocytes cultured 0-24 h in nonadherent conditions (rocking polypropylene tubes) (16,31). Monocytes purified by adherence to plastic are induced to low level expression of M-CSF. This may be due to signals resulting from adherence or from undetectably low levels of LPS or other stimulants. However, M-CSF expression during adherence appears to be self-limited by a PGE-related molecule since inclusion of 10^{-6} M indomethacin greatly increases the level of M-CSF transcripts seen 24 h later (16).

High level export of M-CSF protein from adherent monocytes requires either a classical inducer such as LPS (31) or indomethacin (16). LPS also induces G-CSF and GM-CSF expression in adherent monocytes. PGE2 inhibits levels of M-CSF and GM-CSF transcripts at 24 h of incubation but increases G-CSF transcripts. It blocks secretion of TNF and all CSF proteins (16).

When monocytes are cultured 1 day on plastic, they can no longer be induced for G- or GM-CSF expression. M-CSF expression is maintained. However, in contrast to fresh monocytes, PGE2 is no longer able to inhibit levels of M-CSF transcripts when added at 1 day. Thus, PGE2 differentially regulates cytokine mRNAs depending on the type of cytokine and condition of monocyte culture, and as a separate effect blocks cytokine protein production (Table 6).

A NEW FORM OF HUMAN IL1 RECEPTOR ANTAGONIST (IL1ra) (Table 7)

The IL1ra blocks the stimulatory effects of IL1 on T lymphocytes and fibroblasts by competing for binding to the receptor. The protein has been cloned and is distantly related to IL1 by nucleic acid and protein homology (32-34). We have found a variant of this molecule which uses an upstream exon instead of the first IL1ra exon. The resulting peptide lacks a leader sequence for secretion and is N-terminally extended by 7 amino acids compared to the mature IL1ra. Since the novel form would not be secreted, it is called intracellular IL1ra (icIL1ra). The complete cDNA was cloned from a human blood cell library (35).

TABLE 6. Differential Effects of PGE2 on Cytokine Expression by Plastic-Adherent Human Monocytes (ref. 16)

Time	Inducer	Transcripts Expressed			Protein		
0-24 h	0	(M)					
	I	M^+			M^+		
	LPS	M	GM	G	M	GM	TNF
	LPS + I	M^+	GM^+	G	M^+	GM	TNF^+
	LPS + I + PGE	↓	↓	↑	↓	↓	↓
24-48 h	I	(M)			M		
	LPS + I	M			M		(TNF)
	LPS + I + PGE	↑			↓		↓

Monocytes were purified from blood mononuclear cells by 2 h adherence to plastic. Cells were incubated with 1 μM indomethacine (I), 10 ng/ml LPS or 10 μM PGE2 for 24 h (0-24 h) and secreted protein (M-CSF and GM-CSF by specific Elisa, TNF by bioassay) and mRNA transcripts measured. Parallel cultures were incubated 24 h with I, washed and then pulsed another 24 h with agents (24-48 h). Blanks = not detected, ↓ = inhibition by PGE, ↑ = stimulation.

TABLE 7. The Intracellular IL1 Receptor Antagonist (icIL1ra) (ref. 35)

Complete cDNA from an induced blood cell library at a frequency of 0.001%
Same gene as IL1ra (33), but uses an alternate upstream exon that changes the N-terminus of the protein.
The signal peptide required for secretion is deleted.
Recombinant icIL1ra blocks IL1-induced IL2 and PGE2 production.
Found predominately in epithelial cells.

When recombinantly expressed in monkey COS cells, icIL1ra inhibits IL1-induced IL2 production from the mouse T line LBRM-33, IL1-induced prostaglandin production by human fibroblasts (35), and monocyte binding to IL1-stimulated endothelial cells (D. Liu, unpublished). In keeping with our prediction, icIL1ra is expressed mainly inside COS cells and is not secreted. icIL1ra is required to be present at the time of cell exposure to IL1 to be an effective antagonist.

The icIL1ra was expressed in *E. coli* in the pL system. Induced cells show a highly expressed new protein band at 18-22 kd in both the soluble supernatant and insoluble pellet of cells lysed by sonication in a Tris buffer (V. Wittman, unpublished). The supernatant is active to a dilution of 1:320,000 in suppressing IL1-induced IL2 production compared to a control bacterial preparation. The *E. coli* material also blocks prostaglandin E production stimulated by IL2 in human fibroblasts (unpublished).

mRNA studies of Northern gels and PCR analysis show that icIL1ra is mainly expressed in epithelial cells, including breast, nasal, bronchial, retinal pigment, vaginal and ovary, epithelium, and keratinocytes. No expression is seen in umbilical vein endothelial cells, breast or endometrium stromal cells, or blood lymphocytes, neutrophils or monocytes. The protein is found in keratinocyte lysates but is not secreted (35).

In vitro studies with icIL1ra show that the protein may be a useful pharmacologic drug to counteract the pathologic properties of endogenously produced IL1 in such diseases as rheumatoid arthritis, autoimmunities, graft rejection, graft-versus-host disease, other inflammations, and shock. There are a number of scientific questions about the physiologic role of icIL1ra. What is its intracellular role? There are nuclear receptors for IL1, and exteriorly presented IL1 is translocated in an active form to the nucleus (36-39). The intracellular proform of IL1α is active and found in many cell types, suggesting that it may have a function in that location. Senescence of endothelial cells may be regulated by the intracellular activity of IL1 (40). icIL1ra could thus modulate intracellular effects of exogenous or endogenous IL1.

Why is icIL1ra constitutively expressed predominantly in epithelial cells? These cells are in organs exposed to environmental stimuli. Keratinocytes synthesize but do not secrete appreciable amounts of IL1 (41). They and other epithelial cells may release stored IL1 as an early signal of wounds or infection. icIL1ra may be a self-protective mechanism during IL1 synthesis, or a reflection of continual low-level inflammation in these exposed tissues.

REFERENCES

1. Ralph P, Nakoinz I, Sampson-Johannes A (1990). Ann NY Acad Sci, in press.
2. Turner M, D Chantry, M. Feldmann (1988). Biochem. Biophys Res Comm 156: 830-839.
3. Gaffney EV, CR Stoner, SE Lingenfelter, LA Wagner (1989). J Immunol Meth (Netherlands) 122: 211-218
4. Cochran FR, MB Finch-Arietta (1989). Agents and Actions 27: 271-273.
5. Aderka D, J Le, J Vilcek (1989). J Immunol 143: 3517-3523.
6. Sisson SD, CA Dinarello (1988). Blood 72: 1368-1374.
7. Hart PH, GA Whitty, DS Piccoli, JA Hamilton (1989). Immunol 66:376-383.
8. Molvig J, L Baek, P Christensen, KR Manogue, H Vlassara, P Platz, LS Nielsen, A Svejgaard, J Nerup (1988). Scand J Immunol 27:705-716.
9. Herrmann F, G Gebauer, A Lindemann, M Brach, R Mertelsmann (1989). Clin Exp Immunol 77: 97-100
10. Debets JMH, TJM Ruers, MPMH van der Linder, CJ van der Linden & WA Buurman (1989). Clin Exp Immunol 78: 224-229.
11. Desch CE, NL Kovach, W Present, C Broyles, JM Harlan (1989). Lymphokine Res 8: 141-146.
12. Arenzana-Seisdedos F, J-L Virelizier (1983). Eur J Immunol 13: 437-440.
13. Newton RC (1985). Immunol 56: 441-449.
14. Hurme M, IJT Seppala (1988). Scand J Immunol 27: 725-730.
15. Arend WP, S D'Angelo, FG Joslin (1988). Clin Exp Immunol 74: 377-381.
16. Lee M-T, K Kaushansky, P Ralph, MB Ladner (1990). J Leukocyte Biol 47: 275-282.
17. Szefler SJ, CE Norton, B Ball, JM Gross, Y Aida, MJ Pabst (1989). J Immunol 142: 3985-3992.

18. Hart PH, GF Vitti, DR Burgess, GA Whitty, DS Piccoli, JA Hamilton (1989). Proc Natl Acad Sci USA 86: 3803-3807.
19. Weiss L, N Haeffner-Cavaillon, M Laude, J-M Cavaillon, MD Kazatchkine (1989). Eur J Immunol 19: 1347-1350.
20. Hurme M, T Palkama, M Sihvola (1988). Biochem Biophys Res Comm 157: 861-866.
21. Essner R, K Rhoades, WH McBride, DL Morton, JS Economou (1989). J Immunol 142: 3857-3861.
22. te Velde AA, BA Yard, JPG Klomp, JE De Vries, CG Figdor (1989). IL-4 modulates the phenotype of human monocytes and inhibits IL-1 secretion. *In* Mechanisms of Action and Therapeutic Applications of Biologicals in Cancer and Immune Deficiency Disorders. Pages 95-104. Alan R. Liss, Inc., New York, NY.
23. Donnelly RP, MJ Fenton, DS Finbloom, TL Gerrard (1990). J Immunol 145: 569-575.
24. Chantry D, M Turner, E Abney, M Feldmann (1989). J Immunol 142: 4295-4300.
25. Hurme M, M Sihvola, K Alitalo, J Keski-Oja (1989). J Cell Biochem 39: 467-475.
26. Wahl SH, DA Hunt, LM Wakefield, N McCartney-Francis, LM Wahl, AB Roberts, MB Sporn (1987). Proc Natl Acad Sci USA 84: 5788-5792.
27. Pockley AG, AE Bolton (1990). Immunol 69: 277-281.
28. Flegel WA, A Wolpl, DN Mannel, H Northoff (1989). Infect Immun 57: 2237-2245.
29. Scuderi P, RT Dorr, JD Liddil, PR Finley, P Meltzer, AB Raitano, J. Rybski (1989). Eur J Immunol 19: 939-942.
30. Greve JW, DJ Gouma, WA Buurman (1989). Hepatology 10: 454-458.
31. Haskill S, C Johnson, D Ierman, S Becker, K Warren (1988). J Immunol 140: 1690-1694.
32. Hannum CH, CJ Wilcox, WP Arend, FG Joslin, DJ Dripps, PL Heimdal, LG Armes, A Sommer, SP Eisenberg, RC Thompson (1990). Nature 343: 336-340.
33. Eisenberg SP, RJ Evans, WP Arend, E Verderber, MT Brewer, CH Hannum, RC Thompson (1990). Nature 343: 341-346.
34. Carter DB, MR Deibel Jr, CJ Dunn, CS Tomich, AL Laborde, JL Slighton, AE Berger, MJ Bienkowski, FF Sun, RN McEvan, RP Harris, AW Yem, GA Waszak, JG Chosay, LC Sieu, MM Hardee, HA Zurcher-Neely, IM Reardon, RL Heinrikson, SE Truesdell, JA Shelly, TE Essalu, BM Taylor, DE Tracey (1990). Nature 344: 633-637.
35. Haskill S, G Martin LV Le, J Morris, A Peace, CF Bigler, GF Jaffe, SA Sporn, S Fong, WP Arend, P Ralph (1991). Proc Natl Acad Sci USA, in press.
36. Mizel SB, PL Kiliam, JC Lewis, KA Paganelli, RA CHizzonite (1987). J Immunol 138: 2906-2912.
37. Grenfell S, N Smithers, K Miller, R Solari (1989). Biochem J 264: 813-822.
38. Curtis BM, MB Widmer, P deRoos, EE Qwarnstrom (1990). J Immunol 144: 1295-1303.

39. Qwarnstrom EE, RC Page, S Gillis, SK Dower (1988). J Biol Chem 263: 8261-8269.
40. Maier JAM, P Voulalas, D Roeder, T Maciag (1990). Science 249:1570-1574.
41. Kupper TS, AO Chua, P Flood, J McGuire, U Gubler (1987). J Clin Invest 80:430-436.
42. Han J, P Thompson, B Beutler (1990). J Exp Med 172: 391-394.
43. Poubelle PE, J Grassi, P Pradelles, F Marceau (1990). Immunopharmacology 19: 121-130.
44. te Velde AA, F Rousset, C Peronne, JE de Vries, CG Figdor (1990). J Immunol 144: 3052-3059.
45. Fiorentino DF, MW Bond, TR Mosmann (1989). J Exp Med 170: 2081-2095.
46. Zucali JR, HE Broxmeyer, D Levy, C Morse (1989). Blood 74: 1531-1536.
47. Broxmeyer HE, DE Williams, K Geissler, G Hangoc, S Cooper, DC Bicknell, S Levi, P Arosio (1989). Blood 73: 74-79.
48. Tsoukas CD, D Watry, SS Escobar, DM Provvedini, CA Dinarello, FG Hustmyer, SC Manolagas (1989) J Clin Endocrinol Metab 69: 127-133.
49. Schindler R, P Ghezzi, CA Dinarello (1990). J Immunol 144:2216-2222.
50. Laerum OD, O Sletvold, R Bjerknes, JA Eriksen, JH Johansen, J-S Schanche, T Tveteras, WR Paukovits (1988). Exp Hematol 16: 274-280.
51. Frindel E, J-P Monpezat (1989). Leukemia 3: 753-754.
52. Metcalf D (1987). The molecular nature of stimulators and inhibitors of granulocyte and macrophage production. *In* The Inhibitors of Hematopoiesis. A. Najman, M. Guigon, *et al.*, Eds. Colloque INSERM Vol. 162: 3-8. John Libbey Eurotext Ldt., Paris.
53. Lu L, K Welte, JL Gabrilove, G Hangoc, E Bruno, R Hoffman, HE Broxmeyer (1986). Cancer Res 46: 4357-4361.
54. Sing GK, JR Keller, LR Ellingsworth, FW Ruscetti (1988). Blood 72: 1504-1511.
55. Seckinger P, MT Kaufmann, J-M Dayer (1990). Immunobiol 180: 316-327.
56. Arend WP, HG Welgus, RC Thompson, SP Eisenberg (1990). J Clin Invest 85: 1694-1697.
57. Maliszewski CR, TA Sato, T Bos, S Waugh, SK Dower, J Slack, MP Backmann, KB Grabstein (1990). J Immunol 144:3028-3033.
58. Loetscher H, Y-CE Pan, H-W Lahm, R Gentz, M Brockhaus, H Tabuchi, W Lesslauer (1990). Cell 61: 351-359.
59. Englmann H, D Aderka, M Rubinstein, D Rotman, D Wallach (1989). J Biol Chem 264: 11974-11980.
60. Mosley B, MP Beckmann, CJ March, RL Idzerda, SD Gimpel, T Vanden Bos, D Friend, A Alpert, D Anderson, J Jackson, JM Wignall, C Smith, B Gallis, JE Sims, D Urdal, MB Widmer, D Cosman, LS Park (1989). Cell 59: 335-341.
61. Gewirtz AM, B Calabretta, B Rucinski (1989). J Clin Invest 83: 1477-1486.

62. Maione TE, GS Gray, J Petro (1990). Science 247: 77-79.
63. Hofman FM, M Brock, CR Taylor, B Lyons (1988). J Immunol 141 :1185-1190.
64. Jelinek DF, PE Lipsky (1988). J Immunol 141: 164-173.
65. Defrance T, B Vanbervliet, J-P Aubry, J Banchereau (1988). J Exp Med 168: 1321-1337.
66. Martinze OM, RS Gibbons, MR Garovoy, FR Aronson (1990). J Immunol 144: 2211-2215.
67. Jansen JH, G-JHM Wientjens, WE Fibbe, R Willemze, HC Kluin-Nelemans (1989). J Exp Med 170: 577-582.
68. Rennick D, G Yang, C Muller-Sieburg, C Smith, N Arai, Y Takabe, L Gemmell (1987). Proc Natl Acad Sci USA 84: 6889-6893.
69. Petit-Koskas E, E Genot, D Lawrence, J-P Kolb (1988). Eur J Immunol 18: 111-116.
70. Wahl SM, DA Hunt, HL Wong, S Dougherty, N McCartney-Francis, LM Wahl, L Ellingsworth, JA Schmidt, G Hall, AB Roberts, MB Sporn (1988). J Immunol 140: 3026-3032.
71. deMartin R, B Haendler, R Hofer-Wasrbinek, H Gaugitsch, M Wrann, H Schlusener, JM Seifert, S Bodmer, A Fontana, E Hofer (1987). EMBO J 6: 3673-3677.
72. Ambrus Jr JL, MG Peters, AS Fauci, EJ Brown (1990). J Immunol 144:1549-1553.
73. Van Oers NSC, BL Cohen, RA Murgita (1989). J Exp Med 170: 811-825.
74. Nong Y-H, RG Titus, JMC Ribeiro, HG Remold (1989). J Immunol 143: 45-49.
75. Bermudez LE, M Wu, LS Young (1990). Lymphokine Res. 9: 137-144.
76. Liew FY, S Millott, Y Li, R Lelchuk, WL Chan, H Ziltener (1989). Eur J Immunol 19: 1227-1232.
77. Lehn M, WY Weiser, S Engelhorn, S Gillis, HG Remold (1989). J Immunol 143: 3020-3024.
78. Tsunawaki S, M Sporn, A Ding, C Nathan (1988). Nature 334: 260.
79. TeVelde, AA, RJF Huijbens, JE DeVries, CG Figdor (1990). J Immunol 144: 3046-3051.
80. Kownatzki E, E Liehl, H Aschauer, S Uhrich (1990). Immunopharmacology 19: 139-144.
81. Gimbrone MA Jr, MS Obin, AF Brock, EA Luis, PE Hass, CA Hebert, YK Yip, DW Leung, DG Lowe, WJ Kohr, WC Darbonne, KB Bechtol, JB Baker (1989). Science 246: 1601-1603.
82. Swisher SG, JS Economous, EC Holmes, SH Golub (1990). Cell Immunol 128: 450-461.
83. Spits H, H Yssel, X Paliard, R Kastelein, C Figdor, JE DeVries (1988). J Immunol 141: 29-36.
84. Clark DA, M Falbo, RB Rowley, D Banwatt, J Stedronska-Clark (1988). J Immunol 141: 3833-3840.
85. Ranges GE, IS Figari, T Espevik, MA Palladino Jr (1987). J Exp Med 166: 991-998.
86. Lohoff M, E Marsig, M Rollinghoff (1990). J Immunol 144: 960-963.
87. Gamble JR, MA Vadas (1988). Science 242: 97.

88. Tanaka M, K Lee, J Yodoi, H Saito, Y Iwai, K-M Kim, M Morita, M Mayumi, H Mikawa (1989). Cellular Immunol 122: 96-107.
89. Good DJ, Polverini PJ, F Rastinejad, MM LeBeau, RS Lemons, WA Frazier, NP Bouck (1990). Proc Natl Acad Sci USA 87: 6624-6628.

Cellular and Cytokine Networks in
Tissue Immunity, pages 31-36

ENHANCING AND SUPPRESSING CYTOKINES MODULATE MYELOPOIESIS

Hal E. Broxmeyer

Departments of Medicine and Microbiology/ Immunology, and the Walther Oncology Center, Indiana University School of Medicine, Indianapolis, Indiana 46202-5121

Myeloid blood cell production is stimulated in vitro and in vivo (3-5) by the hematopoietic colony stimulating factors (CSF): Interleukin (IL)-3 (multi-CSF), granulocyte-macrophage (GM)-CSF, G-CSF, M-CSF (CSF-1), IL-5 (Eosinophil CSF) and erythropoietin (Epo). Combinations of the CSFs syngergize in vitro and in vivo (7,17) to enhance myeloid progenitor cell (MPC) proliferation. In fact, a genetically engineered human GM-CSF/IL-3 fusion protein is up to 10 fold more active than the combination of GM-CSF plus IL-3 (14). Additionally, there are a number of cytokines which can enhance and/or suppress the proliferation in vitro of stem (S) cells and multipotential (CFU-GEMM), erythroid (BFU-E) and granulocyte-macrophage (CFU-GM) progenitor cells. These cytokines include: mast cell growth factor (MGF, a c-kit ligand), the other interleukins, thus far numbering 1 to 11, activin, inhibin, the macrophage inflammatory proteins (MIP)-1α, -1β, -2, the interferons (IFN)-α, -β, -γ, the tumor necrosis factors (TNF)-α, -β (lymphotoxin), transforming growth factor (TGF)-β, the E-type prostaglandins (E_1 and E_2), lactoferrin (LF) and H-subunit (acidic) ferritin (2-4). Effects of these cytokines can be direct acting at the level of MPC themselves, and/or they can act indirectly by effects on accessory cells to up or down modulate the production/release of other cytokines, which can themselves have direct or indirect effects on MPC. The cytokines usually manifest pleiotrophic effects, and the same cell population can respond in a phenotypically similar manner to the actions of different molecules. This redundancy may be "nature's" way of protecting the body against simple insults to the network of cytokine interactions. The physiological significance of the cytokines is not entirely clear, although a good case for their relevance can be made from the studies of exogenous administration of cytokines to mice, monkeys and man in which marrow and blood cell responses have been elicited (5,7). This review focuses on the activities of MGF, H-ferritin, MIP-1α, MIP-1β, and MIP-2. The actions of these cytokines are direct ones on MPC (2,8,10,12).

<u>MGF</u>: A number of groups have recently purified and cloned ligands for the c-kit receptor protein (1,16,18,20). MGF is a ligand for the c-kit proto-oncogene product (1,18). This has also been called stem cell factor (SCF) (20) and KL (16). By itself, MGF had some CSF activity for CFU-GM (10,11), but the colonies stimulated were much lower in number and in size than those stimulated by GM-CSF. In combination with GM-CSF, MGF effects were greater than additive for stimulating colony number and colony size. Colonies from the jointly stimulated CFU-GM were macroscopic in size. While MGF did not stimulate colony formation by CFU-GEMM or BFU-E, it did have very potent activity for these MPC in the presence of Epo. MGF was far more active than IL-3 or GM-CSF in stimulating Epo-dependent CFU-GEMM and more active than IL-3 or GM-CSF in enhancing Epo-dependent BFU-E. The large size of the macroscopic colonies opened up the possibility that MGF may have the capacity for enhancing self-renewal.

<u>H-ferritin</u>: The iron-binding protein H-(acidic) ferritin, but not the related L-(basic) ferritin, has been implicated by us (6,9) and others (reviewed in 2) in the negative regulation of human and murine hematopoiesis <u>in vitro</u> and also <u>in vivo</u>. Abnormalities in H-ferritin-cell interactions have been associated with the progression of leukemia and other related blood disorders (2). Suppression occurs during S-phase of the cell cycle (2) and has been associated with a high density distribution of major histocompatibility (MHC) class II antigens (HLA-DR, Ia-antigens) on MPC (reviewed in 2). Evaluation of 10 recombinant (r) human (hu) H-ferritin muteins, obtained by oligonucleotide site-directed mutagenesis, suggested that the suppressive activity resided in the capacity of the molecule to manifest ferroxidase activity (9). Ferroxidase activity converts iron from the ferrous (Fe^{++}) to ferric (Fe^{+++}) form. Iron is necessary for MPC proliferation and

iron-saturated transferrin is a necessary ingredient for their growth. Cellular iron-deprivation, which can be induced by various means including the blocking of transferrin receptors with monoclonal antibodies to the transferrin receptor, has a suppressive effect on cellular proliferation, an effect that can be reversed by added iron. It is possible that H-ferritin acts by preventing the donation of iron from transferrin to the cell, assuming that the cell has receptors for H-ferritin. Since transferrin carries iron in a ferric form, and evidence suggests that donated iron needs to be in a ferrous form, H-ferritin may interfer with this process. This speculation is enhanced by studies showing that transferrin and ferritin are internalized together in coated pits and endosomes, and that transferrin receptor numbers are increased in cycling cells, when H-ferritin suppressive effects are apparent (above effects are reviewed in 9). We have noted that iron supplied to the cell in the non-transferrin form of hemin counteracts the suppression of MPC proliferation by H-ferritin (2).

MIP: The macrophage inflammatory proteins (MIP)-1 and -2 are heparin binding proteins originally identified by their capacity to elicit an inflammatory reaction when put into the footpads of C3H/HeJ mice (19). They represent two families that are structurally related and that may have evolved from a common ancestral gene that duplicated and then diverged (19). Natural (n) MIP-1 is composed of both MIP-1α and MIP-1β. We have shown that nMIP-1, rMIP-1α, rMIP-1β, nMIP-2 and rMIP-2 have enhancing effects for hu and murine (mu) CFU-GM stimulated by either GM-CSF or M-CSF, and that enhancement is most apparent when suboptimal concentrations of the CSFs are used (8,13). In contrast, nMIP-1 and rMIP-1α, but not rMIP-1β, nMIP-2 or rMIP-2 have myelosuppressive activity against progenitor cells stimulated by multiple cytokines (13). This includes CFU-GEMM and BFU-E stimulated by Epo + IL-3 or GM-CSF and CFU-GM stimulated by IL-3 + GM-CSF. MIP-1α reduces colony formation to the level of that seen in the presence of only one CSF. These results were interpreted to suggest that the enhancing effects of MIP-1α, MIP-1β and MIP-2 were on later, more mature and lineage restricted progenitors (e.g. CFU-G, CFU-M and a subpopulation of CFU-GM) and the suppressive effects of MIP-1α were on early, more immature progenitors (13). This latter interpretation was consistent with that from another group (15).Interestingly,

MIP-1β, but not MIP-2, blocks (abrogates) MIP-1α suppression, but MIP-1β has to be at a 2 to 4 fold excess to do this (12). A 1:1 ratio of MIP-1β to MIP-1α does not block MIP-1α inhibition, which explains how nMIP-1, which contains MIP-1α and MIP-1β at a 1:1 ratio can suppress colony formation by MPC. Pulse exposure of cells to MIP-1α gives maximal inhibition which is not overcome by later addition of MIP-1β, but pulse exposure to MIP-1β blocks the suppression by later addition of MIP-1α. This suggests receptor-mediated effects.

Studies on the actions and interactions of the above mentioned cytokines: MGF, H-ferritin, MIP-1α, MIP-1β, and MIP-2 should enhance our understanding of the mechanisms of action involved in the enhancement and suppression of myeloid blood cell production, as well as offer us the possibility of understanding how best to use these molecules in the future for treatment of hematopoietic disorders.

ACKNOWLEDGEMENT

We thank Linda Cheung for typing the manuscript.

REFERENCES

1. Anderson DM, Lyman SD, Baird A, Wignall JM, Eisenman J, Rauch C, March CJ, Boswell HS, Gimpel SD, Cosman D, Williams DE (1990). Molecular cloning of a mast cell growth factor, a hematopoietin that is active in both membrane bound and soluble forms. Cell 63:235-243.
2. Broxmeyer HE (1989). Iron-binding proteins and the regulation of hematopoietic cell proliferation/differentiation. In: deSousa M, Brock JH (eds), "Iron, Immunity, Cancer, and Inflammation," England: John Wiley and Sons, Limited, pp 199-221.
3. Broxmeyer HE (1990). Interacting effects of cytokines on hematopoietic stem and progenitor cells. In: Mertelsmann R, Herrmann F (eds), "Hematopoietic Growth Factors in Clinical Applications," New York: Marcel Dekker, Inc., pp 3-24.
4. Broxmeyer HE, Williams DE (1988). The production of myeloid blood cells and their regulation during health and disease. CRC Crit Rev Oncol/Hematol 8:173-226.
5. Broxmeyer HE, Vadhan-Raj S (1989). Preclinical and clinical studies with the hematopoietic colony

stimulating factors and related interleukins. Immunological Res 8:185-201.

6. Broxmeyer HE, Bognacki J, Dorner MH, deSousa M (1981). The identification of a leukemia-associated inhibitory activity (LIA) as acidic isoferritins: A regulatory role for acidic isoferritins in the production of granulocytes and macrophages. J Exp Med 153:1426-1444.
7. Broxmeyer HE, Williams DE, Hangoc G, Cooper S, Gillis S, Shadduck RK, Bicknell DC (1987). Synergistic myelopoietic action in vivo of combinations of purified natural murine colony stimulating factor-1, recombinant murine interleukin-3, and recombinant murine granulocyte-macrophage colony stimulating factor administered to mice. Proc Natl Acad Sci USA 84:3871-3875.
8. Broxmeyer HE, Sherry B, Lu L, Cooper S, Carow C, Wolpe SD, Cerami A (1989). Myelopoietic enhancing effects of murine macrophage inflammatory proteins 1 and 2 on colony formation in vitro by murine and human bone marrow granulocyte/macrophage progenitor cells. J Exp Med 170:1583-1594.
9. Broxmeyer HE, Cooper S, Levi S, Arosio P (1990). Mutated recombinant human H-ferritins and myelosuppression in vitro and in vivo: A link between H-ferritin ferroxidase activity and interactions with iron. Proc Natl Acad Sci USA. in press.
10. Broxmeyer HE, Cooper S, Lu L, Hangoc G, Anderson D, Cosman D, Lyman SD, Williams DE (1990) Effect of murine mast cell growth factor (c-kit proto-oncogene ligand) on colony formation by human marrow hematopoietic progenitor cells. Submitted.
11. Broxmeyer HE, Hangoc G, Cooper S, Anderson D, Cosman D, Lyman SD, Williams DE (1990). Influence of murine mast cell growth factor (c-kit ligand) on colony formation by mouse marrow hematopoietic progenitor cells. Exp Hematol in press.
12. Broxmeyer HE, Sherry B, Cooper S, Ruscetti FW, Williams DE, Kwon BS, Cerami A (1990). Influence of recombinant murine macrophage inflammatory protein (MIP)-1 on suppression by MIP-1 of human and murine hematopoietic progenitor cells. Submitted.
13. Broxmeyer HE, Sherry B, Lu L, Cooper S, Oh KO, Tekamp-Olson P, Kwon BS, Cerami A (1990). Enhancing and suppressing effects of recombinant murine macrophage inflammatory proteins on colony formation in vitro by bone marrow myeloid progenitor cells. Blood 76:1110-1116.

14. Curtis BM, Williams DE, Broxmeyer HE, Dunn J, Farrah T, Jeffrey E, Clevenger W, de Roos P, Martin U, Friend D, Craig V, Gayle R, Price V, Cosman D, March CJ, Park LS (1990). Enhanced hematopoietic activity of a human GM-CSF/IL-3 fusion protein. Submitted.

15. Graham GJ, Wright EG, Hewick R, Wolpe SD, Wilkie NM, Donaldson D, Lorimore S, Pragnell IB (1990). Identification and characterization of an inhibitor of haematopoietic stem cell proliferation. Nature 344:442-444.

16. Huang E, Nocka K, Beier DR, Chu TY, Buck J, Lahm HW, Wellner D, Leder P, Besmer P (1990). The hematopoietic growth factor KL is encoded by the SL locus and is the ligand of the c-kit receptor, the gene product of the W locus. Cell 63:225-233.

17. Williams DE, Straneva JE, Cooper S, Shadduck RK, Waheed A, Gillis S, Urdal D, Broxmeyer HE (1989). Interactions between purified murine colony stimulating factors (natural CSF-1, purified recombinant GM-CSF, and purified recombinant IL-3) on the _in vitro_ proliferation of purified murine granulocyte-macrophage progenitor cells. Exp Hematol 15:1007-1012.

18. Williams DE, Eisenman J, Baird A, Rauch C, Van Ness K, March CJ, Park LS, Martin U, Mochizuki DY, Boswell HS, Burgess GS, Cosman D, Lyman SD (1990). Identification of a ligand for the c-kit proto-oncogene. Cell 63:167-174.

19. Wolpe SD, Cerami A (1989). Macrophage inflammatory proteins 1 and 2: members of a novel superfamily of cytokines. FASEB J 3:2565-2573.

20. Zsebo KM, Wypych J, Lu HS, Smith KA, Karkare SB, Sachdev RK, Yuschenkoff VN, Birkett NC, Williams LR, Satyagal VN, Tung W, Bosselman RA, Mendiaz EA, Langley KE (1990). Identification, purification, and biological characterization of hematopoietic stem cell factor from buffalo rat liver-conditioned medium. Cell 63:195-201.

Cellular and Cytokine Networks in Tissue Immunity, pages 37-42

ONTOGENY OF EPITHELIAL $\gamma\delta$ T LYMPHOCYTES

Wendy L. Havran and James P. Allison

Cancer Research Laboratory and Department of Molecular and Cellular Biology, University of California, Berkeley, CA 94720

INTRODUCTION

MHC restricted recognition of antigen is mediated by T cell antigen receptors (TCR) composed of α and β chains in association with the CD3 complex (Allison and Lanier, 1987). More recently, an alternate TCR composed of γ and δ chains, also in association with CD3, has been described (Raulet, 1989). A minor population of T cells in the lymphoid organs express the $\gamma\delta$ TCR. The relationship between these two T cell populations and the functional necessity for generating discrete TCR-bearing populations is unclear.

In the mouse, the majority of T cells present in certain epithelial tissues express $\gamma\delta$ TCR (Bonyhadi et al.1987; Itohara et al.1990; Goodman and LeFrancois, 1988). There is a strong correlation between $V\gamma$ gene use and epithelial localization, as well as differences in the potential TCR repertoire in the different epithelial tissues. The use of early fetal V genes and TCR with limited diversity raised the possibility that the early TCR-bearing populations exit the fetal thymus and migrate to distinct peripheral sites, not previously thought to be the domain of T cells, where they take up residence and perform specialized immune functions. These studies were undertaken to analyze the appearance of cells bearing distinct TCR during development and to determine the subsequent localization of the cells in the adult mouse.

RESULTS

Ordered Appearance of TCR During Ontogeny

TCR genes are rearranged and expressed in an ordered manner during the early stages of development with $\gamma\delta$ TCR expression preceeding the appearance of $\alpha\beta$ TCR+ cells in the thymus (Raulet et al.1985; Pardoll et al.1987; Havran and Allison, 1988). Within the γ and δ loci, V gene segments also rearrange and are expressed in an ordered manner, with Vγ3, Vγ4, and Vδ1 transcripts detected first in the early fetal thymus (Raulet et al.1985). Phenotypic analysis of thymocytes from day 14-20 embryos was performed using a panel of monoclonal antibodies directed against CD3 and TCR chains to determine whether the ordered rearrangement was reflected in the expression of TCR on the cell surface (Figure 1). We established that the earliest CD3+ cells to appear in the fetal thymus expressed Vγ3 (Havran and Allison, 1988). Vγ3+ cells decrease as a percentage of CD3+ cells to undetectable levels after day 18 of gestation. Message for Vγ4 and the presence of cells expressing Vγ4 can be detected at day 15 (Garman et al.1986; Itohara et al.1989), demonstrating that the second wave of $\gamma\delta$ TCR-bearing cells use the Vγ4 chain. Vγ2 expressing cells appear next and remain as part of the $\gamma\delta$ TCR+ population in the adult thymus. Cells expressing other $\gamma\delta$ TCR also appear late in ontogeny or shortly after birth. Expression of these early Vγ genes appears in waves and the generation of at least the Vγ3 expressing population is limited to this discrete time in development.

Cells expressing $\alpha\beta$ TCR first appear at day 17 of gestation and rapidly become the major population in the thymus. Analysis using Vβ8, which can be detected at similar levels in fetal and adult $\alpha\beta$ populations, suggests that the α and β TCR genes may not be rearranged and expressed sequentially but probably rearrange randomly with the capability of using any V region present at all times. These studies indicate potential differences in the generation of different TCR populations and raise the possibility that cells generated at different times during ontogeny may have different functions from later appearing T cells.

Tissue Localization of $\gamma\delta$ T cells

Analysis of adult lymphoid organs (thymus, spleen, and lymph node) indicated that these tissues do not contain cells expressing Vγ3 or Vγ4 TCR (Garman et al.1986; Havran and Allison, 1988). In contrast, virtually all of the T cells present in the epidermis of adult mice (Thy-1+ dEC) express homogeneous TCR composed of Vγ3/Vδ1 chains (Kuziel et al.1987; Havran and Allison, 1988; Asarnow et al.1988). Cells expressing Vγ3 were not detected in other epithelial tissues indicating that mouse skin is exclusively the province of cells bearing the Vγ3 TCR.

T cells obtained from female reproductive epithelium were characterized and the $\gamma\delta$ TCR+ cells found to express TCR composed of Vγ4/Vδ1 chains (Itohara et al.1990) (D. Nandi, unpublished results). $\gamma\delta$ cells found in tongue epithelium likewise express homogeneous Vγ4/Vδ1

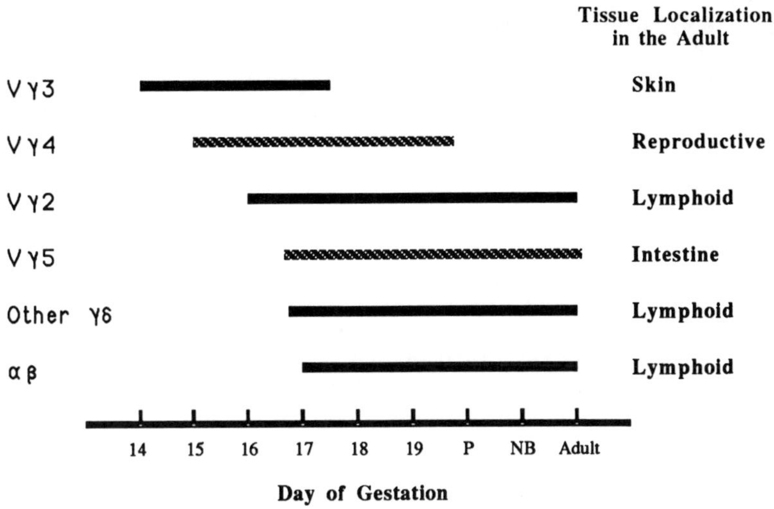

Figure 1. Expression of TCR chains during development and subsequent tissue localization in the adult mouse. Multicolor immunofluorescence analysis was performed on thymocyte suspensions obtained from day 14 of gestation through birth. Monoclonal antibodies used included 500A2 (anti-CD3ϵ) (Havran and Allison, 1988), 536 (anti-Vγ3) (Havran and Allison, 1988), UC3-10A6 (anti-Vγ2) (J. Bluestone), GL3 (anti-pan γ) (Goodman, and LeFrancois, 1989), and H57-597 (anti-pan β) (Kubo et al.1989). Information regarding Vγ4 and Vγ5 were obtained by sequence determination of cDNA amplified by PCR (Garman et al.1986; Itohara et al.1989).

TCR (Itohara et al.1990). Examination of $\gamma\delta$ T cells found in intestinal epithelium indicated that the majority of these cells express the Vγ5 chain (Asarnow et al.1989). These results indicate that $\gamma\delta$ TCR+ populations with restricted Vγ gene use localize in specific epithelial tissues. This raises the possibility that the early waves of $\gamma\delta$ expressing cells may contain precursors which migrate from the fetal thymus and specifically home to different epithelial tissues.

Fetal Thymic Origin of $\gamma\delta$ Cells in the Skin

While the role of the thymus in the generation of the vast majority of T cells is well established, the involvement of the thymus in the generation of the dEC has not been clear. Phenotypic, functional, and molecular analysis of Vγ3+ cells in the early fetal thymus indicated that they have characteristics in common with the Vγ3+ dEC in adult skin. These results raise the possibility that the first receptor-bearing component of the T cell system to appear in ontogeny might give rise to the adult dEC. Cell transfer experiments were performed to directly address this issue.

While Thy-1+ cells are present in the skin of athymic nude mice, they differ from the normal dEC population in that they lack expression of CD3 and associated Vγ3/Vδ1 TCR (Nixon-Fulton et al.1988; Havran and Allison, 1990). Implantation of fetal thymic lobes or injection of Vγ3+ cells purified from fetal thymus give rise to Thy-1+ Vγ3+ cells in the recipient mouse, demonstrating that the Vγ3+ fetal thymic cells can seed the skin (Havran and Allison, 1990). Implantation of newborn or adult thymus lobes into normal or nude recipient mice did not give rise to Thy-1+ Vγ3+ dEC. These studies indicated that cells found in fetal, but not adult thymus lobes were capable of giving rise to the adult dEC cells.

To determine whether the capacity to generate the dEC is limited to early fetal development, mice were treated in utero with anti-Vγ3 antibody to ablate Vγ3+ cells as they appeared in the fetal thymus. Analysis of the skin of the mice 4 months after birth and the last exposure to antibody indicated an absence of Vγ3+ dEC (Havran and Allison, 1990). These results indicate that the dEC precursors arise during a discrete period of ontogeny and the ability to generate them is lost later in development.

In order to test whether the loss of the abiltiy to generate dEC precursors is due to differences between fetal and adult stem cells or changes in the thymic microenvironment, radiation chimeras were constructed. Lethally irradiated normal mice or athymic nude mice were reconstituted with either fetal liver or adult bome marrow cells as a source of stem cells in the presence of a fetal or adult thymus microenvironment. Analysis of the host mice indicated that only mice in which fetal stem cells matured in fetal thymus lobes contained Vγ3+ donor cells in the skin. Maturation of fetal stem cells in an adult thymus microenvironment or adult stem cells in a fetal thymus did not generate donor-derived dEC in the host skin. These studies indicate that both a fetal stem cell population and fetal thymic microenvironment are required to generate the adult dEC.

CONCLUSIONS

These findings indicate that the generation of components of the immune system is temporally programmed by the order of TCR gene rearrangement and suggests that distinct sites in the periphery are seeded with discrete populations of T cells generated at different stages of development. The fetal origin and limited TCR gene use implies a limited repertoire of the adult dEC. It seems unlikely that their function is to recognize diverse foreign antigens in the context of self-MHC products in the same way as peripheral $\alpha\beta$ TCR+ cells. It is currently unknown what role the dEC play in protection from disease but their location and functional capabilities make it likely that these cells function as a first line of defense in the skin.

Based on these results we would propose that thymocyte differentiation may proceed in two broad stages. The earlier stage would involve the generation of cells bearing specific $V\gamma$ and $V\delta$ gene segments and with highly restricted diversity which may directly seed epithelial tissues. The role of these cells may be to recognize common antigens expressed on damaged cells in the epithelium. In the second stage which would occur later in fetal development and proceed in the adult, additional $V\gamma$ and $V\delta$ elements as well as the full complement of α and β genes would be available for use. This second stage provides for random production of T cell antigen receptors with the functional repertoire determined by selection, generating T cells capable of recogntion of diverse antigens.

ACKNOWLEDGEMENTS

We thank J. Bluestone for FITC-UC3-10A6, L. Lefrancois for GL3, and R. Kubo for H57-597 antibody. WLH is a Lucille P. Markey Scholar and this work was supported in part by grants from the Lucille P. Markey Charitable Trust and the N.I.H.

REFERENCES

Allison, J.P., and Lanier, L.L. (1987). Structure, function, and serology of the T-cell antigen receptor complex. Ann. Rev. Immunol. 5, 503-540.

Asarnow, D., Goodman, T., LeFrancois, L., and Allison, J.P. (1989). Distinct antigen receptor repertoires of two classes of murine epithelium-associated T cells. Nature 341, 60-62.

Asarnow, D.M., Kuziel, W.A., Bonyhadi, M., Tigelaar, R.E., Tucker, P.W., and Allison, J.P. (1988). Limited diversity of $\gamma\delta$ antigen receptor genes of Thy-1+ dendritic epidermal cells. Cell 55, 837-847.

Bonyhadi, M., Weiss, A., Tucker, P.W., Tigelaar, R.E., and Allison, J.P. (1987). Delta is the Cx-gene product in the $\gamma\delta$ antigen receptor of dendritic cells. Nature 330, 574-576.

Garman, R.D., Doherty, P.J., and Raulet, D.H. (1986). Diversity, rearrangement, and expression of murine T cell γ genes. Cell 45, 733-742.

Goodman, T., and LeFrancois, L. (1988). Expression of the $\gamma\delta$ T-cell receptor on intestinal CD8+ intraepithelial lymphocytes. Nature 333, 855-858.

Goodman, T., and LeFrancois, L. (1989). Intraepithelial lymphocytes: Anatomical site, not T cell receptor form, dictates phenoype and function. J. Exp. Med. 170, 1569-1581.

Havran, W.L., and Allison, J.P. (1988). Developmentally ordered appearance of thymocytes expressing different T cell antigen receptors. Nature 335, 443-445.

Havran, W.L., and Allison, J.P. (1990). Origin of Thy-1+ dendritic epidermal cells of adult mice from fetal thymic precursors. Nature 344, 68-70.

Itohara, S., Nakanishi, N., Kanagawa, O., Kubo, R., and Tonegawa, S. (1989). Monoclonal antibodies specific to native murine T-cell receptor $\gamma\delta$: Analysis of $\gamma\delta$ T cells during thymic ontogeny and in peripheral lymphoid organs. Proc. Natl. Acad. Sci. USA 86, 5094-5098.

Itohara, S., Farr, A.G., Lafaille, J.J., Bonneville, M., Takagaki, Y., Haas, W., and Tonegawa, S. (1990). Homing of a $\gamma\delta$ thymocyte subset with homogenous T-cell receptors to mucosal epithelia. Nature 343, 754-757.

Kubo, R.T., Born, W., Kappler, J.W., Marrack, P., and Pigeon, M. (1989). Characterization of a monoclonal antibody which detects all murine $\alpha\beta$ T cell receptors. J. Immunol. 142, 2736-2742.

Kuziel, W.A., Takashima, A., Bonyhadi, M., Bergstresser, P.R., Allison, J.P., Tigelaar, R.E., and Tucker, P.W. (1987). Regulation of T-cell receptor γ-chain RNA expression in murine Thy-1+ dendritic epidermal cells. Nature 328, 263-266.

Nixon-Fulton, J.L., Kuziel, W.A., Santerse, B., Bergstresser, P.R., Tucker, P.W., and Tigelaar, R.E. (1988). Thy-1+ epidermal cells in nude mice are distinct from their counterparts in thymus-bearing mice. A study of morphology, function, and T cell receptor expression. J. Immunol. 141, 1897-1903.

Pardoll, D., Fowlkes, B.J., Bluestone, J.A., Kruisbeek, A., Maloy, W.L., Coligan, J.E., and Schwartz, R.H. (1987). Differential expression of two distinct T cell receptors during thymocyte development. Nature 326, 79-81.

Raulet, D.H., Garman, R.D., Saito, H., and Tonegawa, S. (1985). Developmental regulation of T-cell receptor gene expression. Nature 314, 103-107.

Raulet, D.H. (1989). The structure, function, and molecular genetics of the $\gamma\delta$ T cell rceptor. Ann. Rev. Immunol. 7, 175-207.

Cellular and Cytokine Networks in
Tissue Immunity, pages 43-48

STRUCTURE AND FUNCTION OF CUTANEOUS IMMUNE CELLS

J. Wayne Streilein
Department of Microbiology and Immunology
University of Miami School of Medicine
Miami Florida 33136

INTRODUCTION

Immune responses to antigens and pathogens encountered in regionally distinct and functionally diverse organs and tissues of the body are specialized. More than a decade ago this concept was formalized for the skin under the term Skin Associated Lymphoid Tissues or SALT (Streilein 1990). SALT is comprised of skin-seeking lymphocytes, epidermal and dermal antigen presenting cells, specialized dermal endothelial cells, and keratinocytes - the parenchymal cell of the skin. Evidence suggests that the cutaneous microenvironment, generated primarily by keratinocytes (cytokines and cell adhesion molecules) dictates (a) the antigen processing and presenting properties of epidermal Langerhans cells, (b) the ability of endothelial cells to promote the migration of blood lymphocytes into the skin, and (c) modifies the effector functions of T lymphocytes once they have entered the skin. Antigen presenting cells (APC), endothelial cells, and lymphocytes are themselves capable of expressing cell adhesion molecules and secreting cytokines, although the rules of intercommunication with each other and with keratinocytes have yet to be deduced. This paper will focus on recent developments in (a) the roles of cutaneous antigen presenting cells in cutaneous immunity, especially the epidermal Langerhans cell, and (b) the influences of cytokines on Langerhans cell function.

CUTANEOUS ANTIGEN PRESENTING CELLS

The elegant and prescient studies of Macher and Chase (1969) demonstrated conclusively that events within the skin itself, immediately after application of a hapten, governed the nature of the subsequent immune outcome. Thereafter, Silberberg (1973) called attention to the fact that lymphocytes cluster around epidermal Langerhans cells in contact hypersensitivity (CH) skin reactions. The brilliant in vitro studies of antigen presenting potential of Langerhans cell-enriched epidermal cell suspensions by Stingl and his various collaborators (1978) identified the Langerhans cell as the primary antigen presenting cell of skin. In vivo studies revealed that cutaneous surfaces that are naturally deficient, or artificially depleted of Langerhans cells are incapable of supporting the induction of CH to haptens such as dinitrofluorobenzene. Acute, low dose irradiation of skin with ultraviolet B light (UVB) depleted the surface of normal appearing Langerhans cells, and DNFB applied to UVB-treated skin failed to induce CH (Toews et al 1980). It was soon realized that the effect of UVB on induction of CH was not uniform in all individuals, and that the UVB-susceptibility trait was genetically determined (Streilein and Bergstresser 1988). It has now been formally shown (Streilein 1989) that hapten application to cutaneous surfaces rendered completely devoid of Langerhans cells (by tape-stripping, and by excision of epidermis) can still induce CH, implying that cells within the dermis can act as "back-up" APC for skin. The dermis contains at least two types of bone marrow-derived cells that are candidates for this role: conventional macrophages, and dermal dendritic cells (Weber-Matthiesen and Sterry 1990).

LANGERHANS CELLS AND THE INDUCTION OF CONTACT HYPERSENSITIVITY

In vivo evidence that Langerhans cells migrate to draining lymph nodes.

Dermal lymphatic channels of skin that has been painted with hapten contain "veiled cells", which are believed to be migrating epidermal Langerhans cells.. Taking advantage of the capacity of fluorescein isocyathianate (FITC) to function as a hapten, Knight et al (1985) and Kripke and McClendon (1986) have demonstrated that class II MHC positive cells, bearing FITC on their surface, arrive in the draining lymph node within 24 hours after FITC is painted on normal, but not UVB-exposed, epidermis. It has been deduced that the majority of Ia-bearing, FITC-positive lymph node cells are derived from Ia+ epidermal cells that were derivatized in situ by FITC, i.e., Langerhans cells. The immunogenic properties of these cells are impressive; when injected into syngeneic recipients, they induce vigorous FITC-specific CH. By contrast, FITC-positive cells harvested from lymph nodes draining FITC-painted, UVB-exposed skin fail to sensitize their recipients.

Using TNP-specific hybridoma cells that secrete IL-2 when confronted by TNP-derivatized, Ia+ antigen presenting cells, Bigby et al (1989) have detected hapten-bearing cells in draining lymph nodes as early as 6 hours after hapten application to normal epidermis, but they failed to detect hapten-bearing cells in lymph nodes at any time after TNCB is painted on UVB-treated skin. Thus, evidence strongly supports the conclusion that, in the induction of CH, hapten is picked up by epidermal Langerhans cells which then migrate across the dermal-epidermal junction, and follow lymph to the draining lymph node. These hapten-bearing cells come to rest within the parafollicular cortex, attract recirculating lymphocytes from the blood, and present their antigen, thereby initiating T cell activation and differentiation.

In vitro evidence that Langerhans cells exist in two functionally distinct forms.

While the trail-blazing studies of Stingl demonstrated that Langerhans cells prepared from normal epidermis can function as APC, they did not reveal the manner in which this was accomplished. Recent studies have begun to flesh out the interesting, and in some ways surprising, details. Langerhans cells prepared from enzymatically digested epidermis survive poorly in tissue culture, unless keratinocytes are also present (Schuler and Steinman, 1985). Inaba et al (1986) found that such epidermal cell suspensions, cultured in vitro for three days, were extraordinarily active in lymphocyte activation, unlike freshly prepared epidermal cell suspensions. Streilein and Grammer (1989) determined that fresh Langerhans cells were incapable of activating autologous T cells, whereas cultured Langerhans cells were profoundly stimulatory for autologous T cells, implying that the latter are enriched for accessory cell functions. Romani et al (1989) and Streilein and Grammer (1989) have independently determined that antigen processing, as opposed to antigen presentation, is a property that is highly developed in fresh, but not necessarily cultured, Langerhans cells. Thus, fresh and cultured Langerhans cells differ functionally: fresh cells are superior at ingesting and processing native proteins into immunogenic peptide fragments, but display limited accessory cell properties; by contrast, cultured Langerhans cells display elaborate accessory cell functions, but are less efficient at processing native protein antigens. It has been proposed that this division of labor is physiologically relevant and may reflect different functional properties of Langerhans cells located in the epidermis and Langerhans cells that have recently migrated to the draining lymph node, respectively.

LANGERHANS CELL FUNCTION IS DICTATED BY ENVIRONMENTAL CYTOKINES

Heufler et al (1988) demonstrated that keratinocytes sustain Langerhans cell viability in vitro by secreting GM-CSF. Purified Langerhans cells that have been maintained for several days in GM-CSF no longer express CD1 or Fc receptors, and their cytoplasm no longer contains Birbeck granules; however, expression of class I and II MHC molecules is markedly enhanced, and the cells express large amounts of ICAM-1. Koch et al (1990) have recently tested numerous other cytokines for their ability to sustain Langerhans cells in tissue culture. Among the 20 cytokines tested, only tumor necrosis factor-alpha (TNF_a) also kept Langerhans cells alive in tissue culture. But such cells failed to activate resting T cells in oxidative mitogenesis or primary MLR, and they resembled freshly procured Langerhans cells morphologically.

Since the microenvironment plays a critical role in determining Langerhans cell function, Langerhans cells may display different properties when they occupy normal epidermis (dominated by keratinocytes), draining lymph nodes (dominated by T cells), or epidermis that has been perturbed by haptens or UVB.

TNF_a MEDIATES EFFECTS OF UVB RADIATION ON LANGERHANS CELLS AND ON CONTACT HYPERSENSITIVITY

Ultraviolet B radiation (UVB) has numerous biological effects, especially on the skin and the immune system. Alterations in Langerhans cells are prominent after acute, low dose UVB radiation of mouse and human skin, and Yoshikawa and Streilein (in press) have recently reported that UVB might accomplish its immune effects through the induction of TNF_a production in skin: (a) intradermal (ID) injections of TNF_a impair the induction of DNFB-induced CH in a manner similar to UVB, and (b) UVB-impairment of CH induction can be reversed by treating UVB-exposed mice with neutralizing anti TNF_a antibodies immediately prior to hapten application. Thus, TNF_a is an essential mediator of the deleterious effects of UVB on induction of CH. Vermeer and Streilein (manuscript submitted) have explored the possibility that TNF_a may mediate its deleterious effects by acting directly on epidermal Langerhans cells. They found that a single exposure to low dose UVB, as well as a single ID injection of TNF_a, induced identical morphologic changes in Langerhans cells: the cells lose their dendrites and round-up, implying major cytoskeletal rearrangements. Systemic treatment with anti-TNF_a antibodies abrogated both the UVB and TNF_a-induced effects. Thus, local TNF_a mediates UVB-induced changes in Langerhans cells, and these effects occur within the epidermis. These workers also showed that ID injections of TNF_a prevented Langerhans cells from emigrating from skin painted with DNFB, and that local treatment with either TNF_a or UVB promoted the expression of CH. It is suspected that TNF_a directly (and UVB indirectly) alters the cytoskeleton of Langerhans cells such that the cells are transiently immobilized, and are unable to carry hapten to the draining node to initiate the immune response. By the same token, their intraepidermal immobilization ensures that there will be ample hapten-bearing target cells for circulating immune T cells to recognize when CH is expressed in UVB-exposed skin.

SUMMARY

The cellular components of SALT occupy a confined microenvironment potentially containing a wide variety of cytokines. It is proposed that the particular functional program adopted by individual cell types within this microenvironment is dictated in large measure by the local cytokine content. In support of this view, in vitro and in vivo experimental evidence confirms that the functional properties of Langerhans cells are remarkably susceptible to modulation by GM-CSF and TNF_a, and that this modulation has important consequences for immune responses to cutaneous antigens. Further exploration of this idea with other cytokines, and with the other cellular components of SALT should prove scientifically stimulating and may even have clinical and therapeutic benefits for patients suffering from cutaneous diseases.

REFERENCES

Bigby B, Vargas R, Sy M-S (1989). Production of hapten-specific T cell hybridomas and their use to study the effect of ultraviolet B rradiation on the development of contact hypersensitivity. J Immunol 143: 3867-3872.

Heufler C, Koch F, Schuler G (1988). Granulocyte/macrophage colony-stimulating factor and interleukin 1 mediate the maturation of murine epidermal Langerhans cells into potent immunostimulatory dendritic cells. J Exp Med 167:700-705.

Inaba K, Schuler G, Witmer MD, Valinksy J, Atassi B, Steinman RM (1986). Immunologic properties of purified epidermal Langerhans cells. J Exp Med 164:605-613.

Knight SC, Krejci J, Malkovsky M, Colizzi V, Gautam A, Asherson GL (1985). The role of dendritic cells in the initiation of immune responses to contact sensitizers. Cellular Immunol 94:427-434.

Koch F, Heufler C, Kampgen E, Schneeweiss D, Bock G, Schuler G (1990). Tumor necrosis factor$_a$ maintains the viability of murine epidermal Langerhans cells in culture, but in contrast to granulocyte-macrophage colony-stimulating factor, without inducing their functional maturation. J Exp Med 171:159-171.

Kripke ML, McClendon E (1986). Studies on the role of antigen-presenting cells in the systemic suppression of contact hypersensitivity by UVB radiation. J Immunol 137:443-448.

Macher E, Chase MW (1969). Studies on the sensitization of animals with simple chemical compounds. XII. J Exp Med 129:103-114.

Romani N, Koide S, Crowley M, Witmer-Pack M, Livingston AM, Fathman CG, Inaba Y, Steinman RE (1989). Presentation of exogenous protein antigens by dendritic cells to T cell clones. Intact protein is presented best by immature, epidermal Langerhans cells. J Exp Med 169: 1169-1182.

Schuler G, Steinman RM (1985). Murine epidermal Langerhans cells mature into potent immunostimulatory dendritic cells in vitro. J Exp Med 161:526-546.

Silberberg I (1973). Apposition of mononuclear cells to Langerhans cells in contact allergic reactions. Acta Derm Venerol 53:1-9.

Stingl G, Katz SI, Clement L, Green I, Shevach EMN (1978). Immunologic functions of Ia-bearing epidermal Langerhans cells. J Immunol 121:2005-2010.

Streilein JW, Bergstresser PR (1988). Genetic basis of ultraviolet-B effectson contact hypersensitivity Immunogenetics 27:252-258.

Streilein JW (1989). Antigen-presenting cells in the induction of contact hypersensitivity in mice: evidence that Langerhans cells are sufficient but not required. J Invest Derm 93:443-448.

Streilein JW and Grammer SF (1989). In vitro evidence that Langerhans cells can adopt two functionally distinct forms capable of antigen presentation to T lymphocytes. J Immunol 143:3925-3933.

Streilein JW (1990). Skin Associated Lymphoid Tissues (SALT): The Next Generation. in <u>The Skin Immune System (SIS)</u>, edited by J. Bos,CRC Press, Inc., pp. 26-48.

Toews GB, Bergstresser PR, Streilein JW (1980). Epidermal Langerhans cell density determines whether contact hypersensitivity or unresponsiveness follows skin painting with DNFB. J Immunol 124:445453.

Weber-Matthiesen K, Sterry W (1990). Organization of the monocyte/macrophage system of normal human skin. J Invest Derm 95:83-89.

Yoshikawa T, Streilein JW (In Press). On the genetic basis of the effects of ultraviolet light B on cutaneous immunity. Evidence that polymorphisms at the TNF$_a$ and Lps loci govern susceptibility. Immunogenetics.

Cellular and Cytokine Networks in Tissue Immunity, pages 49-54

IMMUNE FUNCTION OF KERATINOCYTES

Shigeyuki Nozaki and Daniel N. Sauder

Department of Dermatology, Showa University, Tokyo Japan and University of Toronto, Toronto, Canada

One of the most remarkable developments in cutaneous biology of the past decade has been the observation that keratinocytes can synthesize and express a variety of cytokineds including various interleukins, colony stimulating factors and growth factors.

KERATINOCYTE IL-1

Studies have demonstrated that biologically active form of IL-1 exists in normal human keratinocyte in the absence of intentional stimuli. Immunoreactive IL-1 can be seen in normal human epidermis. Both membranes and cytosolic IL-1α and IL-1β immunoreactivity was found in all epidermal cell layers including stratum corneum. Cultured normal human keratinocytes produce more IL-1αmRNA than IL-1βmRNA[1]. Pam 212, a murine keratinocyte cell line, produces exclusively IL-1αmRNA[2]. In contrast, COLO16, a human squamous cell carcinoma cell line, contains equivalent amounts of IL-1α and IL-1βmRNA[3]. In addition, molecular characterization of cloned COLO16 completmentary DNA has revealed that COLO16 contains, in addition to IL-1α and IL-1βmRNA, a unique keratinocyte derived IL-1 (termed interleukin 1k)[4].

Keratinocytes produce more biologically active form of IL-1α than IL-1β without stimulation. Blanton et al. have demonstrated that all IL-1 in all lysates from cultured normal human keratinocytes is unprocessed IL-1α by Western blot[5]. IL-1 activity of conditional media from cultured normal human keratinocytes is neutralized by an antibody that neutralizes both IL-1α and IL-1β, but not by an antibody that neutralizes only IL-1β[1]. McKenzie et al. have reported that in

COLO16 cell line all the IL-1 activity in cell lysate was neutralized by antisera to IL-1α and majority of IL-1 activity in cell-conditioned media was also neutralized by anti-IL-1α antibodies[3]. This data suggests that unprocessed IL-1α is the predominant form of cell associated IL-1 and that most of the IL-1 activity found in culture media as well as cell lysates is IL-1α. However, the implication for IL-1α predominance in keratinocytes remains to be elucidated. Both forms of IL-1 are unique for secretory polypeptides in that they lack signal sequence for effective processing. Precise mechanism of processing and release of IL-1 is not known. There is evidence that monocytes possess a specific convertase activity for pre-IL-1β[6]. However, keratinocytes do not appear to contain proteolytic activity to cleave precursor IL-1β to mature IL-1β[7]. The presence of this performed IL-1 in keratinocytes is suited to the concept of epidermis as a barrier against external environment since disruption of skin cause prompt release of IL-1, leading to host defence responses. Although neither form of IL-1 seems to be effectively processed and released, membrane-bound IL-1 was described and found to be biologically active. Membrane-bound IL-1 may account for a significant part of immunoregulatory effects of IL-1 in local tissue reactions, particularly keratinocyte interaction with T cells. Recent observations show that cultured keratinocytes express high-affinity receptors for IL-1[5,8]. Keratinocytes bear in the range of 400-2000 receptors/cell which is more abundant that most of the cell types including T cell. These keratinocyte IL-1 receptors in culture respond to exogenous IL-1 and produce IL-6, IL-8 and GM-CSF[8-10]. IL-1 receptor synthesis is important in regulation of immune and inflammatory reactions.

AUTOCRINE/PARACRINE EFFECTS OF KERATINOCYTE IL-1

Thus keratinocytes, by virtue of their production of IL-1, influence the biology not only of keratinocytes themselves but also of resident cells to skin and inflammatory cells recruited to skin. One of the most important effects of IL-1 on keratinocytes is enhance more production of IL-1 in autocrine mechanism.

Keratinocytes appear to be involved in immune responses characterized by antigen presentation by Langerhans cells to T cells.

The colony stimulating factor granulocyte-macrophage colony stimulating factor (GM-CSF), another IL-1 inducible keratinocyte cytokine, in the presence of IL-1, maintains viability of Langerhans cells and enhances Langerhans cell function. Recent studies suggest that accessary factors involved in T cell activation besides recognition of MHC-antigen complex may include IL-1 and IL-6[11]. Keratinocytes, by virtue of their production of IL-1, IL-6 and GM-CSF, may play an important role in the initiation of immune reaction in skin by modulating Langerhans cell function and providing accessory factors.

Release of keratinocyte IL-1 by disruption of skin appear to be involved in wound healing by synergizing with growth factors and other IL-1 inducible cytokines. Regeneration of blood vessels is regulated by transforming growth factor α (TGF-α) and platelet-derived growth factor (PDGF) which in synergy with IL-1 also induce fibroblast proliferation. Recent data suggests that the mitogenic effect of IL-1 on fibroblasts is mediated by fibroblast PDGF synthesis induced by IL-1[12]. Addition of PDGF to fibroblasts increases IL-1 receptor expressions[13], further activating this paracrine growth factor loop. IL-1, IL-8 and GM-CSF induce migration of inflammatory cells to wound site; these cells may play an important role in cleaning nonviable tissue from the wound. Finally, re-epithelization is enhanced by IL-1 and GM-CSF which induces migration and proliferation of keratinocytes[8,14].

INTERLEUKIN 6

Keratinocytes have been shown to express IL-6 mRNA and synthesize IL-6 protein in vitro upon stimulation[15]. Increased IL-6 levels have been documented in hyperplastic psoriatic tissue[16]. This may be explained by the ability of IL-6 to enhance proliferation of normal human keratinocytes and to activate T-cell and B-cell function. However, it is likely that IL-6 synergize with cytokines such as IL-1 in mediating these effects in local cutaneous environment.

INTERLEUKIN 8

Interleukin 8 (IL-8) is a novel polypeptide neutrophil chemotactic factor, originally described as a product of LPS-stimulated peripheral blood monocytes described in detail in other sections of this symposium. Biologically active IL-8 molecules have been extracted from psoriatic scales[17]. These polypeptides may account for the margination of neutrophils toward psoriatic scales.

COLONY-STIMULATING FACTOR

It has been shown that human keratinocytes produce M-CSF *in vitro* and the production of M-CSF is upregulated by bacterial LPS[18]. IL-3, in addition to its multi-colony-stimulating factor activities, activates mast cells and induces the proliferation of hematopoietic stem cell lines. Although IL-3-like activity has been found in murine neonatal keratinocytes and Pam 212 cells[19], production of IL-3 has not been demonstrated in human keratinocytes. Granulocyte-macrophage colony-stimulating factor (GM-CSF) is a glycoprotein that promotes differentiation of hematopoietic progenitor cells to mature granulocytes and macrophages. Keratinocytes are potent sources of 6M-CSF. Like IL-6, keratinocyte production of GM-CSF can be upregulated by tumour promotor, other cytokines such as IL-1 and TNF, as well as UV irradiation[19]. In addition to its effect on hematopoietic progenitor cells, GM-CSF has profound effects on survival and activation of mature neutrophils, eosinophils and macrophages, including antibody-dependent cell-mediated cytotoxicity, oxidative metabolism and phagocytosis of micro-organism. GM-CSF also inhibits migration of neutrophils. Thus, production of keratinocyte GM-CSF at the site of cutaneous inflammation would promote local retention of granulocytes and activate their function.

TUMOR NECROSIS FACTOR AND LYMPHOTOXIN

Cultured human keratinocytes have been shown to express TNF and mRNA following stimulation with LPS and IL-6.[20] Both LT and TNF are cytostatic for normal human keratinocytes[21]. TNF has been linked to acute cutaneous GVHD[22]. An important function of TNF in skin diseases may be synergism with IL-1, since the effects of IL-1 or TNF are often biologically indistinguishable and when the two cytokines are used together *in vitro*, the net effect often exceeds the additive effect of each cytokine.

SUMMARY

It is now clear that keratinocytes produce a wide range of cytokines which can be regarded as important mediators of intercellular communication. A major emphasis has been placed on IL-1 because of its relations with other cytokines and other differentiated tissues. Dysregulation of IL-1, IL-1 receptor and inhibitory factors for IL-1 may cause inbalance of skin biology, leading to perpetuation of immune and inflammatory events. Interaction of IL-1 with other cytokines *in vivo* are also important in understanding of pathophysiology of skin diseases.

REFERENCES

1. Kupper TS, Ballard DW, Chuo AO et al. Human keratinocytes contain mRNA indistinguishable from monocyte interleukin 1α and βmRNA. *J. Exp. Med.* 164:2095, 1986.
2. Ansel JC, Luger TA, Lowry D et al. The expression and modulation of IL-1α in murine keratinocytes. *J. Immunol.* 140:2274, 1988.
3. McKenzie RC, Arsenault TV, Sauder DN et al. Expression of interleukin 1β in a human keratinocyte cell line. *Lymph. Res.* 9:391, 1990.
4. Arsenault TV, McKenzie RC, Sauder DN et al. Identification and characterization of a partial cDNA expressing interleukin-1-like activity in keratinocytes. (submitted).
5. Blanton RA, Kupper TS, McDougall JK et al. Regulation of interleukin 1 and its receptor in human keratinocytes. *Proc. Natl. Acad. Sci. USA.* 86:1273, 1989.
6. Kostura MJ, Tocci MJ, Limjuco G et al. Identification of a monocyte specific pre-interleukin 1β convertase activity. *Proc. Natl. Acad. Sci. USA.* 86:5227, 1989.
7. Mizutani H, Black R and Kupper TS. Post-translation modulations of IL-1 differ markedly in keratinocytes and monocytes:implication for epidermal biology. *J. Invest. Dermatol.* 92:483 (abstract), 1989.
8. Sauder DN, Orr FW, Matic S et al. Human interleukin 1α is chemotactic for normal human keratinocytes. *Immunol. Lets.* 22:123, 1989.
9. Grossman RM, Krueger J, Yourish D et al. Interleukin 6 is expressed in high levels in psoriatic skin and stimulates

proliferation of cultured human keratinocytes. *Proc. Natl. Acad. Sci. USA.* 86:6367, 1989.

10. Larsen CG, Anderson AO, Oppenheim JJ et al. Production of interleukin 8 by human dermal fibroblasts and keratinocytes in response to interleukin 1 or tumor necrosis factor. *Immunol.* 68:31, 1989.
11. McKenzie D. Alloantigen presentation by B cells requirement for IL-1 and IL-6. *J. Immunol.* 141:2907, 1988.
12. Schmidt JA, Mitzel SB, Cohen D et al. Interleukin 1: a potential regulator of fibroblast proliferation. *J. Immunol.* 128:2177, 1982.
13. Bonin P and Singh JP. Modulation of interleukin 1 receptor expression and interleukin 1 response in fibroblasts by platelet-derived growth factor. J. Biol. Chem. 263:10052, 198.
14. Hancock GE, Kaplan G and Cohn ZA. Keratinocyte growth regulation by the products of immune cells. *J. Exp. Med.* 168:1395, 1988.
15. Kirnbauer R, Köck A, Schwarz T et al. Interferon $\beta 2$, B-cell differentiation factor 2, hybridoma growth factor (interleukin 6) is expressed and released by human epidermal cells and epidermoid carcinoma cell lines. *J. Immunol.* 142:1922, 1989.
16. Grossman RM, Krueger J, Yourish D et al. Interleukin 6 is expressed in high levels in psoriatic skin and stimulates proliferation of cultured human keratinocytes. *Proc. Natl. Acad. Sci. USA* 86:6367, 1989.
17. Schroeder JM and Christophers E. Identification of C5 ades arg and an anionic neutrophil-activating peptide (ANAP) in psoriatic scales. *J. Invest. Dermatol.* 87:53, 1986.
18. Chodakewitz JA, Lacy J, Edwards SE et al. Macrophage colony-stimulating factor production by murine and human keratinocytes. *J. Immunol.* 144:2190, 1990.
19. Luger TA, Köck A, Kirnbauer R et al. Keratinocyte interluekin 3 production. *Ann. N.Y. Acad. Sci.* 548:253, 1989.
20. Köck A, Urbanski A, Lugar TA. mRNA expression and release of tumor necrosis factor-α by human epidermal cells. *J. Invest. Dermatol.* 92:462A, 1989.
21. Symington FW. Lymphotoxin, tumor necrosis factor and gamma interferon are cytostatic for normal human keratinocytes. *J. Invest. Dermatol.* 92:798, 1989.
22. Pignet P-F, Gran GE, Allet B et al. Tumor necrosis factor/cachetin is an effector of skin and gut lesions of acute phage of graft-vs-host disease. *J. Exp. Med.* 166:1280, 1987.

Cellular and Cytokine Networks in Tissue Immunity, pages 55-61

IMMUNOLOGY OF THE INTESTINAL TRACT : ROLE OF ANTIGEN PRESENTING CELLS

Dominique KAISERLIAN

INSERM U80 CNRS URA 1177 UCBL, Pavillon P,
Hôpital E.HERRIOT, 69437 LYON CEDEX 03, FRANCE

INTRODUCTION

The large surface area of the gastrointestinal (GI) tract, which represents an important interface between the external environment and internal milieux, is protected by a number of mechanisms. In addition to innate defense factors, including gastric acid, proteolytic enzymes, lyzosyme, lactoferin and mucin, large amounts of specific antibodies mainly of the IgA isotype, are secreted into the lumen and contribute to antigenic exclusion. Most of the IgA found in external secretions is synthetized locally in the gut mucosa by IgA-producing plasma cells (10^{10} cells/meter of human gut). Thus the intestine contains more Ig-producing cells than all other lymphoid and hematopoietic tissues combined. immunocompetent cells within the gut lymphoid tissues are comprised in two compartments. Diffuse leucocytes are interspersed in the vascular and lymphatic rich connective tissues of the lamina propria of the villi and distributed within the epithelium (intraepithelial leucocytes). Organized lymphoid formations such as the Peyer's patches (PP) and the mesenteric lymph nodes contain leucocytes distributed in T and B cell compartments. The term GALT (gut-associated lymphoid tissues) is used exclusively for PP. The intestinal immune system is a tightly regulated system which protects the host against environmental pathogens, and at the same time avoids deleterious hypersensitivity reactions, harmfull for the host. However, uncontrolled events may disturb these powerful immune control mechanisms, resulting in unexpected tissue damage and immune response against self components as those seen in inflammatory bowel disease.

Our laboratory has been involved for several years in the understanding of the gut immune paradigm : oral immunity versus oral tolerance. We provided evidence that initiation of a local immune response in the gut is not restricted to PP, and that gut villi may be an alternative site of antigen presentation. We propose that initiation of a local immune response in the villi may be the basis for the oral tolerance phenomenon and for some pathological disorders of the GI tract. In this paper, we will first give a short review of the current knowledge of intestinal immunology ; in the second part, we will discuss our data on the characteristics of antigen presenting cells (APC) in the gut villi.

I- THE INTESTINAL IMMUNE SYSTEM

Three major features characterize the gut immune system:

1) the immune response to luminal pathogens, 2) oral tolerance to dietary protein and commensal bacteria, and 3) disorders of intestinal immunity.

1) The intestinal immune response to luminal antigens.

Initiation of a local immune response is thought to take place in the PP after antigen entry (especially particulate antigens and macromolecules) through M cells (i.e specialized phagocytic epithelial cells of the doma region), and transport to underlying immunocompetent cells of PP (1). Antigen presentation to local T cells by interdigitating dendritic cells, results in specific T cells activation and B cell commitment to IgA isotype (2). Once activated T and B cell blasts migrate through efferent lymph to mesenteric nodes, then circulate through lymph and blood to lamina propria and distant mucosal sites (3) and home to both intestinal and extra-intestinal mucosal sites where terminal differentiation into IgA plasma cells occurs ; this generalized mucosal system : MALT (i.e mucosal-associated lymphoid tissues) (4) provides that immunization by the oral route can protect from possible infections occuring at other mucosal sites. The tissue localisation of these emigrant cells and gut homing mechanisms seem to depend on the presence of homing receptors, i.e. adressins on post capillary veinules of PP, lymph nodes and lamina propria. (5). A number of immune mechanisms are involved in the regulation of intestinal immunity. Interactions of T cells with dendritic cells in the PP is required for B cell IgM to IgA switch (6).

Cytokines produced by both T cells and non T cells also influence the isotype switching process (TGF-beta (7), IL-4, IL-5, IL-6 (8). Finally IgA binding factor is also implicated in negative feedback regulation of IgA synthesis (8). Non immune factors may also be involved. They include neuroendocrine regulation by intestinal pepetides, such as VIP, Substance P, Somatostatine, locally produced by nerves ending in the lamina propria, and which affect PP lymphoid cell proliferation and differentiation in vitro (9). Other factors such as the gut microflora and nutrition are also important during ontogeny and for the development and maintenance of intestinal immunity during adult life.

2) Oral tolerance

Certain types of antigens, especially dietary proteins and commensal bacteria, are not immunogenic by the oral route. Instead they induce a state of specific tolerance called "oral tolerance", characterized by the absence of both secretory and systemic immune responses (10), and mediated by specific circulating T cells (11). Furthermore oral encounter with such antigens prevents systemic IgG and IgE responses and delayed type hypersensitivity (DTH) reactions to the same antigen subsequently administered systemicallY. Oral tolerance can be induced by challenge with high dose of antigen and/or prolonged antigenic exposure. Oral immunity and oral tolerance are both associated with the induction of circulating antigen-specific T cells. Depending on the type of antigen (particulate or soluble protein), and maybe on the site of antigen entry (PP versus Villi), T cell activation will be associated intestinal immunity or oral tolerance. Therefore we hypothesized that antigen processing/presentation through the gut could play an important role in the generation of tolerogenic T cells. The consequences of oral tolerance are beneficial for the host ; they prevent undesired allergic reactions to food antigens mostly, and prevent autoimmune reactions which may occur as a result of the cross reactivity between some bacterial antigens and self components. Interestingly, in celiac disease, abrogation of oral tolerance to gluten results in a severe gluten enteropathy.

3) Disorders of the gastrointestinal (GI) tract.

Immunological disorders of the GI tract include primarily

celiac disease (CD) (12), and inflammatory bowel diseases (IBD) (13). CD is a strongly HLA-linked gluten enteropathy, considered as an autoimmune reactivity to gut epithelium. This disease induces villus atrophy, crypt hyperplasia and massive infiltration of the lamina propria and the epithelium with activated T cells. As a result of inflammation, crypt epithelial cells are DR+ and villus epithelial cells express both DR and DQ molecules. The direct role of these cells in CD is supported by the recent data that Ia+ gut epithelial cells can present soluble antigen to activated T cells in an MHC restricted manner, (14), the genotypic association with class II in CD may result in impaired local immune response through expresion of the susceptibility HLA molecules. Therefore unexpected presentation of gluten by enterocytes, through expression of particular class II molecules, may explain abrogation of oral tolerance to gluten characteristic of this disease. IBD comprise a spectrum of disorders marked by chronic inflammation of the GI tract, which cannot be ascribed to a specific pathogen. The most typical IBD include Crohn's disease and Ulceritive colitis. Both diseases present acute phases and relapses, and are characterized by a massive infiltration of the lamina propria with activated T cells and macrophages. The ethiology of IBD is unknown but the bottom line is a focal destruction of the epithelium, and it has been proposed that they might represent an autoimmune reaction to inflammed gut epithelium of the large bowel, through unusual class II molecules expression.

II-ANTIGEN PRESENTATION IN THE INTESTINAL VILLI

APC which initiate antigen recognition by T cells may play an important role in the way T cell recognize antigen (sensitization phase), and this may have important implication in the effector phase of the response : immunity versus tolerance. The rationale for the hypothesis that gut epithelial cells from the gut villi could be involved in presentation of oral antigen is based on the following observations. Enterocytes, which cover 95% of the whole intestinal mucosa, are in direct contact with environmental antigen ; they are capable of antigen transport and degradation, and most importantly express MHC class II molecules. In recent studies we have reported that gut epithelial cells bear markers in common with dendritic cells (15), and constitutively express functional intercellular adhesion molecule-1 (ICAM-1) allowing adhesion of enterocytes to activated T cells (D.Kaiserlian, submitted for publication). Furthermore we demonstrated that enterocytes express functional Ia molecules, and can present antigen to CD4+ T cell hybridoma in an MHC-restricted way (16). These data pointed out a new role for enterocytes as intestinal antigen-presenting cells, besides their fuction in the transepithelial transport of polymeric IgA and production of secretory IgA. Thus it may be suggested that initiation of an immune response can take place within intestinal villi at distance from PP, and that antigen specific T cell may be activated in situ, following interaction with enterocytes. It is interesting to note that phenotypic differences between villus enterocytes and epithelial cells covering the PP dome region have been observed in the mouse. At variance with enterocytes, PP dome epithelium is class II negative in the mouse, does not express dendritic cell markers (15), and therefore is an unlikely candidate as intestinal APC. Instead several lines of evidence indicate that the major APC type in PP is the interdigitating dendritic cells, which initiate priming of virgin T cells. We recently observed evidence that enterocytes from the mouse small intestine express Ia molecules antigenically distinct from those of conventional APC. Indeed, of a large panel of anti-Ia antibodies, each of which stained 50% of splenocytes, only 2 strongly reacted with enterocytes, whereas none out of 20 allogeneic anti-Ia monoclonal antibodies tested recognized Ia on gut epithelial cells (although they stained splenocytes as expected). This lack of reactivity was not due to non specific steric hindrance by sialic acid, and was not restored after gamma interferon treatment in vivo. The molecular basis for these findings are currently being investigated. Our data support the view that molecular signals transmitted to T cells upon interaction with enterocyte Ia might not be identical to those transduced after interaction with conventional APC, and that incomplete or altered T cell activation pathway may lead to T cell anergy. Intraepithelial cells, which are in close contact with enterocytes, and lamina propria T cells, are both likely candidates for such lymphoepithelial interactions. In addition, enterocyte Ia may be the target of autoimmune reactions to gut epithelium such as those occuring in CD and in IBD.

REFERENCES

1. Owen R., Pierce N., Apple R. and Cray W. 1986. M cell transport of Vibrio Cholera from the intestinal lumen into Peyer's patches. J.Infect.Dis. 153 : 1108-1118.

2. George A., Kerlin R., Schrader C. and Cebra J. 1990. A clonal microculture that supports IgA expression by murine B cells. In "Advances in Mucosal immunology. Proceedings of the fifth International Congress of Mucosal Immunology". Klewer Acad. Publishers, London, pp 136-141.

3. Guy-Grand D. and Vassali P. 1987. Origin and traffic of gut mucosal lymphocytes and mast cells. In "Migration and homing of lymphoid cells". Vol II. Alan J.Husband Ed. CRC Press Inc. Florida pp 100-110.

4. Mestecky J. 1987. The common mucosal immune system and current strategies for induction of immune responses in external secretions. J.Clin.Immunol. 7:265-276.

5. Duijvestijn A. and Hamann A. 1989. Mechanisms and regulation of lymphocyte migration. Immunol.Today. 10:23-28.

6. Spalding D., Williamson S., Koopman W. and McGhee J. 1984. Preferential induction of polyclonal IgA secretion by murine Peyer's patch dendritic cell-T cell mixture. J.Exp.Med. 160:941-946.

7. Lebman D. Lee F. and Coffman R. 1990. Mechanism for transforming growth factor beta and IL-2 enhancement of IgA expression in LPS-stimulated B cell cultures. J.Immunol. 144:952-959.

8. McGhee J., Mestecky J. Elson C. and Kiyono H. 1989. Regulation of IgA synthesis and immune response by T cells and Interleukins. J.Clin.Immunol. 9:175-199.

9. Stanisz A., Bienenstock J. and Agro A. 1989. Neuromodulation of mucosal immunity. Regional Immunol. 2:414-419.

10. Mowat A. 1987. The regulation of immune responses to dietary protein antigens. Immunol.Today. 8:93-98.

11. MacDonald T. 1982. Immunosuppression caused by antigen feeding. I. Evidence for the activation of a feedback suppression pathway in the spleens of antigen fed mice. Eur.J.Immunol. 12:767-773.

12. Kagnoff M. 1988. Celiac disease: a model of an immunologically mediated intestinal disease. In "Immunology and allergy clinics of north america". Ed. by M.Kagnoff. W.B. Saunders Company, London. Vol 8 pp 505-520.

13. MacDermott R. and Stenson W. 1988. The role of the immune system in inflammatory bowel disease. In "Immunology and allergy clinics of north amarica". Ed. by M. Kagnoff. W.B. Saunders Company, London. Vol 8 pp 521-542.

14. Mayer L. and Shlien R. 1987. Evidence for function of Ia molecules on gut epithelial cells in man. J.Exp.Med. 166:1471-1483.

15. Vidal K., Kaiserlian D. and Revillard J.P. 1989. Hetero geneity of murine gut epithelium : three subsets defined by dendritic cell markers. Regional Immunology. 2:360-365.

16. Kaiserlian D., Vidal K. and Revillard J.P. 1989. Murine enterocytes can present soluble antigen to specific class II- r estricted $CD4^{+}$ T cells. Eur.J.Immunol. 19:1513-1516.

Cellular and Cytokine Networks in Tissue Immunity, pages 63-68

IMMUNOLOGY OF THE LOWER RESPIRATORY TRACT: A MODEL OF IMMUNE MEDIATED FIBROSIS IN THE LUNG.

Joan Stein-Streilein, Luisa Salter-Cid, Hernando Garcia and Judy Guffee.

Departments of Medicine and Microbiology/Immunology, University of Miami School of Medicine, Miami, Florida 33101.

INTRODUCTION.

It is accepted that the immune response in peripheral blood may not be representative of local immune responses within particular organs or tissues. The lung is representative of an organ in which immune responses may be uniquely local or in certain circumstances originate systemically as well (1,2). Antigenic challenge may originate in the airways from external stimuli or exit into pulmonary parenchyma from the vasculature. Unlike other internal organs, the lung can be sampled by lavage and both cellular and humoral aspects of the immune response can be monitored without extirpation of tissue (3). Because of this property, immune models of hypersensitivity that have previously been studied in external organs such as the skin can be studied in the lung. The capacity to sample from within the organ extends the capability of studies beyond that which can be done in the skin.

Contact hypersensitivity is induced experimentally by skin painting with hapten in carrier on a laboratory animal's abdomen five days prior to challenging on the ear (4). The assay is read by measuring the amount of swelling induced by the challenge. This phenomenon has been shown to be T lymphocyte dependent and includes an inflammatory response with associated fibrosis. Using this model of contact hypersensitivity, we modified the challenge site to the airways of the lung and observed a T dependent inflammatory response that resulted in non-resolving fibrosis in the challenged animals that were also immune. A non-specific inflammatory response with an accompanying fibrosis that healed by day 14 was observed in the challenge-only animals.

Pulmonary Fibrosis is characterized by a progressive increase in connective tissue in the lung parenchyma (5). Fibrosis has long been associated with conditions that are a consequence of cell-mediated responses including graft-versus-host disease, delayed type hypersensitivity reactions and granulomas. The hapten-immune hamster model for Pulmonary Interstitial Fibrosis correlates the non-resolving fibrosis observed in the lung parenchyma directly with the animal's prior immunization to the hapten.

The non-resolving nature of the fibrosis in the challenged-immune animal was supported by histologic examination by light microscopy and morphometric analysis of paraffin fix sections (6,7). Increased collagen deposition was shown with specific staining of collagen with Masson's trichrome. Both challenge-only and immune-challenged animals showed diffuse collagen deposition on day 7, but by day 14 the amount of collagen in the challenged control animals approached that seen in the unmanipulated animals. The Fibrosis was non-resolving in the experimental animals and was documented morphometrically in lungs of animals who were challenged as long as *six months previously (7).

The collagen deposition was measured biochemically by amino acid analysis of hydroxyproline content and results supported the histological data (6). Work reported at this meeting pertains to current studies that have adapted the model to *in vitro* analysis of the hypersensitivity and attempts to define a role for the T lymphocyte in the induction of non-resolving fibrosis in the hamsters.

Two questions are addressed: What is the nature of the collagen that is produced in the immune animals that are challenged? What lymphokines are uniquely present in the lungs of the immune-challenged hamsters?

Fibroblasts were cultured from all treatment groups. After two passages, aliquots were tested for collagen productions or served as a source for cellular RNA. Fibroblast cultures that were assayed for collagenase sensitive protein confirmed previous data that more collagen was deposited from cells harvested from primed animals that were challenged than by challenged-only or unmanipulated hamsters.

Slot hybridization studies were performed to quantitate the amounts of mRNA for procollagen I and procollagen III that were present in the fibroblasts from lung in each treatment group. The ratio for these messages was approximately 1:1 in total RNA harvested from control and challenge-only lung fibroblasts. The ratio for mRNA procollagen I:III approached 2:1 or greater in the challenged/immune treatment group. Interestingly, the mRNA for procollagen I was increased in both challenge groups that were challenged procollagen III was also increased but in the challenge-only treatment group. Since collagen III fibrils have been implicated in the termination of the collagen I fibrils (8), it is possible that collagen I continues to be deposited and/or resistent to breakdown when the quantity of collagen III is inadequate to regulate the termination of the fibril. Since both mRNA procollagen I and III

TABLE 1
Hapten Challenge of Immune Hamster alters mRNA ratio
Procollagen I : III in Lung Fibroblasts

Group	Experimental[a] Treatment Skin Paint	IT Chal.	Days Post Challenge	Pro-α 1(I) U/ug RNA	%	Pro-α 1(III) U/ug RNA	%	Type I:III Collagen mRNA Ratio[b]
A	+	+	2	6.1	95	7.5	93	1.22
			7	10.6	145	7.6	87	2.09
			14	15.4	220	11.0	117	2.10
			21	10.1	164	9.6	133	1.58
B	-	+	2	6.0	93	8.7	107	1.04
			7	11.2	153	12.6	144	1.33
			14	11.4	163	14.5	155	1.18
			21	8.1	132	9.9	131	1.28
C	-	-	2	6.5	100	8.1	100	1.19
			7	7.3	100	8.8	100	1.25
			14	7.0	100	9.4	100	1.12
			21	6.2	100	7.2	100	1.28

a Skin Painting: 100 μl of 7% TNCB in carrier to shaved abdomen. Challenge: 100 μl of 3% TNBS was inoculated intratracheally five days post sensitization.

b The amount of Procollagen I mRNA was adjusted from number chains detected by cDNA probe (2/3) by multiplying by 1.5.

are increased in the challenged-only animals, the immune response in the experimental animals may contribute to down regulating procollagen III transcription rather than inducing up regulation of procollagen I mRNA.

Studies to elucidate the lymphokine that may directly or indirectly influence the quality of the collagen made in the model showed that only lymphocytes from the immune-challenged animals expressed mRNA and function for IL2 and TNF β (lymphotoxin). Animals from all treatment groups were subjected to bronchoalveolar lavage at the time of harvesting the lung cells for fibroblast culture or recovering of plastic adherent or non-adherent lung mononuclear cells. The fluid recovered from 3 ml of PBS (Ca++ and Mg++ free) used for lavage was used for lymphokine analysis in a bioassay using the MTT method. CTLL-2 cells were the target for IL2 proliferation and WEHI.164 were the target cells for TNF activity. While TNF activity was increased in both challenged-only and immune-challenged lavage fluid, the activity was consistently greater in the fluid from the lungs of the immune hamsters (data not shown).

Because a specific antibody that discriminates between TNF α and β is not available in the hamster, we used cDNA probes specific for mRNA for TNF α and TNF β to performed Northern blot analysis of total cellular RNA for isolated from plastic adherent and non-adherent bronchoalveolar lavage cell populations from the various treatment groups (Figure 1). These studies also identified the cellular source

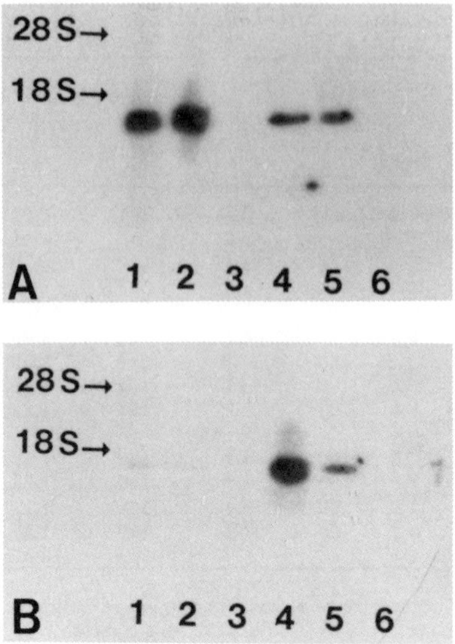

Fig. 1. Northern blot analysis of mRNA for TNF α, TNF β. Total RNA harvested from plastic adherent (lanes 1,2,3) and plastic non-adherent (lanes 4,5,6) subpopulations from collagenase digested lung mononuclear cells dissociated from treatment group A, challenged-immune (lanes 1,4); group B, challenged only (lanes 2,5); group C, age-matched controls (lanes 3,6). After electrophoresis on 1% agarose formaldehyde gels RNA was transferred to Nytro Nylon membranes (baked 2 h, 80°C) prehybridized (2 h, 42°C, 50% Foramide, 5% Denhardt media, 0.1% SDS, 5% SSPE, 10% Dextran Sulfate, 0.2 mg/ml sheared salmon sperm DNA) and hybridized to denature ^{32}P-DNATNF α, (Fig. 1A) or TNF β (Fig. 1B) probe that were added to the prehybridization fluid (16-10 h, 42°C) washed filters were exposed Kodak Xormat film for 6-24 h at -70°C with an intensifying screen.

source of the lymphokines as follows: 1) the adherent cells (macrophages) from both challenged-immune and challenged-only hamsters expressed TNF α mRNA; 2) non-adherent cells (lymphocytes) from the challenged-immune hamsters expressed small amounts of the TNF α mRNA but were unique in the expression of TNF β.

We also observed that IL2 was released into the airways and could be sampled by lavage of the hamsters in the challenged-immune treatment group. The proliferation of CTLL-2 cells induced by the lavage fluid was completely inhibited by the addition of specific antibody to IL2 but not by antibody to IL4. RIL2 (Genzyme Corp., Boston, MA) was used as a standard and units were calculated according to a linear regression analysis software program.

Activated T cells can mediate a change in fibroblast function and collagen formation in the lung by secretion of lymphokines. Such lymphokines can act directly on the fibroblasts (9) or can regulate their cellular function indirectly by inducing monokine (IL1) secretion which in turn can affect collagen synthesis (10-12). It is known that TNP is a small reactive chemical representative of hapten that can covalently bind to soluble or membrane bound proteins (13). Such haptenated antigens can persist within the lung and perpetuate the activation of the immune T cells; this chronic T cell activation may mediate the fibrosis by selectively increasing the type of collagen that is deposited. Activated T cells have been implicated in the mechanisms that mediates renal fibrogenesis (14). It is known that T lymphocytes promote classical contact hypersensitivity diseases (4) which may often involve an element of fibrosis (15-16). The experimental model of hapten-induced pulmonary interstitial fibrosis may be a model for pulmonary disease induced by industrial or environmental chemicals. Simple chemicals with spontaneous reactivity comparable to TNCB are probably, many, ubiquitous, and largely unrecognized as causing lung disease. One example known of a hapten causing lung disease is trimellitic anhydride (TMA), a reactive low molecular weight compound that is considered an industrial hazard in the plastic industry (17). TMA rapidly combines with human serum or with human erythrocytes to form antigens against which numerous types of antibodies can be detected (18). However, cell-mediated immunity to TMA has not been examined well.

In conclusion, the results from these studies show that the immune hamsters that were challenged with the immunizing hapten differed from the other treatment groups in the production of unique lympho-kines (IL2, TNF ß) and in the phenotype of mRNA that was tran-scribed for the procollagen protein. Lung fibroblasts cultured from hapten-immune hamsters that were challenged with the immunizing hapten transcribed more mRNA for procollagen I than procollagen III, thereby increasing the mRNA ratio. The mechanism by which the immune response alters the quality of the collagen produced and induces the non-resolving fibrosis may be related to increased levels of IL2 and TNF β of activated T lymphocytes in the pulmonary environment.

ACKNOWLEDGEMENTS.

The authors thank Dr. Francisco Ramirez, Mount Sinai School of Medicine, New York, NY, for his generous gift of cDNA probes procollagen I and III, and Dr. Nancy Ruddle, Yale University, New Haven, CT, for the cDNA probe for TNF β. Ms. Fatima DeFreitas is acknowledged for her devotion to the technical aspects of culturing fibroblasts and measuring collagen protein. We thank Aleida E. Name for her preparation of this manuscripts. We appreciate Dr. T. Jeff Powell, ImmuLogic Pharmaceuticals Corporation, Palo Alto, CA, for his expertise in the development of the software program used to calculate cytokine units in the MTT assay.

REFERENCES.

1. Mann DW, Sonnenfeld G, Stein-Streilein J (1985). Pulmonary Compartmentalization of Interferon and Natural Killer Cell Activity. Proc Soc Exp Biol Med 180:224-230.
2. Pitchenik AE, Guffee J, Stein-Streilein J (1987). Lung natural killer and Interleukin-2 activity in lung cancer. A pulmonary compartment of augmented natural killer activity occurs in patients with Bronchogenic Carcinoma. Am Rev Respir Dis 136: 1327-1332.

3. Reynolds HY (1987). Bronchoalveolar lavage. Am Rev Respir Dis 135:250-263.
4. Polak L (1980). Immunological aspects of contact sensitivity: an experimental study. Monographs in Allergy 15:1-170.
5. Crystal RG, Gadek JE, Ferrans VJ, Fulmer JD, Line BR, Hunninghake GW (1981). Interstitial lung disease: current concepts of pathogenesis, staging and therapy. Am J Med 70:542-66.
6. Stein-Streilein J, Lipscomb MF, Fisch H, Whitney PL (1987). Pulmonary Interstitial Fibrosis induced in hapten immune hamsters. Am Rev Respir Dis 136:119-123.
7. Altman N, Roberts B, Stein-Streilein J (1990). A histomorphometric analysis of Pulmonary Interstitial Fibrosis induced in hapten-immune hamsters. Proceedings of the 1990 Miami Biotechnology Winter Symposia, ICSU Short Reports, 10:202.
8. Fleischmayer R, Perlish JS, Timpl R (1985). Collagen fibrillogenesis in human skin. Ann NY Acad Sci 4608:246-257.
9. Johnson RL, Ziff M. (1976). Lymphokine stimulation of collagen accumulation. J Clin Invest 58:240.
10. Hadden JW, Sadek JR, Warfel AH (1981). Characterization of lymphokines acting on the macrophage (Hadden JW, Stewart WE, II. eds) In: *The Lymphokine*, The Humana Press, NJ p. 73.
11. Dinarello CA (1984). Interleukin I. Rev Infect Dis 6:51-95.
12. Wahl SM (1985). The role of lymphokines and monokines in fibrosis. In: Fleischmayer R, Olsen BR, Kuhn K, eds. *Biology chemistry and pathology of collagen.* Ann NY Acad Sci 460:225-31.
13. Good AH, Wofsy L, Henry C, Kimura J. (1980) Preparation of hapten-modified protein antigens. In: Mishell B, Shiigi S, eds. *Selected methods in cellular immunology.* Freeman, WH & Co, San Francisco, p. 345.
14. Neilson EG, Jimenez SA, Phillips SM. (1980) Cell mediated immunity in interstitial nephritis. III. T lymphocyte-mediated fibroblast proliferation and collagen synthesis: An immune mechanism for renal fibrogenesis. J Immunol 125:1708-1714.
15. Ulich T, Ahmed AR (1985). Inflammation. In: Stone J, ed, *Dermatology immunology and allergy.* CV Mosby Co, St Louis, p 103-110.
16. Roupe G, Rideu B (1979). The cellular infiltrate in contact hypersensitivity to picryl chloride in the mouse. Acta Dermato Vener (Stockholm) 59:191-95.
17. Zeiss CR, Patterson R, Pruzansky JJ, Miller M, Rosenberg M, Levitz D (1977). Trimellitic anhydride induced airway syndromes clinical and immunological studies. J Allergy Clin Immunol 60:96-103.
18. Zeiss CR, Levitz D, Chacon R, Walkansky P, Patterson R, Pruzansky J (1980). Quantitation and new antigenic determinant specificity of antibodies induced by inhalation of trimellitic anhydride in man. Int Arch Allergy Appl Immunol 61:380-388.

Cellular and Cytokine Networks in
Tissue Immunity, pages 69-75

PROLACTIN, GROWTH HORMONE, AND IMMUNE HOMEOSTASIS

Edward Bernton and Jitendra Dave

Neuropharmacology Br., Dept. of Medical Neuroscience, Div. of Neuropsychiatry, Walter Reed Army Institute of Research, Washington D.C. 20307-5100

INTRODUCTION

The complexities of the *in vivo* integration of immunologic function so as to assure the organism's adaptation to infectious and inflamatory stressors have recieved increased attention over the past decade. Yet the mechanisms by which the immunologic system both regulates and is regulated by non-immunologic physiologic processes remain to be clarified. The highest level of integration of physiologic stimuli and responses occurs at the level of the central nervous system, utilizing two afferent and two efferent pathways, the endocrine system and the autonomic nervous system.

Among the endocrine pathways linking immune and central nervous system, the ability of interleukin-1 to regulate body temperature, sleep, and the secretion of adreno-corticotropic hormone (ACTH) from the pituitary is a striking demonstration of the immune-CNS axis. Conversely, the neuroendocrine system, via the release of ACTH and the consequent secretion of adrenal glucocorticosteroids, has well-known regulatory effects on immunologic and inflammatory responses. Although the mechanisms by which glucocorticoids effect lymphocyte function are incompletely understood, (see Daynes and Aeneo, this volume) these hormones are widely utilized clinically and experimentally as immunosuppresives.

Recently, the immunoregulatory role of two trophic pituitary hormones, growth hormone (GH) and prolactin (PRL), has recieved increased attention. Treatment of mice with bromocryptine, which inhibits pituitary prolactin secretion, increases lethality of infection with L. *monocytogenes*, abrogates T-cell-dependent macrophage activation, and suppresses T-cell mitogenic responses. (1) These effects are prevented by administration of exogenous PRL. Hypophysectomy or treatment with bromocryptine abrogates delayed hypersensitivity responses, adjuvant-induced arthritis, and humoral responses to T-dependent antigens in rats. (2) Treatment with growth hormone or implantation of GH and PRL-secreting adenomas restores thymic cellularity and T-cell mitogenic responses in aged rats (3). Remarkably, treatment of rats with exogenous PRL or drugs stimulating release of endogenous PRL also antagonizes the suppression of T-cell function by cyclosporine. (4) Prolactin treatment, both in vivo and in vitro, increases production of thymulin by thymic epithelial cells. (5) Induction of arthritis in rats injected with Freund's adjuvant is associated with increased nocturnal PRL secretion; when this is blocked by treatment with bromocriptine, arthritis does not develop. (6) Such data all suggest that prolactin and growth-hormone are significant modulators of immune function in vivo.

However, the interaction of the mainly immuno-suppresive glucocorticoids and the immuno-trophic or -stimulatory lactogenic hormones (GH and PRL) has recieved little study. In studies of immunosuppresion due to chronic morphine treatment of mice, which was glucocorticoid-mediated, we found PRL treatment reversed morphine-induced suppression of T-cell functions. Subsequently, the immuno-regulatory interactions of glucocorticoids and lactogenic hormones were systematically studied.

METHODS

Groups of male or female C3H/HeN mice were implanted subcutaneously with Alzet mini-osmotic pumps or with cholesterol-methyl cellulose pellets (Innovative Research, Toledo Ohio) continually releasing varying amounts of corticosterone (CS) or vehicle. The resulting serum levels of CS, as measured by RIA, ranged from 3- to 10-fold above the basal levels in control mice, and were comparable to CS levels measured in mice chronically-stressed with resulting immunosuppression. Mice also recieved either ovine PRL, recombinant monkey PRL, recombinant human growth hormone (which binds as an agonist at PRL receptors) or recombinant bovine growth hormone (which does not bind to PRL receptors. The effects of treatment with CS and lactogenic hormones, individually or in combination, on spleen lymphocyte proliferation in vitro to mitogens and on specific PRL binding in liver microsomal membranes preparations (see 7), was determined. Lymphocytes were cultured in serum-free media supplemented with 2-beta-mercaptoethanol.

RESULTS

Three days of treatment with pellets releasing 50 ug/day of corticosterone resulted in consistent suppression of spleen lymphocyte responses to T-cell mitogens. (**Figure 1**) Simultaneous treatment with either ovine prolactin (PRL), recombinant human growth hormone (rhGH), or bovine growth hormone (bGH) significantly reversed this suppression. These hormones were delivered at a dose of 1ug/hour from a subcutaneous minipump.

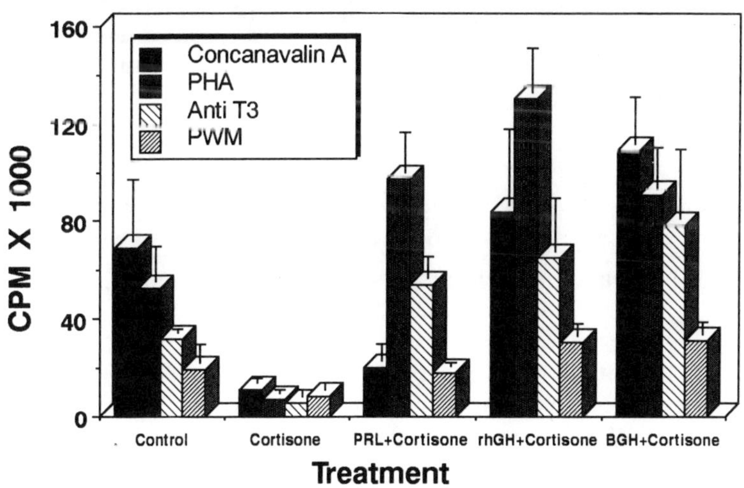

Figure 1. - Proliferation of T-cells assessed by radio-thymidine incorporation. Bars represent mean and SEM for 3 groups of 2 pooled mice spleens for each treatment. This experiment utilized male C3H/HeN mice.

In further experiments the same 3-day corticosterone treatment was again immunosuppressive and was found to suppress prolactin receptors in the liver, measured as specific binding of iodinated PRL to liver microsomal membrane preps. Simultaneous reatment with recombinant human GH was found to upregulate prolactin receptors while reversing suppressed T-cell proliferation. (**Fig 2**) Thymic atrophy due to CS treatment was not antagonized by GH.

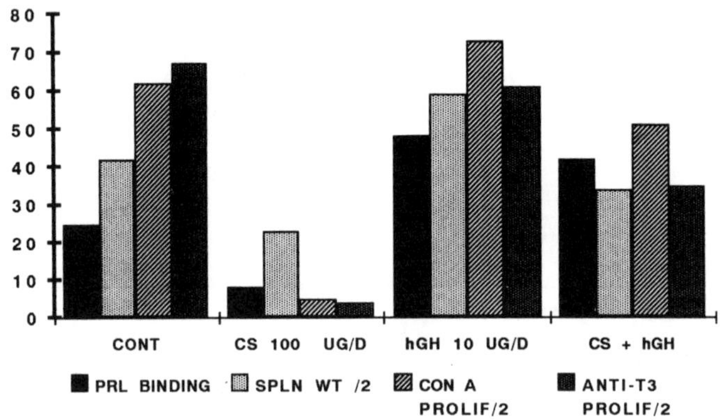

Figure 2. - Vertical scale represents CPM x 10^{-3} of radio-thymidine incorporation, CPM x 10^{-3} per mg.of PRL specific binding to hepatic membranes, and spleen weight in mg.

Treatment of mice for three days with continuously-released corticosterone at doses ranging from 10 to 250 ug/day was found to result in a dose-dependent down-regulation of liver prolactin receptors, without changes in liver growth hormone receptors. Female mice, which had higher circulating PRL levels and up to three-fold greater liver PRL-binding than untreated males, were more resistant to absolute and relative decreases in liver prolactin receptors following CS treatment.. This correlated with a lesser sensitivity to suppression of T-cell proliferation by corticosterone treatment. Measurement of serum corticosterone levels following treatment revealed a highly significant inverse correlation between CS levels and liver PRL specific binding. (**Figure 3**).

Other studies compared the efficacy of daily or twice daily injections or PRL or GH versus continual infusion of hormone for the reversal of CS immunosuppression. These revealed that 20-40 fold higher doses of hormone were required when given by twice daily sc injection compared to continual infusion, for equivalent effect. (Data not shown.) This suggests that maintenance of elevated steady state hormone concentrations are necessary for glucocorticoid antagonism.

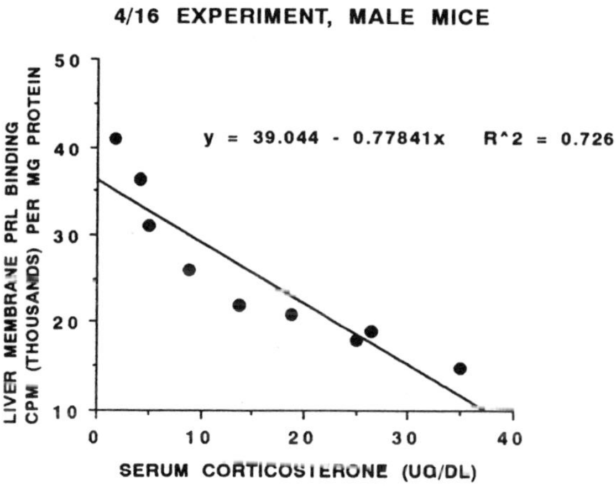

Figure 3. - 9 Groups of 3 male mice recieved varying doses of corticosterone for three days. Specific PRL binding was determined for the 20,000 G liver microsomal membrane preparations and expressed per mg. protein. (7) Corticosterone was measured by RIA. Each point represents the mean values for a group of three mice.

DISCUSSION

Lactogenic hormones were found to antagonize suppression of T-cell mitogenic responses following treatment of mice with quantities of glucocorticoids which elevated blood levels into or somewhat beyond the high physiologic range. The specificity of this effect included prolactin, human GH, which is a PRL-receptor agonist, and bovine GH which does not bind to the PRL receptor. All these lactogenic hormones specifically up-regulated liver PRL receptors, and prevented their downregulation by gluco-corticoid treatment. While prolactin and growth hormone secretion is normally pulsatile and episodic, moderate but sustained elevations of either of these hormones most effectively up-regulated liver prolactin receptors and antagonized glucocorticoid effects on lymphocyte proliferation. Such sustained elevation of lactogenic hormones occurs naturally during pregnancy, and we hypothesize may protect the fetus from the imunosuppressive and neurotoxic effects of high circulating levels of glucocorticoids which also occur at that time, especially close to parturition.

The question remains as to whether changes in liver PRL-receptors directly effect T-lymphocyte function, or simply represent a correlate of changes in PRL receptors occurring in lymphoid tissue compartments. PRL receptors of high affinity but extremely low number have been reported on human and murine lymphocytes (8) and on human large granular lymphocytes (9). Intriguingly, lymphocyte PRL-binding can be antagonized in vitro by the immunosuppressant peptide cyclosporine A.(10) We are unable to date to demonstrate significant lymphocyte PRL-binding using classic radio-ligand receptor binding assays, and thus to examine changes following treatments which modulated liver receptors. However, PRL-receptors have recently been identified on murine T-cell lines using flourescent-activated flow cytometry and a monoclonal antibody to PRLr (11).

We hypothesize that the coordinate regulation of T-cell proliferation by glucocorticoids and lactogenic hormones, may be due to these hormones' effects on lymphocyte PRL receptors. Of interest, lymphocytes have been found to produce a PRL-immunoreactive protein during proliferation (12,13), and antibodies to pituitary PRL can inhibit proliferation of lymphocytes and IL-2 dependent cell lines.(14) Thus both secretion of an autocrine PRL-like protein and the endocrine regulation of PRL receptors may be involved in regulation of lymphocyte function in vivo.

REFERENCES

1. Bernton, E. W., Meltzer, M. S., & Holaday, J. W. (1988). Suppression of macrophage activation and T-lymphocyte function in hypoprolactinemic mice. *Science*, 239(4838), 401-4.

2. E. Nagy, I. Berczi, G. E. Wren, S. L. Asa, K. Kovacs, Modulation of immune function by bromocriptine. *Immunopharm.* 6, 231-238 (1983).

3. Kelley, K. W., Brief, S., Westly, H. J., Novakofski, J., Bechtel, P. J., Simon, J., & Walker, E. B. (1986). GH3 pituitary adenoma cells can reverse thymic aging in rats. *PNAS* 83(15), 5663-7.

4. Hiestand, P. C., Mekler, P., Nordmann, R., Grieder, A., & Permongkol, C. (19861986). Prolactin as a modulator of lymphocyte responsiveness provides a possible mechanism of action for cyclosporine. *PNAS*, 83, 2599-2604.

5. Dardenne, M., Savino, W., Gagnerault, M., Itoh, T., & Bach, J. F. (1989). Neuroendocrine control of thymic hormonal production. I. Prolactin stimulates in vivo and in vitro the production of thymulin by human and murine thymic epithelial cells. *Endocrinology*, 125(1), 3-12.

6. Neidhart, M. (1989). Bromocryptine microcapsules inhibit ornithine decarboxylase activity induced by Freund's complete adjuvant in lymphoid tissues of male rats. *Endocrinology*, 125(6), 2846-2852.

7. Dave, J., Brown, N., and Knazek, R. (1982) Prolactin modifies the prostaglandin synthesis, prolactin binding and fluidity of mouse liver membranes. *Biochem. Biophys. Res. Commun.* 108(1), 193-198.

8. Russell, D. H., Kibler, R., Matrisian, L., Larson, D. F., Poulos, B., & Magun, B. E. (1985). Prolactin receptors on human T and B lymphocytes: antagonism of prolactin binding by cyclosporine. *J. Immunol.* 134(5), 3027-31.

9. Matera, L., Muccioli, G., A, C., Bellussi, G., & Geneazzani, E. (1988). Prolactin receptors on large granular lymphocytes: dual regulation by cyclosporin A. *Brain, Behavior and Immunity*, 2, 1-10.**10.** Russell, D. H., Kibler, R., Matrisian, L., Larson, D. F., Poulos, B., & Magun, B. E. (1985). Prolactin receptors on human T and B lymphocytes: antagonism of prolactin binding by cyclosporine. *J. Immunol.* 134(5), 3027-31.

11. Clevenger, C. V., Russell, D. H., Appasamy, P. M., & Prystowsky, M. B. (1990). Regulation of interleukin 2-driven lymphocyte proliferation by prolactin. *Proc. Natl. Acad. Sci. USA*, 87, 6460-6464.

12. J. R. Kenner, J. W. Holaday, E. W. Bernton, P. F. Smith, (1990) Prolactin-like protein in murine splenocytes: morphological and biochemical evidence. *Prog. NeuroEndocrinImmunol.* **3**, 188-195 .

13. Montgomery, D. W., et al (1987). Concanavalin-A stimulated lymphocytes produce a factor with prolactin-like bioactivity and immunoreactivity. *Biochem. Biophys Res Commun.* 145, 692-697.

14. Hartmann, D. P., Holaday, J. W., & Bernton, E. W. (1989). Inhibition of lymphocyte proliferation by antibodies to prolactin. *FASEB J.* 3(10), 2194-202.

Cellular and Cytokine Networks in
Tissue Immunity, pages 77-82

REGULATION OF T-CELL FUNCTION BY STEROID HORMONES

Raymond A. Daynes and Barbara A. Araneo

**Dept. of Pathology, Univ. of Utah Medical School
Salt Lake City, Utah 84132**

Introduction

The organized lymphoid tissues of warm-blooded animals, which include the lymph nodes, Peyer's patches, spleen, etc., may actually have evolved as a consequence of the differential needs of distinct tissues with regards to the most suitable forms of immunologic intervention required to afford them protection. Immunity against infection of the skin, lungs, gut, or genitourinary tract is best facilitated through distinct types of immune effector responses with cellular immunity generally predominating responses to antigens presented through the skin, while humoral immunity, including the generation of antigen-specific secretory IgA, representing the type of immunity required to effectively protect mucosal tissues.

T cells, which have evolved to recognize antigen peptides in the context of self major histocompatibility complex molecules, are considered by most immunologists to represent the central cell type within the immunologic universe. T cells possess the capacity to influence development of all forms of adaptive immunity, and are also capable of recirculating freely between the blood and the various types of lymphoid tissues. Lymphocyte recirculation provides resting T cells with accessibility to all secondary lymphoid compartments.

What processes control the ability of individual T cells within the recirculating pool to accurately guide the development of the various types of immune effector responses? Functionally, T cells stimulated through their T-cell receptor can be induced to synthesize and secrete a number of lymphokines (LK), each exhibiting pleiotropic activities and being capable of exerting their biologic responses through autocrine, paracrine, or sometimes endocrine routes. Individual species of LK can display either additive, synergistic, antagonistic, or even agonistic influences with other LK on a particular tissue or target cell (1). Therefore, the pattern of LK secreted by T cells in response to stimulation is just as important as the quantity of any individual LK secreted. Collectively these molecules appear to be essential for the intracellular communication needed to promote or inhibit the various types of immunologic responses (2).

What mechanisms might serve to regulate the capacity of T cells to produce a particular repertoire of lymphokines following antigen-specific activation? This represents a central question in contemporary immunobiology, with the probability that such controlling influences are being provided at many distinct levels. It has recently been determined that T-cell-associated CD3 complexes can exhibit a degree of heterogeneity in their polypeptide composition. Such differences directly correlate with the type of signal transduction mechanism capable of being stimulated (3). Since the transcriptional regulation of the various LK genes are not coordinately controlled, variations in the signal transduction mechanisms employed are certainly involved in selective activation of particular lymphokine genes. Further, there exist a number of additional observations demonstrating that the mere physical presence of one species of LK can inhibit or promote the production and/or secretion of other LK species (4,5).

For the past two years our laboratory has been questioning the influences exerted by various species of steroid hormones on the ability of activated T cells to produce particular species of lymphokines. We have recently found that many species of steroid hormones exist that have profound influences on T-cell function. These hormones can be divided into 2 distinct categories: those that mediate their influence through endocrine mechanisms, and those that modify the potential of susceptible target cells primarily through paracrine routes.

The glucocorticoids (GCS) represent a class of steroid hormones whose characteristics place them in the first category. Released by the adrenals, the GCS are known to affect many lymphocyte functions. In addition to their well characterized depressive influences on IL-2 and γIFN synthesis, we recently discovered that the synthesis and secretion of IL-4 is greatly augmented by T cells exposed *in vitro* or *in vivo* to low doses of GCS (6 and Table 1). Based on reports which describe a number of anti-inflammatory properties of IL-4, it is possible that some of the immunologic changes which are associated with elevations in plasma GCS levels (endogenous or therapeutic) might be secondary to their ability to promote IL-4 synthesis (6).

As our work proceeded, we determined that at least three additional species of naturally occurring steroid hormones were also able to exert very fundamental regulatory influences on T-cell function. These hormones, which include dehydroepiandrosterone, dihydrotestosterone, and 1,25-dihydroxyvitamin D_3, share the common property of primarily existing within the circulation in an inactive precursor form (e.g., DHEA sulfate, testosterone, and 25-hydroxyvitamin D_3). Further, these hormone precursors are each capable of being enzymatically converted to their respective active species within a particular tissue or cell, providing a very simple mechanism to achieve site specificity to their regulatory activities.

Dehydroepiandrosterone (DHEA) Augments the Potential for T Cells to Produce IL-2 and γIFN Following Activation.

DHEA represents the major species of steroid hormone produced by most warm-blooded animals and is efficiently sulfated to DHEAS prior to its release from the adrenals. When T cells (both $CD4^+$ and $CD8^+$) are exposed to the effects of DHEA *in vitro* and then activated, their ability to secrete IL-2 and γIFN is significantly enhanced, with no effect being observed on the synthesis and secretion of IL-4 or IL-5 (7 and Table 1). DHEAS was found to be incapable of altering the capacity of activated T cells to produce lymphokines (7). We also determined that macrophages, but not B cells, express the enzyme DHEA-sulfatase, and can effectively provide DHEA-mediated influences to T cells during the process of antigen presentation (e.g., augment their potential to produce IL-2 and γIFN) when DHEAS is present (8).

We feel that the ability to anatomically localize the desulfation of DHEA may represent a fundamental regulatory mechanism for this hormone. Such a mechanism would provide an attractive means to control the potential for given T cells, residing within a particular lymphoid compartment, to produce selected LK. This concept is supported by our observation that T cells resident within lymphoid compartments which receive their primary drainage from nonmucosal tissues produce high levels of IL-2 and low levels of IL-4 following activation, while activated T cells derived from lymphoid compartments receiving their predominant drainage from mucosal tissues produce IL-4 as the major species of T-cell growth factor (9). Furthermore, these phenotypic observations could be directly correlated to the quantity of DHEA sulfatase activity present within the various lymphoid compartments (9).

Additional correlative information on the importance of DHEA and DHEAS to normal immune function has recently been obtained from an analysis of the immune systems of aged mice. We observed that T cells derived from all lymphoid compartments of animals older than 13 months show a marked increase in the production of IL-4 that parallels the clearly described decrease in their capacity to produce IL-2 following activation (10). Since it is known that endogenous production of DHEA and its sulfated derivative exhibits an age-dependence, with older individuals possessing a marked depression in the ability to synthesize this steroid hormone, we questioned whether dietary supplementation with DHEAS would influence the T-cell function of older animals. By providing old animals with DHEAS, we were able to completely reverse the age-associated changes in T-cell lymphokine production. T cells from DHEAS-supplemented animals were able to consistently generate young-adult levels of IL-2, γIFN and IL-4 (10). We conclude that a striking relationship exists between the age-related reduction in the capacity of T cells from old animals to produce certain species of lymphokines and the well-documented loss in their capacity to endogenously produce the steroid hormone DHEA.

Dihydrotestosterone Affects the Capacity of Stimulated T Cells to Produce IL-4, IL-5, and γIFN.

Testosterone represents the naturally occurring androgen steroid found in the circulation of all warm-blooded animals, and has been implicated to possess immunoregulatory properties from studies which determined that testosterone treatment of rodents can provide protection against certain types of autoimmune diseases (11). Testosterone must be converted by the enzyme, 5α-reductase, to dihydrotestosterone (DHT) before it is able to influence susceptible cellular targets. We have determined that DHT, but not testosterone, is capable of significantly influencing the ability of activated T cells to produce certain species of lymphokines (12). Secretion of IL-4, IL-5, and γIFN is depressed following the DHT treatment of murine T cells, while their capacity to produce IL-2 remains unaffected (Table 1). Furthermore, incubation of macrophages with testosterone prior to their use *in vitro* as antigen presenting cells for T-cell clones or T-cell hybridomas, resulted in a change in T-cell lymphokine production which was consistent with their ability to convert this androgen steroid to DHT (12). These findings suggested to us that DHT, which is able to be locally produced from its circulating precursor, might play a significant and natural role in regulating the capacity of activated T cells to produce some of the lymphokine species required for optimal antibody production (e.g., IL-4 and IL-5).

1,25-Dihydroxyvitamin D_3 Augments the Capacity of T Cells to Produce IL-4 and IL-5.

1,25-dihydroxyvitamin D_3 [1,25$(OH)_2D_3$] represents a steroid hormone which historically has been directly implicated in thc control of numerous cellular genes (13). This hormone has also been reported to depress the capacity of treated T cells to produce γIFN and IL-2, but its underlying role in the natural regulation of T-cell function has not yet received considerable attention. We have recently discovered that 1,25$(OH)_2D_3$ is capable of greatly augmenting the ability of activated T cells to produce IL-4 and IL-5 when they are exposed to very low concentrations of this hormone (Table 1). Far greater concentrations of 1,25$(OH)_2D_3$ were needed to cause a reduction in the ability of T cells to produce γIFN and IL-2, indicating that the mechanisms responsible for upregulating lymphokine gene function was far more sensitive than those responsible for causing the inhibition in synthesis of other lymphokines. Once again, macrophages were found to be capable of effectively converting 25-hydroxyvitamin D_3 to 1,25$(OH)_2D_3$ *in vitro*, an effect which could be completely blocked with ketoconazole, a 1α-hydroxylase inhibitor (8).

Table 1.

Steroid Treatment of T Lymphocytes	Change in Lymphokine Activity IL-2	IL-4	IL-5	γIFN
Glucocorticoids[b]	↓ (0.1-0.5)[a]	↑ (150-300)	N.C.	↓ (0.1-0.5)
DHEA[c]	↑ (150-400)	N.C.	N.C.	↑ (125-300)
DHT[d]	N.C.	↓ (0.1-0.5)	↓ (0.1-0.5)	↓ (0.3-0.6)
1,25(OH)D_3[e]	↓ (0.25-0.75)	↑ (175-400)	↑ (200-500)	↓ (0.25-0.75)

a. Arrows indicate direction of change from control values in production of the indicated lymphokines. N.C. indicate no change from control values and the parentheses () indicate the range in percent change.
b. Effective dose range to mediate changes in lymphokine production: Stimulation (10^{-11} M - 10^{-8} M); Inhibition (10^{-8} M - 10^{-6} M).
c. Effective dose range = 10^{-10} M- 10^{-7} M.
d. Effective dose range = 10^{-10} M - 10^{-7} M.
e. Effective dose range: Stimulation (10^{-11} - 10^{-9}); Inhibition (10^{-6} M - 10^{-7} M).

Conclusion

Our studies into the control of T-cell lymphokine production by steroid hormones are presently at a stage where their biologic effects are still being defined. Therefore, any conclusions drawn from this work remains highly speculative at this time. Our determination, that an immunomodulatory role exists for a number of distinct steroid hormones, whose circulating precursors require site-specific metabolism for effective conversion to their bioactive species, implicates their involvement in the most basic aspects of lymphokine gene regulation.

References

1. Mosmann TR, Coffman RL (1989). TH1 and TH2 cells: different patterns of lymphokine secretion lead to different functional properties. Ann Rev Immunol 7: 145-173.

2. Miyajima A, Miytake S, et al. (1988). Coordinate regulation of immune and inflammatory responses by T cell-derived lymphokines. FASEB J 2: 2462-2473.
3. Ashwell JD, Klausner RD (1990). Genetic and mutational analysis of the T cell antigen receptor. Ann Rev Immunol 8: 139-168.
4. Finkelman FD, Holmes J, et al. (1990). Lymphokine control of *in vivo* immunoglobulin isotype selection. Ann Rev Immunol 8: 303-334.
5. Peleman R, Wu J, et al. (1989). Recombinant interleukin 4 suppresses the production of interferon γ by human mononuclear cells. J Exp Med 170: 1751-1756.
6. Daynes RA, Araneo BA (1989). Contrasting effects of glucocorticoids on the capacity of T cells to produce the growth factors interleukin 2 and interleukin 4. Eur J Immunol 19: 2319-2325.
7. Daynes RA, Dudley D, et al. (1990). Regulation of murine lymphokine production *in vivo*. II. Dehydroepiandrosterone is a natural enhancer of IL-2 synthesis by helper T cells. Eur J Immunol 20: 793-802.
8. Daynes RA, Meikle AW, et al. (1990). Locally active steroid hormones may facilitate compartmentalization of immunity by regulating the types of lymphokines produced by helper T cells. Res Immunol Forum (in press).
9. Daynes RA, Araneo BA, et al. (1990). Regulation of murine lymphokine production *in vivo*. III. The lymphoid tissue microenvironment exerts regulatory influences over T helper cell function. J Exp Med 171: 979-996.
10. Araneo BA, Terui T, et al. (1990). The age-related alterations in murine T-cell potential for lymphokine synthesis are linked to endocrine output of adrenal androgen steroid hormones. Mech Aging Devel (submitted).
11. Theofilopoulos AN, Dixon FJ (1985). Murine models of systemic lupus erythematosus. Adv Immunol 37: 269-390.
12. Araneo BA, Dowell TA, et al. (1990). Dihydrotestosterone exerts a depressive influence on the production of IL-4, IL-5, and γIFN but not IL-2 by activated murine T cells. Blood (submitted).
13. Minghetti P, Norman AW (1988). 1,25$(OH)_2$-Vitamin D_3 receptors: gene regulation and gene circuitry. FASEB J 2: 3043-3053.

Cellular and Cytokine Networks in Tissue Immunity, pages 83-89

INTERACTION BETWEEN INFLAMMATORY CELLS AND NERVES IN THE GASTROINTESTINAL MUCOSA. EVIDENCE FOR A MAST CELL RELAY.

Ron H. Stead

Department of Pathology, McMaster University, Hamilton, Ontario, Canada.

INTRODUCTION

For many years the immune and nervous systems have been viewed as different and independent physiological entities, both with respect to each other and with reference to somatic homeostatic mechanisms in general. However, during the past decade, considerable effort has gone into trying to elucidate biochemical pathways which are common to both the immune and nervous systems, in an attempt to provide a molecular basis for cross-talk between the two. It is now known that several interleukins are synthesized within the central nervous system (although most of this data relates to glial populations) and that inflammatory cells are able to synthesize and secrete a range of molecules that have usually been termed neuropeptides. Additional evidence suggests that lymphokines, such as interleukin (IL)-1, IL-2, IL-3 and IL-6 affect nerve growth and, conversely, that 2.5S nerve growth factor may also act on hematopoietic lineages. Yet other studies have shown that immune responses can be modified using Pavlovian conditioning, providing some substance to the older anecdotal observations that an individual's psychological state can affect disease processes. The reader is referred to a recent text for detailed descriptions and references in this general area (Ader *et al.*, 1990).

That different "physiological" systems produce or are affected by the same regulatory molecules does not provide a basis for communication between immune and neural cell types. Such data would, however, be more pertinent if inflammatory cell populations were shown to be innervated. The pre-requisites for neuro-effector junctions between peripheral nerve terminals and immune cells include: 1) close apposition of preterminal axons and the target cells; 2) localization of appropriate neurotransmitter(s) in the nerve terminals; 3) release of the transmitter(s) upon nerve stimulation; 4) appropriate receptors on the target cells; and 5) activation of the target by applied neurotransmitter(s). Similar criteria could be defined for a sensory relationship of inflammatory cells and nerves.

Of the diverse immune cell types, the predominantly paravascular, connective tissue-based mast cells are certainly candidates for direct communication with nerves. Many investigators consider such interactions to be involved in neurogenic inflammation and the axon-reflex to noxious stimuli.[1] The substantial body of evidence for this has been reviewed elsewhere (Stead *et al.*, 1990b). My own studies have focused on the gastrointestinal tract, where several of the prerequisites for the innervation of mast cells have been determined (Stead *et al.*, 1990a; Stead, Bienenstock, 1990). The reader is referred to these last three reviews for references not included in the following.

INNERVATION OF MAST CELLS IN THE GASTROINTESTINAL MUCOSA

Microanatomical Evidence for the Association of Mast Cells and Nerves

Two or three earlier publications alluded to a close association between intestinal mucosal mast cells (IMMC) and nerves, and Newson *et al.* (1983) provided electron-microscopical evidence for bouton-like synapses between two mast cells and nerves in the rat ileum. However, enteric nerves, like autonomic fibres, do not necessarily form such tight synaptic structures with their targets and separations of 250nm or more are considered acceptable for neurotransmission. Accordingly, light- and electron-microscopical studies of rat and human intestines were performed (Stead *et al.*, 1987; Stead *et al.*, 1988; Stead *et al.*, 1989). In the normal rat jejunum, about one-half of the mucosal mast cells were apposed to neuron-specific enolase-containing nerves and this increased to approximately two-thirds in animals infected 35 days previously with *Nippostrongylus brasiliensis*. Equivalent light-microscopical determinations in the human, in relatively normal mucosa, revealed a similar range of associations (47% to 77%) of mucosal mast cells with PGP9.5-immunoreactive nerves. Electron microscopy confirmed this association, with between 4% and 8% of mast cells in the rat jejunum exhibiting membrane/membrane (20nm) apposition with preterminal axons. Arizono *et al.* (1990) have also recorded mast cell/nerve associations in rat intestines, although they found smaller proportions of IMMC close to nerves at the ultrastructural level.

Presence of Neurotransmitter Substances in Nerves Apposed to Mast Cells

I have also reported ultrastructural evidence for peptider-

---

(1) Although recent reports indicate that mast cells in the skin are not readily activated by nerve stimulation, the readout of mast cell degranulation in such experiments may not be a sufficiently sensitive indicator, especially when large numbers of mast cells appear partially degranulated, even in control animals (Kowalski & Kaliner 1988; Daranluk et al 1990).

gic nerves associated with mast cells, as well as immunohistochemical data for both substance P (SP) and calcitonin gene-related peptide in nerves adjacent to IMMC (Stead *et al.*, 1987; Stead *et al.*, 1988). Yonei and colleagues published ultrastructural evidence for cholinergic-type vesicles in nerves apposed to mast cells in the gastrointestinal mucosa (Yonei, 1987; Yonei *et al.*, 1985). Studies in other tissue sites have also shown SP-containing nerves apposed to mast cells.

Release of Neurotransmitters from Nerves Adjacent to Mast Cells

Although direct nerve stimulation studies have not been done to address this question, Bani-Sacchi *et al.* (1986) have shown that field stimulation of the ileum causes a diminution of mast cell granularity, accompanied by histamine and acetylcholine release. These effects were reduced by both tetrodotoxin and atropine, suggesting cholinergic-induced secretion from mast cells. Evidence also exists in the rat stomach, where, after sectioning the vagus nerve, mast cells exhibited increased granularity, with some presumably related changes in histamine levels (Ganguly, Gopinath, 1979; Ganguly *et al.*, 1978).

Additional physiological data suggests that there might be two-way comunication between mast cells and nerves in the gastrointestinal mucosa. This has been derived from Ussing chamber studies of epithelial short-circuit current, which increases in response to antigen challenge in previously sensitized animals. These changes involve mediators which may be mast cell-derived, such as histamine, serotonin and arachidonic acid metabolites, and can be diminished by pretreatment with doxantrazole (which stabilizes mucosal mast cells). More importantly, the antigen-induced increase in short circuit current can also be inhibited by tetrodotoxin, which blocks sodium channels in nerves (see Stead *et al.*, 1990b).

Neurotransmitter Receptors on Mast Cells in the Gastrointestinal Mucosa

Definitive evidence for the presence of neurotransmitter receptors on mast cells in the gastrointestinal mucosa is not yet available, although pharmacological studies on peritoneal mast cells suggest that these may have SP (NK_1) (Devillier *et al.*, 1985) and muscarinic receptors (see Stead *et al.*, 1990b). Immunohistochemical and hybridization studies are currently underway in my laboratory to look for the expression of neurokinin and acetylcholine receptors on mucosal mast cells. Preliminary experiments using an antiserum raised against the third extracellular domain of the rat SP receptor (provided by Dr. D. G. Payan, San Fransisco) suggest that IMMC from *Nippostrongylus brasiliensis*-infected rats have SP receptor-immunoreactivity.

Response of Mast Cells to Applied Neurotransmitters

Although connective tissue mast cells, especially those isolated from the peritoneal cavity, are well known to release histamine in response to a range of neuropeptides, to date only SP has been shown to cause histamine release from rat IMMC (Shanahan *et al.*, 1985). The classical transmitters acetylcholine and noradrenaline also affect mast cell function, although the literature in this area is somewhat contradictory (Stead *et al.*, 1990b).

CONSEQUENCES OF NEUROCRINE MAST CELL ACTIVATION

Mast cell activation is generally thought of in terms of the binding of IgE to high affinity receptors and the subsequent effects of challenge with antigen, resulting in immediate-type hypersensitivity reactions and allergy. However, mast cells may also be activated by a variety of other stimuli including heat, cold, pressure and chemicals (such as neurochemical). It is well established that activated mast cells produce arachidonic acid metabolites, in addition to the preformed, granule-based mediators, such as histamine, proteoglycans and proteases. These substances have a diverse range of biological activities including vasodilation or vasoconstriction, increased vascular and epithelial permeability, recruitment of other granulocytes, and disruption of connective tissues. Recent data derived from cultured mast cell lines suggest a plethora of other activities associated with several cytokines which are rapidly generated after mast cell activation. These include interleukins 3 to 6, granulocyte/monocyte colony stimulating factor and tumour necrosis factor α (see Stead, Bienenstock, 1990).

Importantly, mast cell activation may not necessarily result in degranulation, and the different preformed and newly generated mediators are not necessarily all produced in concert. In this context the reader should note that the majority of studies looking at mast cell stimulation have employed histamine release to indicate a response. Recently, more attention has been paid to the possibility of differential release of mast cell mediators. For example, Levi-Schaffer and Shalit (1989) studied the actions of antigen, SP, neurotensin and bradykinin on peritoneal mast cells maintained in fibroblast cultures. Challenge with antigen caused histamine release and significant production of prostaglandin D_2; however, SP, neurotensin and bradykinin were effective histamine releasers but had minimal or no effect on the synthesis of the arachidonic acid metabolite. This type of data suggests that neurocrine (SP?) activation of mast cells might have different phsyiological effects to challenge with antigen.

REMODELLING OF NERVES DURING INFLAMMATION

When considering the possibility of innervation of

migratory inflammatory cells, the tendency is to think of the nerve component as a static phase. However, in classical nerve/target relationships, such as voluntary muscle, alterations in the target density are accompanied by parallel changes in the innervation. Similar interactions between autonomic nerves and their targets have also been documented (see Stead, Bienenstock, 1990). I hypothesized, therefore, that if cells of the mucosal immune system (especially mast cells) were innervated, changes in the density of the local innveration might occur during inflammation and repair.

To test this hypothesis, I used the *Nippostrongylus brasiliensis* model (Stead *et al.*, submitted). During the acute inflammatory phase in the jejunum, which occurs between one and two weeks post-infection, the mucosal innervation underwent a phase of degeneration. This was evidenced by increased cross-sectional area of the mucosal nerves resulting from axonal dilation; apparent leakage of neuron-specific enolase into the lamina propria; and ultrastructural changes including damaged axonal profiles with myelin bodies. Subsequently, after about two-and-a-half weeks, there was a rapid increase in the number of IMMC, which persisted for several weeks, and the acute inflammatory changes subsided. During this recovery phase the mucosal neuronal population regenerated, evidenced by a marked increase in the proportion of small diameter GAP-43-immunoreactive fibres (2-fold greater than controls and 4-fold greater than the number present during the degenerative phase). At seven weeks post-infection the number of GAP-43-immunoreactive nerves was approximately 30% greater than controls ($p<0.001$). It is not yet known if any particular subpopulation of mucosal nerve fibres was affected, nor if the nerve changes are related to mast cell density. However, there is other circumstantial evidence for co-ordinate changes in mast cell and nerve density in the gastrointestinal tract (Stead *et al.*, 1990c). Experiments designed to study the mechanism of nerve remodelling during inflammation are currently underway.

WHAT IS A MAST CELL?

In the mid to late 1800's, when mast cells were first identified by von Recklinghausen and named by Ehrlich, it was recognized that this extremely pleomorphic cell type could be found throughout connective tissues, often associated with blood vessels and nerves (see Selye, 1965). At that time, mast cells were considered to be true connective tissue elements, perhaps involved in homeostasis through the action of their secreted products on the vasculature and other connective tissue cells. A century later, Ishizaka *et al.* (1972) described the release of histamine from mast cells by cross-linking bound IgE; and Kitamura *et al.* (1977) adoptively transferred beige mouse bone marrow cells into irradiated normal recipients, to show that mast cells can be derived from the bone marrow. This modern data and the importance of mast cells in anaphylaxis has resulted in research on this cell type being focused on immunological mechanisms. Nevertheless, the older visions of these connective tissue cells are still plausible. Perhaps mast cells serve a primary homeostatic function through interactions with nerves and other somatic elements; yet through the provision of immunoglobulin receptors they also respond to appropriately primed antigenic challenge. It seems surprising to me that most epithelia, but not connective tissues, are provided with cells of the diffuse neuroendocrine system. Does the mast cell subserve such a role?

REFERENCES

Ader R, Felten DL, Cohen N (1990). "Psychoneuroimmunology II." Orlando: Academic Press, in press.

Arizono N, Matsuda S, Hattori T, Kojima Y, Maeda T, Galli SJ (1990). Anatomical variation in mast cell nerve associations in the rat small intestine, heart, lung, and skin: Similarities of distances between neural processes and mast cells, eosinophils, or plasma cells in the jejunal lamina propria. Lab Invest 62:626-634.

Bani-Sacchi T, Barattini M, Bianchi S, Blandina P, Brunelleschi S, Fantozzi R, Mannaioni PF, Masini E (1986). The release of histamine by parasympathetic stimulation in guinea-pig auricle and rat ileum. J Physiol 371:29-43.

Baraniuk JN, Kowalski ML, Kaliner MA (1990). Relationships between permeable vessels, nerves, and mast cells in rat cutaneous neurogenic inflammation. J Appl Physiol 68:2305-2311.

Devillier P, Renoux M, Giroud J-P, Regoli D (1985). Peptides and histamine release from rat peritoneal mast cells. Eur J Pharmacol 117:89-96.

Ganguly AK, Sathiamoorthy SS, Bhatnagar OP (1978). Effect of sub-diaphragmatic vagotomy on gastric mucosal mast cell population in pylorus ligated rats. Quart J Exp Physiol 63:89-92.

Ganguly AK, Gopinath P (1979). Vagus nerves and the gastric tissue histamine concentration in pylorus ligated albino rats. Quart J Exp Physiol 64:1-6.

Ishizaka T, Ishizaka K, Tomioka H (1972). Release of histamine and slow reacting substance of anaphylaxis (SRS-A) by IgE-anti-IgE reactions on monkey mast cells. J Immunol 108:513-520.

Kitamura Y, Shimada M, Hatanaka K, Miyano Y (1977). Development of mast cells from grafted bone marrow cells in irradiated mice. Nature 268:442-443.

Kowalski ML, Kaliner MA (1988). Neurogenic inflammation, vascular permeability, and mast cells. J Immunol 140:3905-3911.

Levi-Schaffer F, Shalit M (1989). Differential release of histamine and prostaglandin D_2 in rat peritoneal mast cells activated with peptides. Int Arch Allergy Appl Immunol 90:352-357.

Newson B, Dahlstrom A, Enerback L, Ahlman H (1983). Suggestive evidence for a direct innervation of mucosal mast cells. An electron microscopic study. Neuroscience 10:565-570.

Selye H (1965). " The mast cells." London: Butterworths.

Shanahan F, Denburg JA, Fox J, Bienenstock J, Befus D (1985). Mast cell heterogeneity: effects of neuroenteric peptides on histamine release. J Immunol 135:1331-1337.

Stead RH, Tomioka M, Quinonez G, Simon GT, Felten SY, Bienenstock J (1987). Intestinal mucosal mast cells in normal and nematode-infected rat intestines are in intimate contact with peptidergic nerves. Proc Natl Acad Sci USA 84:2975-2979.

Stead RH, Dixon MF, Bramwell NH, Riddell RH, Bienenstock J (1989). Mast cells are closely apposed to nerves in the human gastrointestinal mucosa. Gastroenterology 97:575-585.

Stead RH, Bienenstock J (1990). Cellular interactions between the immune and peripheral nervous systems. A normal role for mast cells?. In: Burger MM, Zinkernargel RM (eds.), "Cell to Cell Interactions," Basel: S.Karger, in press.

Stead RH, Tomioka M, Riddell RH, Bienenstock J (1988). Substance P and/or calcitonin gene-related peptide are present in sub-epithelial enteric nerves apposed to intestinal mucosal mast cells. In: MacDermott RP (ed.), "Inflammatory bowel disease: current status and future approach," Amsterdam: Elsevier, pp 43-48.

Stead RH, Tomioka M, Pezzati P, Marshall J, Croitoru K, Perdue M, Stanisz A, Bienenstock J (1990a). Interaction of the mucosal immune and peripheral nervous systems. In: Ader R, Felten DL, Cohen N (eds.), "Psychoneuroimmunology II," Orlando: Academic Press, in press.

Stead RH, Perdue MH, Blennerhassett MG, Kakuta Y, Sestini P, Bienenstock J (1990b). The innervation of mast cells. In: Freier S (ed.), "The neuroendocrine-immune network," Boca Raton: CRC Press Inc., pp 19-37.

Stead RH, Franks AJ, Goldsmith CH, Bienenstock J, Dixon MF (1990c). Mast cells, nerves and fibrosis in the appendix: a morphological assessment. J Pathol 161:209-219.

Yonei Y, Oda M, Nakamura M, Watanabe NH, Tsuskada N, Komatsu HK, Akaiwa Y, Ichikawa E, Kaneko K, Asakura H, Fujiwara T, Tsuchiya M (1985). Evidence for direct interaction between the cholinergic nerve and mast cells in rat colonic mucosa. J Clin Electron Microscopy 18:560-561.

Yonei Y (1987). Autonomic nervous alterations and mast cell degranulation in the exacerbation of ulcerative colitis. Jap J Gastroenterol 84:1045-1056.

Cellular and Cytokine Networks in Tissue Immunity, pages 91-98

CYTOKINES IN INFLAMMATORY BRAIN DISEASES

Karl Frei, David Nadal, Peter Ralph and Adriano Fontana
Section of Clinical Immunology and Department of Neurosurgery, University Hospital (K.F., A.F.), Division of Infectious Diseases and Immunology, University Children's Hospital (D.N.), Zürich, Switzerland and Cetus Corp. (P.R.), Emeryville, California 94608

INTRODUCTION

Acute bacterial and viral meningitis remain relatively common diseases worldwide. Paradoxically, the case fatality rate and the risk of permanent neurologic sequelae being observed mainly in bacterial meningitis have not changed over 30 years despite the availability of advanced medical intensive care and of continued improvement in antibiotics (Dodge, 1986; Smith, 1988). Furthermore, in meningitis the establishment of the causative agent can still be difficult. Cultures of blood and cerebrospinal fluid (CSF) for detection of the etiologic agent have the drawback of the time required to become positive. In addition, measurements of cell counts and concentrations of protein and glucose in the CSF may not always be absolutely diagnostic as the ranges of the data in bacterial meningitis overlap significantly with those in viral meningitis (Weinstein, 1985; Bolan and Barza, 1985).

There is increasing evidence that cytokines, in addition to their known effects in the periphery during bacterial and viral infections mediate many host responses in infectious diseases of the central nervous system (CNS). In this paper we demonstrate the production of tumor necrosis factor-α (TNF-α), interleukin-1β (IL-1β), interleukin-6 (IL-6) and macrophage colony-stimulating factor (M-CSF) in the CSF of patients with infectious meningitis.

RESULTS

Compared to viral meningitis the CSF of bacterial meningitis showed a higher degree of pleocytosis as well as higher protein levels (Table 1).

TABLE 1. Cerebrospinal Fluid Protein Concentrations and Cell Counts in Patients with Infectious Meningitis

CSF	Bacterial Meningitis (n = 10)	Viral Meningitis (n = 20)	Controls (n = 20)
Cell Count[a]			
Mean ± SEM ($x10^6$/L)	6,305±1,318	185 ± 38	1.5 ± 0.2
Range	23 - 12,500	24 -461	0 - 4
Protein[b]			
Mean ± SEM (mg/L)	3,011 ± 376	300 ± 41	234 ± 18
Range	450 - 4,350	50 -760	119 - 459

[a]Normal value <4

[b]Normal value <400

As shown in Figure 1 TNF-α was only found in CSF of patients with bacterial meningitis. The concentrations of TNF-α ranged from 65 - 20,235 pg/ml (mean ± SEM: 6,383 ± 2,281 pg/ml). Thus, bacterial and viral meningitis can be distinguished from each other in the TNF-α assay.

IL-1β was detected in CSF in 9 of 12 patients (75%) with bacterial meningitis, and in 5 of 20 patients (25%) with viral meningitis; none of 20 controls contained IL-1β. The controls consisted of tension headache patients. The mean values for bacterial and viral meningitis were 460 ± 195 pg/ml and 105 ± 10 pg/ml, respectively. The values ranged from 15 to 2080 pg/ml in bacterial meningitis and 15 to 150 pg/ml in viral meningitis.

IL-6 was demonstrated in 18/20 samples (90%) from patients with viral and in all 8 samples tested from patients with bacterial meningitis. However, the mean values in the two groups were very different: in viral meningitis 1,288 ± 340 U/ml (range: 5-6,400) and in bacterial meningitis 67,520 ± 4,904 U/ml (range: 10,880-120,000), respectively.

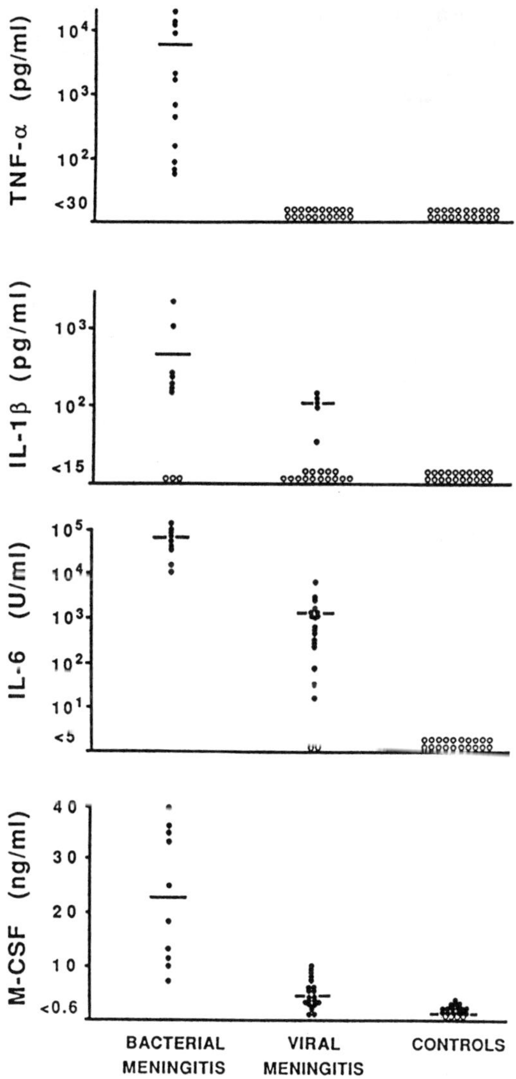

FIGURE 1. Levels of TNF-α, IL-1β, IL-6 and M-CSF in CSF of patients with infectious meningitis. The horizontal bars denote the mean values. Open circles represent values below the detection limit of the assays.

M-CSF was observed in all patient groups. Highest values were seen in samples of patients with bacterial meningitis with a range of 7.2-39.9 ng/ml (mean $\pm$ SEM: 23 $\pm$ 3.9, followed by samples of viral meningitis ng/ml (mean $\pm$ SEM: 4.8 $\pm$ 0.6) and low but still detectable values in control patients 0.6-3.6 ng/ml (mean $\pm$ SEM: 1.4 $\pm$ 0.2).

The protein concentration and cell count in the CSF were analyzed for correlations between these parameters and the levels of cytokines in the CSF. In bacterial meningitis the levels of TNF-α, IL-1β and protein correlated with each other by significantly positive ($p < 0.025$) Spearman's correlation coefficients between 0.37 and 0.58. In addition, the levels of IL-1β and M-CSF correlated significantly ($p < 0.025$) by a correlation coefficient of 0.33, but only the IL-1β level correlated with the cell count ($r = 0.27$, $p < 0.025$). In viral meningitis the only correlation was found between the levels of IL-6 and M-CSF ($r = 0.1$, $p < 0.025$).

DISCUSSION

In recent years, the role of TNF-α and IL-1β in the pathogenesis of meningeal inflammation has been investigated intensively. Studies in different animal models have provided evidence of their local production within the CNS. The TNF-α activity has been documented in the CSF of mice injected intracerebrally with *Listeria monocytogenes* (Leist et al., 1988) in the CSF of rabbits inoculated intracisternally either with *H. influenzae* type b (Mustafa et al., 1989) or meningococci (Waage et al., 1989) or *S. pneumoniae* (Saukonen et al., 1990). Likewise IL-1 has been detected in the CSF of rabbits after intracisternal inoculation of meningococcal LPS (Waage et al., 1989). Human patients with bacterial meningitis show intrathecal synthesis of both, TNF- and IL-1 (Leist et al., 1988; Nadal et al.,1989; McCracken et al., 1989; Mustafa et al., 1989). Unlike TNF-α, IL-1 is found not only in bacterial meningitis but also in the CSF of patients with viral meningitis (Ramilo et al., 1990). Our observation of absence of TNF-α in the CSF of viral meningitis patients (Leist et al., 1988; Nadal et al., 1990) was confirmed by others (Gallo et al., 1989; Ramilo et al., 1990). Thus, the examination of CSF for TNF-α may be helpful in differentiating between bacterial and viral meningitis in patients with acute disease.

Viral diseases of the CNS are characterized by intrathecal synthesis of immunoglobulins (Ig) by B lymphocytes having infiltrated the brain tissue (Moench and Griffin, 1984; Link, 1987). The mechanisms leading to activation of B cells and enhancement of their capacity to secrete Ig in the CNS are not yet understood. In general, the terminal differentiation of activated B-cells into Ig-producing plasma cells depends on T cell-derived signals such as IL-6 (Kishimoto, 1989). In recent experiments we have shown that IL-6 is produced in the CNS in mice infected intracerebrally with lymphocytic choriomeningitis virus (LCMV) (Frei et al., 1988) or vesicular stomatitis virus (VSV) (Frei et al., 1989). IL-6 was detected in CSF of mice with acute LCMV disease. However, in athymic mice which do not develop LCMV disease, no IL-6 becomes measurable in the CSF. A T cell independent pathway for IL-6 production is shown in athymic mice with acute VSV infection, the amounts of IL-6 being up to 60 times higher in CSF compared to serum (Frei et al., 1989). These observations suggest that in the brain synthesis of IL-6 may take place not only by invading T cells but also by parenchymal cells. Indeed, both cultured astrocytes and microglial cells of newborn mice secrete IL 6 when infected with virus in vitro (Frei et al., 1989). IL-6 was detected also in humans in 18 of 20 patients with viral meningitis (Frei et al., 1988; Houssiau et al., 1988; Gallo et al., 1989).

Like TNF-α, IL-6 is also produced by activated monocytes/macrophages (Aarden et al., 1987). Accordingly, the identification of IL-6 in TNF-α positive samples from patients with bacterial meningitis would not be surprising. Indeed, all the 12 CSF of patients with bacterial meningitis were positive for IL-6. Other investigators have demonstrated similar findings (Houssiau et al., 1988; Helfgott et al., 1989; Waage et al., 1989). Whereas the role of IL-6 in the antibacterial host response is not clear yet, IL-6 produced in the course of viral diseases by glial cells and/or by T cells/monocytes, which have invaded the brain parenchyma or meninges, may serve as an amplifier for the maturation of infiltrating virus-immune B-lymphocytes to secrete high levels of antiviral antibodies, which prevent further spread of cytopathic virus. Furthermore, IL-6 was found to induce the synthesis of nerve growth factor by astrocytes (Frei et al., 1989) and thus may lead to neurotrophic support in areas of virus-caused cell damage in the CNS.

Interestingly, M-CSF was detected in the CSF of patients with bacterial and viral meningitis. M-CSF being produced by activated monocytes, fibroblasts and endothelial cells acts on both progenitor and mature cells of the macrophage lineage. Moreover, it stimulates release of cytokines such as IL-1 (Moore et al., 1980), TNF-α (Warren and Ralph, 1986) and interferons (Fleit and Rabinovitch, 1981) and increases resistance to viral infections (Lee and Warren, 1987). In conclusion, the analysis of the production of cytokines in the brain compartment offers a strategy which in general will help to define the role of cytokines in inflammatory reactions. Furthermore, the demonstration of cytokine production in immune deficient animals e.g. intrathecal synthesis of IL-6 in athymic nude mice offers the advantage to dissect the cellular sources such as T cell derived versus non T cell derived (e.g. brain parenchymal cells) produced of the respective cytokines.

REFERENCES

Aarden L, De Groot E, Schaap O, Lausdorp P (1987). Production of hybridoma growth factor by human monocytes. Eur J Immunol 17:1411-1416.

Bolan G, Barza M (1985). Acute bacterial meningitis in children and adults. A perspective. Med Clin N Am 69: 231-241.

Dodge PR (1986). Sequelae of bacterial meningitis. Pediatr Infect Dis J 5:618-620.

Fleit HB, Rabinovitch M (1981). Interferon induction in marrow-derived macrophages: regulation by L cell conditioned medium. J Cell Physiol 108:347-352.

Frei K, Leist TP, Meager A, Gallo P, Leppert D, Zinkernagel RM, Fontana A (1988). Production of B cell stimulatory factor-2 and interferon γ in the central nervous system during viral meningitis and encephalitis. J Exp Med 168: 449-453.

Frei K, Malipiero UV, Leist TP, Zinkernagel RM, Schwab ME, Fontana A (1989). On the cellular source and function of interleukin 6 produced in the central nervous system in viral diseases. Eur J Immunol 19:689-694.

Gallo P, Frei K, Rordorf C, Lazdins J, Tavolata B, Fontana A (1989). Human immunodeficiency virus type 1 (HIV-1) infection of the central nervous system: an evaluation of cytokines in cerebrospinal fluid. J Neuroimmunol 23: 109-116.

Helfgott DC, Tatter SB, Sauthanam U, Clarick RH, Bhardwaj N, May LT, Sehgal PB (1989). Multiple forms of IFN-β2/IL-6 in serum and body fluids during acute bacterial infection. J Immunol 142:948-953.

Houssiau FA, Bukasa K, Sindic CJM, Van Damme J, Van Snick J (1988). Elevated levels of the 26K human hybridoma growth factor (interleukin 6) in cerebrospinal fluid of patients with acute infection of the central nervous system. Clin Exp Immunol 71:320-323.

Kishimoto T (1989). The biology of interleukin-6. Blood 74: 1-10.

Lee MT, Warren MK (1987). CSF-1-induced resistance to viral infection in murine macrophages. J Immunol 138:3019-3022.

Leist TP, Frei K, Kam-Hansen S, Zinkernagel RM, Fontana A (1988). Tumor necrosis factor alpha in cerebrospinal fluid during bacterial but not viral meningitis. J Exp Med 167: 1743-1748.

Link H (1987). Cerebrospinal fluid in immunological CNS diseases. In: Aarli JA, Behan WMH, Behan PO (eds.), "Clinical Neuroimmunology", Oxford: Blackwell Scientific Publications, pp 444-466.

Mc Cracken GH, Mustafa MM, Ramilo O, Olson KD, Risser RC (1989). Cerebrospinal fluid interleukin 1-beta and tumor necrosis factor concentrations and outcome from neonatal Gram-negative enteric bacillary meningitis. Pediatr Infect Dis J 8:155-159.

Moench TR, Griffin DE (1984). Immunocytochemical identification of the mononuclear cells in the cerebrospinal fluid, meninges, and brain during acute viral meningoencephalitis. J Exp Med 159:77-82.

Moore RN, Oppenheim JJ, Farrar JJ, Carter CS, Waheed A, Shadduck RK (1980). Production of lymphocyte activating factor (interleukin 1) by macrophages activated with colony stimulating factors. J Immunol 125:1302-1307.

Mustafa NM, Lebel MH, Ramilo O, Olsen KD, Reisch JS, Beutler B, McCracken GH (1989). Correlation of interleukin-1β and cachectin concentrations in cerebrospinal fluid and outcome from bacterial meningitis. J Pediatr 115: 208-213.

Nadal D, Leppert D, Frei K, Gallo P, Lamche H, Fontana A (1989). Tumor necrosis factor-α in infectious meningitis. Arch Dis Child 64:1274-1279.
Ramilo O, Mustafa MM, Porter J, Sáez-Llorens X, Mertsola J, Olsen KD, Luby JP, Beutler B, McCracken GH (1990). AJDC 144:349-352.
Saukonen K, Saude S, Cioffe C, Wolpe S, Sherry B, Cerami A, Tuomanen E (1990). The role of cytokines in the generation of inflammation and tissue damage in experimental Gram-positive meningitis. J Exp Med 171:439-448.
Smith AL (1988). Neurologic sequelae of meningitis. N Engl J Med 319:1012-1014.
Waage A, Halstensen A, Shalaby R, Brandtzaeg P, Kierulf P, Espevik T (1989). Local production of tumor necrosis factorα, interleukin 1 and interleukin 6 in meningococcal meningitis. J Exp Med 170:1859-1867.
Warren MK, Ralph P (1986). Macrophage growth factor CSF-1 stimulates human monocyte production of interferon, tumor necrosis factor, and colony stimulating activity. J Immunol 137:2281-2285.
Weinstein L (1985). Bacterial meningitis. Med Clin N Am 69: 219-229.

Cellular and Cytokine Networks in Tissue Immunity, pages 99-104

OLIGODENDROCYTE GROWTH FACTORS PRODUCED BY LYMPHOCYTES

Jean E. Merrill

Department of Neurology, Reed Neurological Research Center, UCLA School of Medicine, Los Angeles, California 90024

INTRODUCTION

There is now substantial evidence that the immune response, leukocytes, and their secreted cytokines may play a role in the central nervous system during embryogenesis, neonatal development, trauma, and disease. Not only do leukocytes traffic in and out of the brain on a regular basis but they also secrete mono- and lymphokines that alter morphology and function of brain cells. The mature brain contains both bipotential precursor cells as well as mature glial cells capable of undergoing proliferation and further differentiation in response to stimuli as a result of injury or disease. The significance of cytokine effects on glia is supported by several facts: 1) the presence of leukocytes in brain during embryogenesis, fetal development, and adult life; 2) induction of proliferation and differentiation of glial cells _in vitro_ in response to T cell-derived growth factors; and 3) proliferation of and remyelination by oligodendrocytes in adult CNS after trauma and disease.

Having demonstrated hematogenously-derived cells in brains of normal human embryo and fetuses of 10 weeks or younger, Choi (1981) concluded that hematogenous cells in neural tissue is a ubiquitous developmental phenomenon. While it has been suggested that developmental migration of such cells would be prevented by the blood brain barrier, brain Ia+ cells in normal adult are derived from a bone marrow precursor. Indeed, Wekerle and his colleagues (1986) have evidence that the nervous system is constantly patrolled by low number of activated T cells. Several laboratories have demonstrated activated T lymphocytes in the CSF of patients with MS and other neurological diseases (OND) (Merrill et al., 1984a; Hafler et al., 1985). Activated T cells in CNS brain tissue, secreted cytokines and their surface receptors have also been demonstrated. We have shown IL2 secreting and IL2 receptor bearing cells in frozen sections of MS brain but not in tissues of some OND controls. These T cells produce gamma interferon (IFNγ) (Hofman et al., 1986).

Simulated leukocytes will secrete factors that induce both astrocytes and oligodendrocytes to proliferate. Several groups have demonstrated effects of interleukins on glial cells, in particular oligodendroglia. IL2, for example, has been shown to inhibit proliferation and enhance differentiation of precursor oligodendrocytes while stimulating both proliferation and differentiation of mature oligodendrocytes (Benveniste and Merrill, 1986; Benveniste et al., 1987). In experimental models of CNS demyelination _in vitro_ and _in vivo_, adult oligodendrocytes have been shown to both proliferate and remyelinate (Ludwin, 1979; Seil and Blank, 1981; Arenella and Herndon, 1984). The major pathological abnormality in MS is the occurrence of areas of demyelination in the CNS which are thought to be responsible for the clinical manifestations. The myelin producing cells, oligodendrocytes, initially proliferate at the plaque edge though they are ultimately lost from the plaque area and undergo ultrastructural changes in partially demyelinated areas and areas distant from plaques (Prineas and Connell, 1979). Some remyelination does occur resulting in thinly remyelinated axons and shadow plaques. These studies _in vitro_ and _in vivo_ indicate that mature oligodendrocytes do have proliferative potential and may be induced to remyelinate following CNS trauma or disease (Powell and Lampert, 1983).

METHODS AND RESULTS

In our first attempts to identify T cell-derived oligodendrocyte growth factors, we purified a 30 kd glycoprotein from supernatants of a T lymphoblast cell line Mo. This lymphokine, called Glial Growth Promoting Factor (GGPF), was the first characterized cytokine which specifically induced growth of oligodendrocytes and not other glial cells (Benveniste et al., 1985).

The Mo cell line has been grown continuously in culture for several years. Using 50 liter batch cultures, we were unsuccessful in purifying significant quantities of GGPF for sequencing but were still able to detect growth factor activity. We have now discovered several biochemical differences in the properties of this new positive activity compared to GGPF. While GGPF eluted off a lentil lectin column, this new activity was found in the flow through. On an ACA44 Ultrogel column, GGPF activity eluted at 30,000 MW while the new activity eluted at 12-15,000 MW and 20-22,000 MW. Low amounts of biological activity at 30,000 MW implied GGPF was still present as a trace factor in these new supernatants. GGPF was a basic, hydrophobic protein while the new activity is negatively-charged and acidic, eluting off a Mono Q anion exchange column. Fractions from FPLC have been run over a C-8 reverse phase HPLC column. On SDS PAGE under reduced and non-reduced conditions, Factor A appears to be a 17 Kda protein and Factor B, a 14 Kda protein. Both factors have biological activity in the nanomolar range.

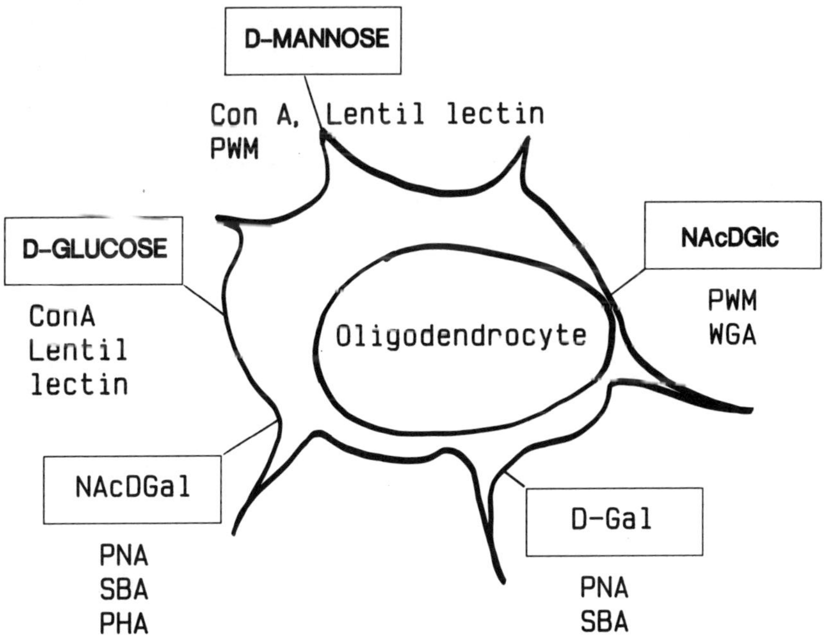

Figure 1. Carbohydrates on Oligodendrocyte Membranes. High density sugars (bold) and lower density sugars (nonbold) determined by FITC-conjugated lectins listed below each sugar.

While it is clear by biochemical and immunological criteria that the new oligodendrocyte growth factors are not any known lymphokines, it is also certain that crude Mo supernatants contain several growth factors as well as inhibitory factors. We have previously shown that rat oligodendrocytes have the capacity to bind ConA, WGA, lentil lectin, and, to a lesser degree or not at all, PNA, PHA, and soybean agglutinin (Merrill et al., 1984b). This means their membranes are rich in mannose, N-acetylD-glucosamine, and glucose containing proteins or lipids (bold type) and contain low amounts of galactose or its derivatives such as N-acetylD-galactosamine (nonbold type, Fig. 1). Using the crude Mo supernatants, we have found the Mo activity is inhibited by L-fucose (but not D-fucose) and mannose. The activity is also inhibited by ConA lectin (Fig. 2). The specificity of ConA is α-D-mannose; lentil lectin also binds mannose. Since the bioactivity flows through the mannose-binding lentil lectin column, our data suggest that the oligodendrocyte receptor for the growth factor activity contains mannose. The fact that L-fucose but not D-fucose inhibits Mo activity on oligodendrocytes and that these cells do not bind asparagus pea lectin which recognizes fucose suggests that the Mo factor contains L-fucose. This information will be of value in isolation and characterization of the receptor and the recombinant protein(s). In addition, the factor activity is enhanced by galactose and N-acetylD-glucosamine suggesting crude Mo supernatants contain one or more inhibitors of this new oligodendrocyte growth factor activity.

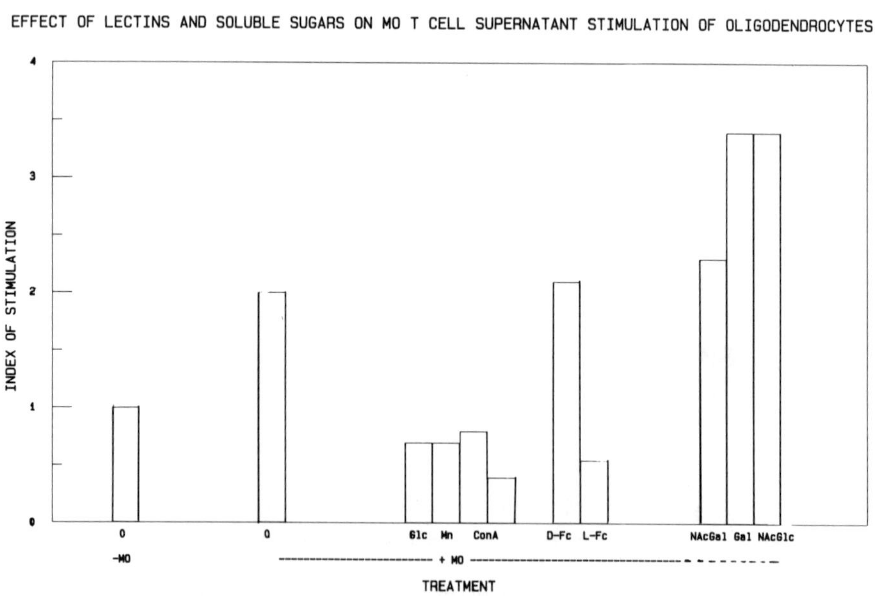

Figure 2. Glc = glucose; Mn = mannose; NAcGal = N-acetyl-D-galactosamine; NAcGlc = N-acetylD-glucosamine; Gal= galactose; Fc = fucose (at 3-6 mM); ConA at 5 & 50μg/ml.

Oligodendrocytes proliferate in response to several known growth factors. Using polyclonal antibodies to TGFα and β, PDGF, IL6, IL2, and IGF-I, we were unable to inhibit Mo factor activity in our crude supernatants. The effects of interactions of the crude Mo supernatant factor with other growth-inducing cytokines, TGFβ and IL2 were examined (Fig. 3). TGFβ stimulates proliferation of oligodendrocytes at 1 ng/ml. IL2 induces proliferation at 150 u/ml but not 50 u/ml. However, TGFβ and IL2 or Mo supernatants do not synergize with each other to produce a greater than additive effect. In contrast, a non-inducing concentration of IL2 (50u/ml) synergizes with optimal concentrations of crude Mo supernatant. Clearly, the crude supernatants may have several positive and negative factors that affect the oligodendrocyte growth. Definitive studies on synergy or tandem effects of Mo activity with IL2 or IGF-1 must await purification of large enough amounts of homogenous proteins or cloning of these proteins from Mo T cell supernatants. This work is in progress.

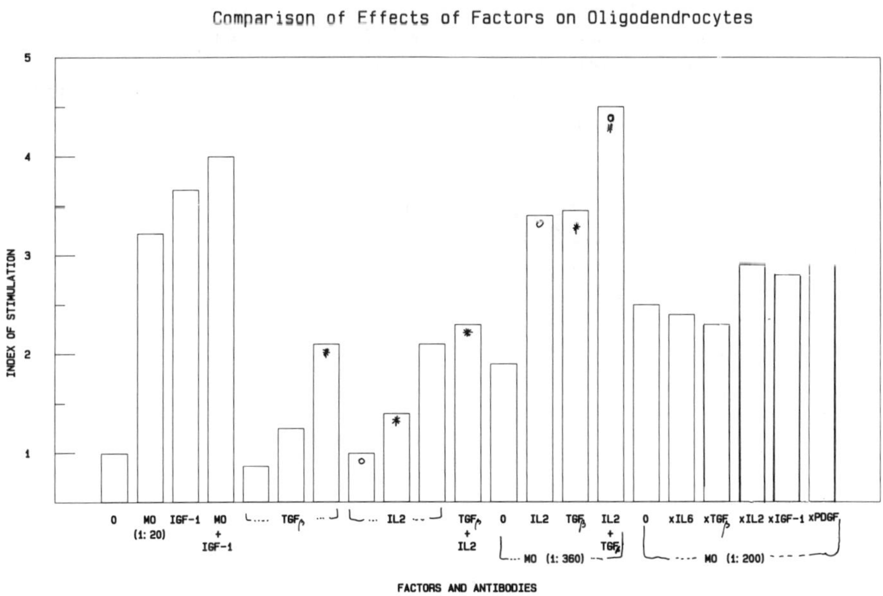

Figure 3. IGF-1 = insulin-like growth factor-1 (0.2mg%); TGFβ = transforming growth factor beta (* 1 ng/ml); IL2 (o 50U/ml; * 100 U/ml); antibodies at 1:500-1000.

REFERENCES

Arenella LS, Herndon RM (1984). Mature oligodendrocytes. Division following experimental demyelination in adult animals. Arch Neurol 41:1162-1165.

Benveniste EN, Herman PV, Whitaker JN (1987). Myelin basic protein specific RNA levels in interleukin-2 stimulated oligodendrocytes. J Neurochem 49:1274-1279.

Benveniste EN, Merrill JE (1986). Stimulation of oligodendroglial proliferation and maturation of interleukin-2. Nature 321:610-613.

Benveniste EN, Merrill JE, Kaufman SE, Golde DN, Gasson JC (1985). Purification and characterization of a human T lymphocyte derived glial growth promoting factor. Proc Natl Acad Sci 82:3930-3934.

Choi BH (1981). Hematogenous cells in the central nervous system of developing human embryos and fetuses. J Comp Neurol 196:683-694.

Hafler DA, Fox DA, Manning ME, Schlossman SF, Reinherz EL, Weiner HL (1985). In vivo activated T lymphocytes in the peripheral blood and cerebrospinal fluid of patients with multiple sclerosis. N Engl J Med 312:1405-1411.

Hofman F, VanHanwher R, Dinarello C, Mizel S, Hinton D, Merrill JE (1986). Immunoregulatory molecules and IL2 receptors identified in multiple sclerosis brain. J Immunol 136:3239-3245.

Ludwin SK (1979). An autoradiographic study of cellular proliferation in remyelination of the central nervous system. Am J Pathol 95:683-696.

Merrill JE, Mohlstrom C, Uittenbogaart C, Kermani-Arab V, Ellison, Myers LW (1984a). Response to and production of interleukin 2 by peripheral blood and cerebrospinal fluid lymphocytes of patients with multiple sclerosis. J Immunol 133:1931-1937.

Merrill JE, Kutsunai S, Mohlstrom C, Hofman F, Groopman J, Golde DW (1984b). Proliferation of astroglia and oligodendroglia in response to human T cell derived factors. Science 224:1428-1430.

Powell HC, Lampert PW (1983). Pathology of Multiple Sclerosis. In: JP Antel (ed.), "Symposium on Multiple Sclerosis, Philadelphia: WB Saunders & Co., pp 631-644.

Prineas JW, Connell F (1979). Remyelination in multiple sclerosis. Ann Neurol 5:22-27.

Seil FJ, Blank NK (1981). Myelination of central nervous system axons in tissue culture by transplanted oligodendrocytes. Science 212:1407-1408.

Wekerle H, Linington C, Lassmann H, Meyermann R (1986). Cellular immune reactivity within the CNS. TINS 9:271-277.

Cellular and Cytokine Networks in
Tissue Immunity, pages 105-110

HUMAN KERATINOCYTES SYTHESIZE AND RELEASE NEUROPEPTIDES SUCH AS αMSH AND ACTH

Andreas Köck, Elisabeth Schauer,
Thomas Schwarz and Thomas A. Luger

LBI-DVS, Laboratory of Cellbiology at Department of Dermatology II, University Vienna (A.K, E.S., T.S., T.A.L.), Department of Dermatology, Hospital Lainz, Vienna, Austria (T.S.), Department of Dermatology, University Münster, FRG (T.A.L.)

Alpha melanocyte stimulating hormone (αMSH) is a 13 amino acid peptide, one of the several proopiomelanocortin (POMC) derived molecules synthesized in the pituitary gland, named originally for its ability to stimulate pigmentation (Eberle, 1988). More recently, αMSH has been shown to exhibit other functions, i.e. modulation of immune/inflammatory processes in particular to modulate contact hypersensitivity in mice, to inhibit some biological activities of interleukin 1 (IL -1) and tumor necrosis factor α and to function as an antipyrogen (Cannon et al., 1986; Rheins et al., 1989). Although αMSH was initially isolated from the pituitary gland it has been extracted from a variety of other tissues including the skin (Thody et al., 1983). Although circulating MSH peptides are likely to be responsible for peripheral and consequently also for cutaneous effects, it was investigated whether human keratinocytes which exhibit a broad immunosecretory capacity (Luger and Schwarz, 1990) can function as a source for MSH peptides.

Normal human keratinocytes (HNK) and the human epidermoid carcinoma cell line A431 were cultured for 48 hours and supernatants tested for αMSH in a αMSH specific RIA. Both HNK and A431 cells constitutively released detectable amounts of αMSH which could be induced by addition of PMA, IL-1 or by irradiation with UVB-light (Table 1).

TABLE 1:

	α MSH (pg/ml)	
Stimuli	A431	HNK
untreated	38	6
PMA (10ng/ml)	104	16
IL-1α (10 U/ml)	91	n.t.
UVB-light (120 J/m^2)	58	n.t.

n.t. = not tested

In order to study whether the protein detected with the RIA is biologically active, A431 conditioned medium was subjected to HPLC gel filtration and fractions tested in a αMSH specific bioassay (tyrosinase assay). Biological activity eluted in the low m.w. fractions corresponding to the m.w. of αMSH (Figure 1).

αMSH is a POMC derived peptide which is intracellularly cleaved into several active fragments including ACTH, CLIP, ß-endorphin etc. Therefore epidermal cell supernatants were also tested for ACTH using an ACTH specific RIA. A431 conditioned medium contained significant amounts of ACTH which were found increased upon stimulation with PMA and IL-1 (data not shown). Furthermore, Northern blot analysis using a cDNA probe encoding for POMC revealed specific transcripts at 1.1 kB in A431 cells (data not shown). In summary, these data demonstrate both at the protein and mRNA level that epidermal cells produce and secrete POMC derived neuropeptides such as αMSH and ACTH.

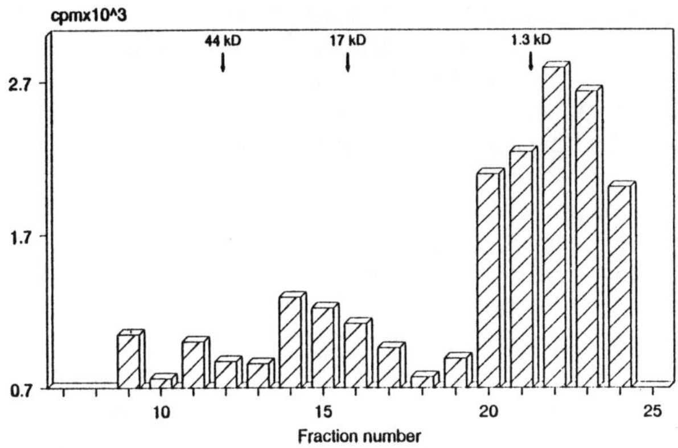

Figure 1. A431 supernatant was subjected to HPLC gel filtration (TSK 125) and fractions tested in the tyrosinase bioassay.

Keratinocytes are well known to release a variety of cytokines and biolgical activities affecting immune functions (Luger and Schwarz, 1990). Previously it was demonstrated that epidermal cells release a factor enhancing the activity of natural killer (NK) cells (Luger et al., 1985) which as recently shown was most due to IL-6 (Kirnbauer et al., 1988). However, as NK-cells were also stimulated by low m.w. fractions of epidermal cell supernatants it was addressed whether that activity could be due to keratinocyte derived αMSH. Therefore nonadherent PBMC were incubated with αMSH and tested in a K562 Cr-release assay. Treatment with αMSH resulted in a significant induction of NK-cell activity. The effect, however, does not appear to be direct but via induction of IL-2, since addition of an IL-2 antibody completely reversed the NK inducing activity of αMSH (Figure 2).

In addition, keratinocytes previously have been demonstrated to release a low m.w. factor reducing major histocompatibility class I (MHC) antigen expression on the macrophage like cell line U937 (Schwarz et al., 1988). The time kinetics of the release and the m.w. were similar to the behaviour of epidermal cell derived αMSH. Thus U937 cells were incubated with αMSH which resulted in a significant reduction of MHC class I and ß2-microglobulin expression as demonstrated by FACS analysis (Figure 3). In addition, the MHC modulating activity present in A431 conditioned medium could be absorbed via a protein A-sepharose coupled with an αMSH antibody. At present, it is not known how αMSH affects MHC class I expression. This could be due to suppression of de novo synthesis, increased internalization, shedding or masking of MHC class I molecules.

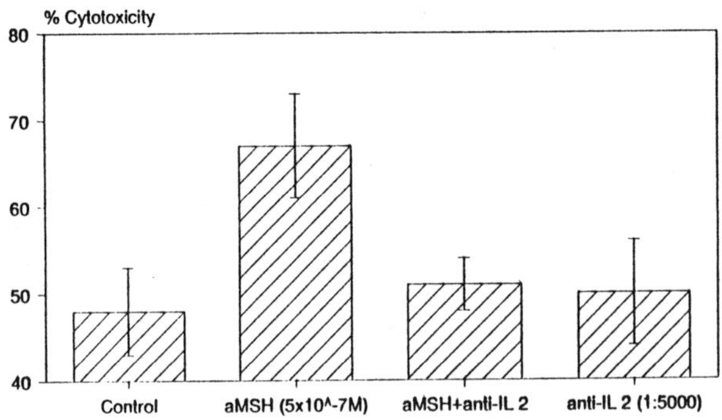

Figure 2. Nonadherent PBMC were incubated overnight with αMSH in the absence or presence of an IL-2 antibody and tested in a K562 Cr-release assay at a E:T ratio of 20:1.

These data demonstrate that human keratinocytes in addition to the production of cytokines and eicosanoides also exhibit the capacity to release neuropeptides such as αMSH and ACTH. Local release of αMSH in the epidermis may be of interest with regard to the pigment system although the role of αMSH in melanogenesis in the human system is still regarded as controversial (Friedmann et al., 1990). Probably of more importance may be the capacity of keratinocytes to influence immunologic and inflammatory reactions within the skin by secretion of these mediators which can modulate certain activities of cytokines (Cannon et al., 1986), influence lymphocytes, monocytes and NK-cells and affect surface marker expression on both immune and non-immune cells. These findings further support the concept that there is a link between the neuroendocrine and the immune system (Bateman et al., 1989) and points out that keratinocytes through their immunosecretory capacity may actively participate in immunologic and inflammatory reactions.

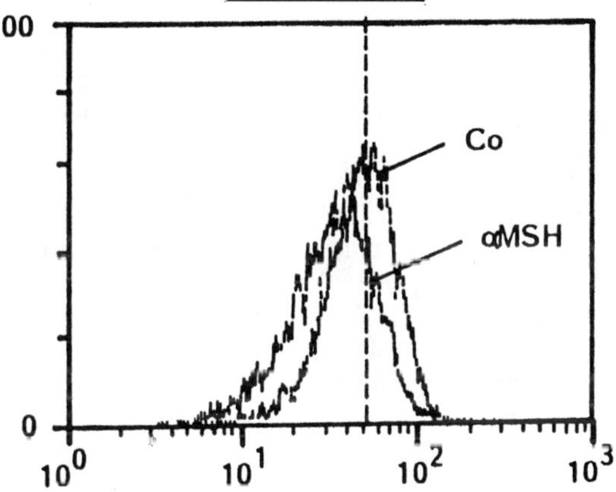

Figure 3. U937 cells were left untreated (Co) or incubated with αMSH ($1x10^{-9}$M) and evaluated for MHC class I antigen expression by FACS analysis using an antibody directed against a monomorphic determinant of MHC class I.

ACKNOWLEDGEMENT

We wish to thank Mrs. M. Bednar for her expert secretarial assistance and Mrs. I. Assmann (Division of Immunobiology, I. Department of Dermatology, Univ. Vienna) for performing FACS analysis.

REFERENCES

Bateman A, Singh A, Kral T, Solomon S (1989).

The immune-hypothalamic-pituitary adrenal axis. Endocrine Reviews 10: 92-111.
Cannon JG, Tatro JB, Reichlin S, Dinarello CA (1986). α melanocyte stimulating hormone inhibits immunostimulatory and inflammatory actions of interleukin 1. J Immunol 137: 2232-2236.
Eberle AN (1988). The Melanotropins. Karger, Basel
Friedmann PS, Wren F, Buffey J, MacNeil S (1990). αMSH causes a small rise in cAMP but has no effect on basal or ultraviolet-stimulated melanogenesis in human melanocytes. Br J Dermatol 123: 145-151.
Kirnbauer R, Köck A, Schwarz T, Micksche M, Luger TA (1988). Epidermal cell natural killer cell activity augmenting factor (ENKAF) is closely related to interleukin 6 (IL 6). J Invest Dermatol 91: 401.
Luger TA, Uchida A, Köck A, Colot M, Micksche M (1985). Human epidermal cells and squamous carcinoma cells synthesize a cytokine that augments natural killer cell activity. J Immunol 134: 2477-2483.
Luger TA, Schwarz T (1990). Epidermal cell derived cytokines. In: Bos J (Ed) The Skin Immune System. CRC Press, Boca Raton FL, pp 257-291.
Rheins LA, Cotleur AL, Kleier RS, Hoppenjans WB, Sauder DN, Nordlund JJ (1989). Alpha-melanocyte stimulating hormone modulates contact hypersensitivity responsiveness in C57/BL6 mice. J Invest Dermatol 95: 511-517.
Schwarz T, Danner M, Schauer E, Kirnbauer R, Urbanski A, Luger TA (1988). Regulation of MHC class I and II antigen expression by different epidermal cytokines. J Invest Dermatol 90: 607.
Thody AJ, Ridley K, Penny RJ, Chalmers R, Fisher C, Shuster S (1983). MSH peptides are present in mammalian skin. Peptides 4: 813-816.

This work was supported by "Fonds zur Förderung der Wissenschaftlichen Forschung" and "Medizinisch-Wissenschaftlicher Fonds des Bürgermeisters der Bundeshauptstadt Wien".

Cellular and Cytokine Networks in Tissue Immunity, pages 111-116

Melanoma Growth Stimulatory Activity--A Modulator of Melanocyte Proliferation, Neutrophil Chemotaxis, and Tumor Progression

Rebecca L. Shattuck, Eddy G. Balentien and Ann Richmond

Department of Cell Biology, Vanderbilt University and Department of Veterans Affairs, Nashville, TN 37232

INTRODUCTION:

A family of cytokines with homology to B-thromboglobulin have recently been characterized (1). Certain of these cytokines are transcriptionally activated by a number of factors including platelet derived growth factor, interleukin 1, tumor necrosis factor, thrombin, lipopolysaccharide, plant lectins, epidermal growth factor, cycloheximide, and the cytokines themselves (2-6). Many of the members of this family of cytokines are highly chemotactic for neutrophils and lymphocytes (1). Thus, it appears that these proteins provide a first line of defense by recruiting white cells into wounded area in response to growth factors and inflammatory modulators. We have shown that keratinocytes of the stratum spinosum, stratum germinativum and the stratum granulosum contain immunoreactive melanoma growth stimulatory activity (MGSA), one of the B-thromboglobulin related cytokines which is highly chemotactic for neutrophils (7,8). This led us to speculate that keratinocytes might serve as a reservoir for MGSA, which upon wounding, would release MGSA to recruit neutrophils and lymphocytes into the wounded area.

In addition to being chemotactic for neutrophils, MGSA is also capable of stimulating the growth of melanocytes as a single agent and in combination with insulin and phorbol ester (9). MGSA promotes the growth of serum free cultures of human malignant melanoma cells in vitro and antibodies to MGSA block the growth of high density cultures of Hs294T melanoma cells (10,11). Thus, in vivo MGSA probably stimulates melanocytes to proliferate, enabling newly healed skin to have the same pigmentation as neighboring, non-wounded tissue. Over-expression of MGSA might also lead to melanocyte tumor progression. In this communication we will review that data which suggest that the MGSA protein is a cytokine with growth regulatory activity. We also will show that overexpression of MGSA in immortalized melancytes is associated with tumor formation.

METHODS:

MGSA Bioassay: Cultures of normal human epidermal melanocytes (Clonetics) were cultured in 24 well plates at a density of 5000 cells per well. After initial plating in serum containing MCDB 151 medium, cells were placed on serum free medium and assayed for response to growth factors as previously described (4).
Transfection of MGSA into Melan-a Mouse Melanocytes: Melan-a cells were the kind gift of Ian Hart. The CMV-MGSA vector and the transfection protocol was identical to that described earlier (10). Five G418 selected clones were analyzed for growth in soft agar, growth in monolayer, and/or ability to form tumors in nude mice.
Soft Agar Assays: One-hundred thousand cells were plated in DMEM medium containing 200nM phorbol ester, 20% FBS, and 0.3% noble agar onto underlayers containing the same medium with 0.5% agar. Cultures were fed once per week and counted on an automated colony counter after 2.5 weeks.
Tumor Formation in Nude Mice: 5×10^6 cells from each of the mel-a clones carrying either the neo marker were injected into each of nine nu/nu mice. Mice were followed for 3 months at which time tumors were removed, fixed, sectioned and stained for marker studies. Mice were also examined for metastasis to internal organs.

RESULTS:

Normal human epidermal melanocytes respond to both insulin (5 ug/ml) and exogenous MGSA (0.6-6.0 ng/ml) with increased incorporation of (^{3}H)-thymidine into DNA (Fig.1). In combination, these two factors give an additive effect, stimulating the incorporation of (^{3}H)-thymidine into DNA approximately 321% of unstimulated controls. Addition of phorbol ester(200nM) did not augment this response to insulin and MGSA. These responses were equivalent to that produced by a combination of insulin, bFGF, and phorbol ester. Thus, MGSA, together with insulin or other progression factors, may serve as a normal regulator of melanocyte growth.

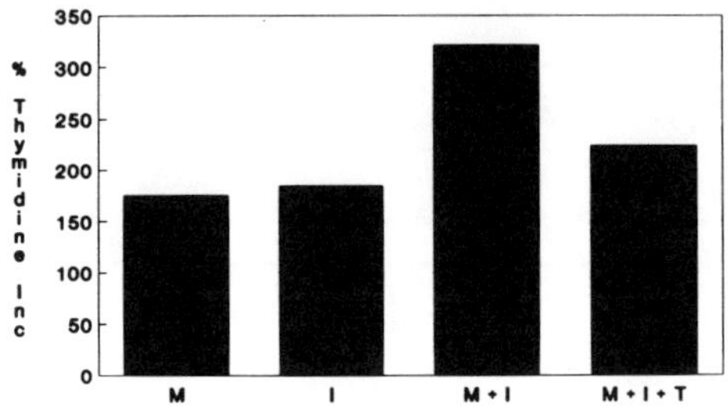

FIGURE 1

Effects of 0.6mg/ml MGSA (M) 5ug/ml insulin (I) and 200nM TPA (T) or combinations of these factors on the incorporation of ^{3}H-thymidine into normal human epidermal melanocytes.

When the melan-a immortalized mouse melanocytes were transfected with the human MGSA gene placed under the control of the CMV promoter/enhancer, melanocyte clones expressing the MGSA transgene mRNA exhibited several properties of the transformed state. These MGSA expressing clones formed large colonies in soft agar (Table 1) and one of the strong MGSA expressors formed tumors in nude mice (Table 2). Nine of nine mice injected with Mel-a-6 cells expressing the MGSA transgene formed tumors in nude mice, while only one of the neomycin control transfectants formed a tumor. One clone expressing a very low level of the MGSA transgene was equivalent to the neomycin control in its tumor forming ability. The tumors which formed in the MGSA transgene expressing melanocytes (mel-a-6) exhibited a histopathology compatible with that of melanoma. The mel-a-6 tumors made less S-100 protein, were positive for the melanoma specific antigen, HMB45, and produced a reduced amount of melanin. There was a small percentage of aneuploidy in the tumors expressing the MGSA transgene, though no aneuploidy was noted in the clone prior to injecting into the nude mice. Thus there may be some tumor progression after injection into the mice. We were unable to detect differences in the angiogenic potential of the clones expressing the MGSA transgene as compared to neomycin control transfectants (Ed Yang, personal communication). These data suggest that indeed MGSA can contribute to the transformation of immortalized melanocytes.

TABLE I

COLONIES IN SOFT AGAR EXPRESSED AS % NEOMYCIN CONTROL

Colony Size	Mel-a-1	Mel-a-6
50um	94	428
60um	133	738
70um	167	994
80um	284	1725
90um	234	1463
100um	245	1583

TABLE 2

TUMOR FORMING CAPACITY OF MGSA TRANSFECTED MELANOCYTES

Cell Type	Number of Mice Injected	Number of Mice with Tumors
mel-a-neo	9	1
mel-a-1	9	1
mel-a-6	9	9

CONCLUSIONS:

We have previously shown that normal keratinocytes contain a large quantity of immunoreactive MGSA. MGSA has been purified from psoriatic scale, macrophages and fibroblasts (12). In this report we have shown that MGSA stimulates the proliferation of normal melanocytes and contributes to the transformation of immortalized melanocytes. Thus there appears to be a clear correlation between expression of the MGSA transgene in immortalized melanocytes and tumor formation. Since the MGSA transgene expressors did not grow faster in monolayer than the neo controls, (data not shown) we suspect that either MGSA acts to stimulate the production of a second factor which promotes growth in agar and tumor formation, or that the tumor inducing capacity of MGSA is separate from its growth stimulatory capacity.

Another potential mechanism for MGSA affecting tumor formation is associated with its capacity to recruit neutrophils and lymphocytes into the site, therefore enhancing the inflammatory response (13). These neutrophils are subsequently activated, release granules, and super-oxide ions are generated, thus further contributing to the tumorigenic process. Thus it seems clear that at least one member of the B-thromboglobulin super family can effect melanocyte tumor progression as well as modulate the inflammatory response.

Acknowledgement:

This work was supported by NCI grant CA34590 (AR) the Department of Veterans Affairs (AR) and NIH AR07491 (RLS).

References:

1. Westwick J., Li Sw, Camp RD (1989). Novel neutrophil-stimulatory peptides. Immunol Today 10:146-147.
2. Bordoni R, Thomas HG, Richmond A (1989). Interaction of melanoma growth stimulatory activity with other growth factors and regulation of messenger RNA expression in melanoma cells. J. Cell. Biochem. 39:421-428.
3. Anisowicz A, Bardwell L, Sager R (1987). Constitutive overexpression of a growth-regulated gene in transformed Chinese hamster and human cells. Proc Natl Acad Sci USA 84:7188-7192.
4. Richmond A, Balentien E, Thomas HG, Flaggs G, Barton DE, Spiess J, Bordoni R, Francke U, Derynck R (1988). Molecular characterization of melanoma growth stimulatory activity, a growth factor structurally related to B-thromboglobulin. EMBO J. 7: 2025-2033.
5. Wen D, Rowland A, Derynck R (1989). Expression and secretion of gro/MGSA by stimulated human endothelial cells. EMBO J 8:1761-1766.
6. Anisowicz A, Zajchowski D, Stenman G, Sager R. (1988). Functional diversity of gro gene expression in human fibroblasts and mammary epithelial cells. Proc Natl Acad Sci USA, 85: 9645-9649.
7. Richmond A and Thomas HG (1988). Melanoma growth stimulatory activity. Isolation from human melanoma tumors and characterization of tissue distribution.J Cell Biochem 36:185-198.

8. Balentien E, Han JH, Thomas HG, Wen D, Samantha AK, Zachariae CO, Griffin PR, Brachmann R, Wong WL, Matsushima K, Richmond A, Derynck R (1990). Recombinant expression and biochemical characterization of the human MGSA/gro protein. Biochem. in press.
9. Bordoni R, Fine R, Murray D, Richmond A (1990). Characterization of the autocrine role of MGSA in normal melanocytes, nevocytes and malignant melanomas. J. Cell Biochem. in press.
10. Richmond A, Lawson DH, Nixon DW (1986). Purification of melanoma growth stimulatory activity. J. Cell Physiol 129:375-384.
11. Lawson DH, Thomas HG, Roy RGB, Gordon DJ, Chawla RK, Nixon DW and Richmond A. (1987). Preparation of a monoclonal antibody to a melanoma growth-stimulatory activity released into serum-free culture medium by Hs294 malignant melanoma cells. J. Cell. Biochem., 31:169-185.
12. Schroder J-M, Person NLM, Christophers E (1990). Lipopolysaccharide- stimulated human monocytes secrete, apart from neutrophil-activating peptidel/interleukin 8, a second neutrophil-activating protein. J. Exp. Med. 171:1091-1100.
13. Moser B, Clark-Lewis I Zwahlen R, Baggiolini M (1990). Neutrophil- activating properties of the melanoma growth-stimulatory activity. J. Exp. Med. 171:1797-1802.

Cellular and Cytokine Networks in
Tissue Immunity, pages 117-124

IMMUNOREGULATORY EFFECTS OF PLATELET FACTOR 4.

Irene R. Katz, Marjorie B. Zucker and G. Jeanette Thorbecke

Department of Pathology and Kaplan Cancer Center
New York University Medical Center,
New York, NY, 10016

Platelet factor 4 is a 7800 D protein that is secreted from the α-granules of activated blood platelets (Niewiarowski and Paul, 1981). PF4 is readily purified by absorption to heparin-agarose and elution at >1 M NaCl. Its sequence is: EAEEDGDLQCLC VKTTSQVRPRHITSLEVIKAGPHCPTAQLIATLKNGRKICLDLQAPLYKKIIKKLLES, determined by amino acid sequencing and by isolation of the human gene (Barone et al, 1988; Park et al, 1990). The molecule has two disulfide bonds and forms a tetramer at physiologic ionic strength (Cowan et al, 1986). PF4 shares about 50% structural homology with platelet basic protein, the precursor of ß-thromboglobulin (ß-TG) and connective tissue activating peptide III (CTAP-III), and 30-40% homology, mostly at the amino terminus, with IL-8.

PF4 is chemotactic for neutrophils, monocytes and fibroblasts and inhibits receptor-mediated internalization of fMLP in neutrophils (Goldman et al, 1985). It also suppresses megakaryopoiesis in bone marrow cultures (Gewirz et al, 1989). Recombinant human PF4 and its C-terminal dodecapep- tide inhibit angiogenesis in chicken chorioallantoic membranes (Maione et al, 1990). PF4 suppresses growth of murine melanoma and of human colon carcinoma in athymic mice (Sharpe et al, 1990).

The ability of PF4 to reverse T-cell mediated suppression of anti-SRBC responses in mice was discovered by accident: normal mouse serum reversed immunosuppression, whereas serum derived from clotted plasma did not (Katz et al, 1985). We used the following assay for our in vivo experiments. On day -1, mice were injected iv with a suppressive agent, usually Con A, and with an antisuppressive agent, usually PF4. The antigen, sheep erythrocytes, was injected iv on day 0, and PFC/spleen were assayed 5 days later.

The presence of the immunoregulatory (IR) factor in serum and its absence from plasma suggested that platelets were involved in its generation. Since relatively few components of platelet releasates are absent from plasma, the active material was readily identified as PF4. CTAP III had some activity, whereas platelet-derived growth factor had none (Katz et al, 1986b). Recombinant (r) PF4 prepared at Repligen was as active as the native material; as little as 0.01 μg per mouse counteracted suppression. As with serum or platelet releasates, the biological activity of rPF4 was abolished by absorption with normal spleen cells, but not by absorption with cells from athymic mice (Katz et al, 1985; Barone et al, 1988). Fractionation of the spleen cells by treatment with specific monoclonal antibodies and complement showed that $CD4^-,CD8^+$ T cells were responsible for removing the IR activity (Katz et al, 1986a).

Portions of the PF4 molecule were also tested. Amino acids 1-28 were synthesized by Repligen. Native PF4 was digested with S. aureus V8 protease to prepare three approx. equal pieces, and the C-terminal tridecapeptide P13S was synthesized (gift from Dr. Niewiarowski, Temple U., and from Repligen). Only the C-terminal portion of the PF4 molecule was active (Table 1).

Table 1.
Immunoregulatory activity of portions of the PF4 molecule

Peptides of PF4	% of control PFC/spleen after injection of Con A alone	Con A + peptide
aa 1-28	54	63
aa 8-28	25	39
aa 29-54	39	35
aa 55-69	62	162
aa 58-70 (P13S)	55	91

Adapted from: Zucker et al, 1989;
(Each value represents the mean of several experiments)

We also showed that injection of 1 μg of three unrelated peptides of about 13 amino acids each could not reverse Con A-induced suppression. Next we studied fragments of P13S, called peptides H1, H2 and H3, which were enzymatically cleaved from P13S (Fig. 1) (Zucker et al, 1989). All three fragments of P13S were active, as well as P18D, the C-terminal 18 amino acid peptide of ß-TG and CTAP-III, which is similar to the C-terminal 13 amino acids of PF4. Activity was also present in an analog of P13S in which lysine molecules were replaced with arginine and the last two amino acids were omitted ("ARG,"gift from Dr. D.A. Walz, Wayne State U.) and in P13S in which the amino groups of lysine were reacted with fluorescamine (Zucker et al, 1989).

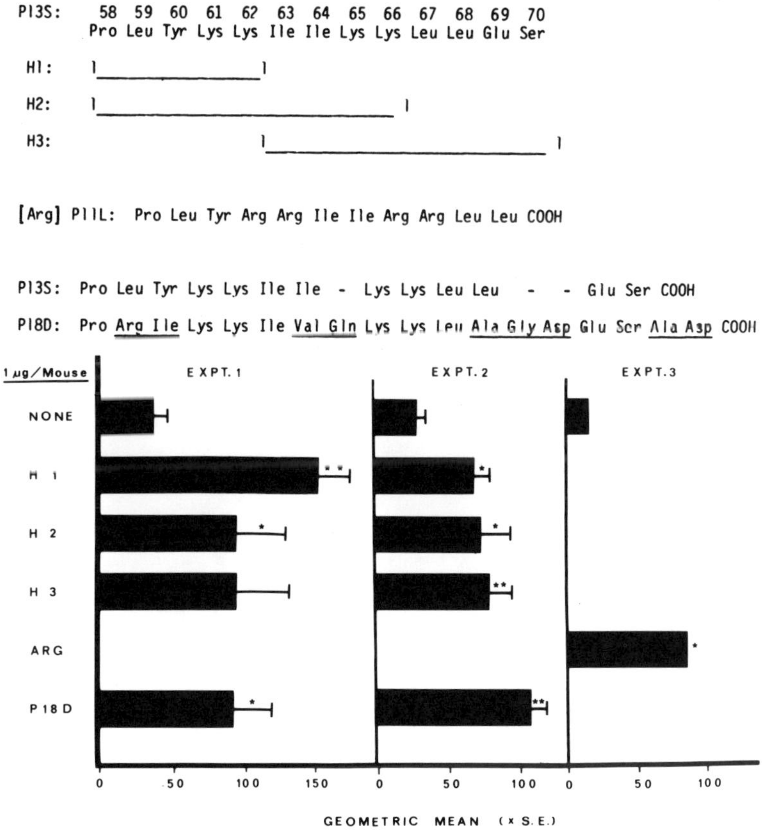

Figure 1: Structure and immunoregulatory activity in vivo of 1 μg of peptides: P13S, its fragments, P18D, and "ARG."
$^*P < 0.05$; $^{**}P = 0.01$.

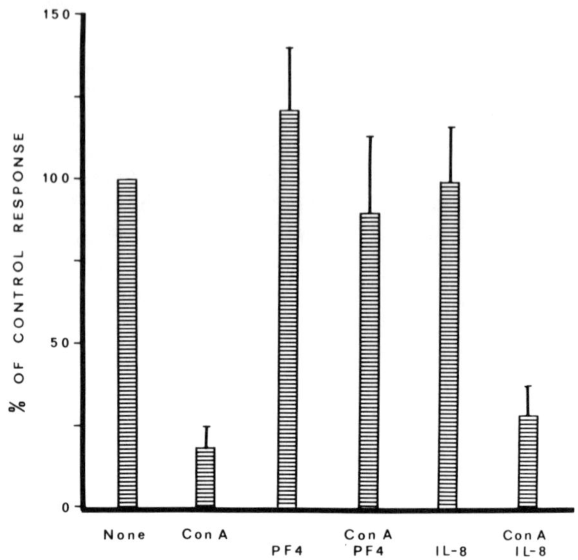

Figure 2: Lack of effect of IL-8 on Con A-induced suppression, compared to suppression abrogation by rPF4.

IL-8 does not alleviate Con A-induced suppression (Fig. 2), probably due to lack of structural homology with PF4 at the C-terminal end (Matsushima et al, 1988). Neither IL-8 nor PF4 show a significant effect on the unsuppressed response.

We also determined whether PF4 could reverse antigen-specific suppression. Mice were immunized with pneumococcal polysaccharide (PPS) type 14 on day 0. On day -3, some mice received a low tolerance-inducing dose of PPS 14, and other mice received rPF4 as well. Serum antibody titers were determined on day 10. Figure 3 shows that rPF4 prevented the tolerance-induced decrease in IgG and IgM antibody titers (Yin et al, 1988).

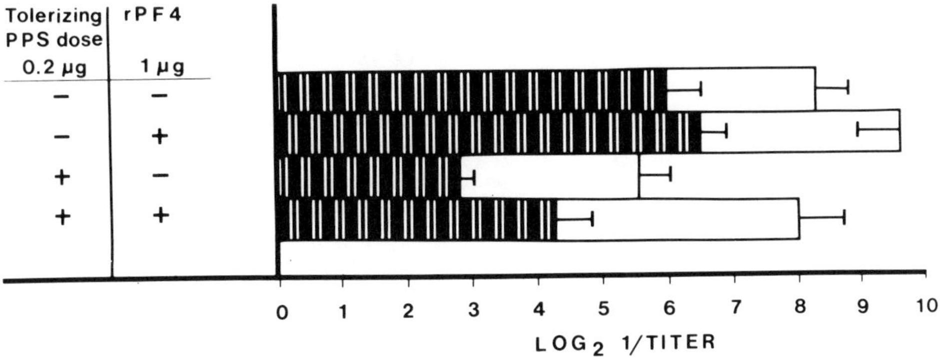

Figure 3: Effect of rPF4 on induction of tolerance to pneumococcal polysaccharide type 14. Entire bars represent IgM + IgG, the shaded bars only the IgG antibody titer reciprocals.

To avoid the complex *in vivo* environment, we developed an *in vitro* assay of the IR activity of PF4. We used the Mishell-Dutton 4 day culture system, with $5x10^6$ spleen cells/dish, obtained from mice primed *in vivo* with SRBC. Suppression was induced by adding $5x10^5$ Con A blasts, produced by culturing spleen or splenic T cells with Con A for 48 h. This suppression was mediated by $CD4^-$,$CD8^+$ cells, and was not due to competition for IL-2, since it was not affected by addition of 500 U of exogenous IL-2. As in our *in vivo* results, both rPF4 and P13S reversed this *in vitro* suppression in a dose-dependent fashion.

To test whether the suppression observed *in vitro* was due to prostaglandin production, we added 0.2-2 µM indomethacin to the cultures. Elimination of prostaglandin production by indomethacin increased background responses, but if anything, increased the % suppression. The effect of PF4 decreased, but was still significant in individual experiments. The data suggest that PF4 may need the production of prostaglandins for its effect.

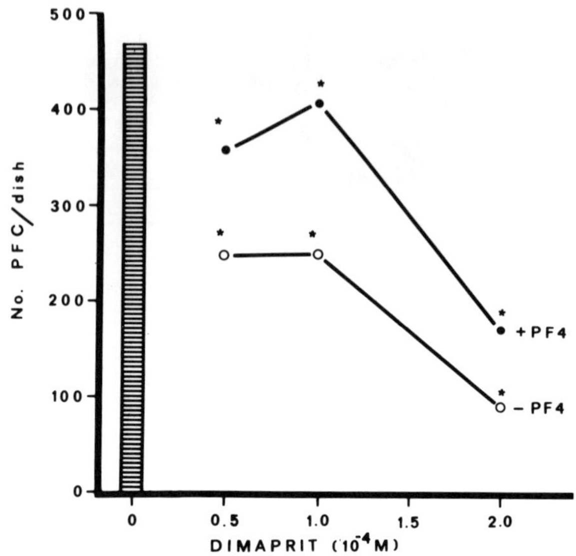

Figure 4: Suppression of % PFC response *in vitro* by three concentrations of dimaprit and its alleviation by rPF4.

To further delineate the mechanism of PF4 action we asked whether PF4 might act by causing production of IL-1. If that were so, addition of IL-1 would prevent Con A-blast induced suppression. In fact, although addition of 10-100 U/ml of exogenous IL-1 raised background responses, the cytokine did not alter the percent of suppression or the effect of PF4.

Since histamine has been described as a signal for suppressor cell activation, we added $2x10^{-4}$M cimetidine, an H2 receptor antagonist, to the culture. Cimetidine reduced the background response somewhat, but completely prevented suppression by Con A blasts. If blocking the H2 receptor prevents suppression, one might expect that stimulation of this receptor would induce suppression. To determine whether this was so, we tested the effect of dimaprit, a synthetic analog of histamine which acts as an H2 receptor agonist. Figure 4 shows the suppressive effect of dimaprit as well as the anti-suppressor effect produced by addition of rPF4. Under study now is the mechanism of PF4's ability to alleviate this suppression. We have observed that, to be active, PF4 must be added during the first 20 h of culture.

In summary: PF4 counteracts Con A-induced and antigen-specific suppression *in vivo*. The activity resides in the C-terminal end of the molecule. $CD8^+$ cells remove the immunoregulatory activity from PF4. PF4 activity *in vitro* reflects its *in vivo* action. It seems to be independent of IL-1 and IL-2, but may need prostaglandin production. Con A blast-induced suppression is inhibited by cimetidine. Dimaprit, an H2-receptor agonist, also induces suppression, which is counteracted by PF4.

REFERENCES

Barone, AD, Ghrayeb, J, Hammerling, U, Zucker, MB, Thorbecke, GJ (1988). The expression in Escherichia coli of recombinant human platelet factor 4, a protein with immunoregulatory activity. J Biol Chem 263:8710-8715.

Cowan,SW, Bakshi, EN, Machin, KJ, Isaacs, NW. (1986). Binding of heparin to human platelet factor 4. Biochem J 234:485-488.

Gewirz AM, Calabretta, B, Rucinski, B, Niewiarowski, S, Xu, WY (1989). Inhibition of human megakaryocytopoiesis in vitro by platelet factor 4 (PF4) and a synthetic COOH-terminal PF4 peptide. J Clin Invest 83:1477-1486.

Goldman, DW, Hannah, AL, Goetzl, EF (1985). Inhibition of human neutrophil receptor mediated uptake of N-formyl-met-leu-phe by platelet factor 4 (59-70). Immunology 54:163-172.

Katz, IR, Hoffmann, MK, Zucker, MB, Bell, MK, Thorbecke, GJ (1985). A platelet-derived immunoregulatory serum factor with T cell affinity. J Immunol 134:3199-3203.

Katz, IR, Bell, MK, Hoffman, MK, Thorbecke, GJ (1986a). Reversal of Con A-induced suppression by a platelet-derived factor which binds to activated suppressor T cells. Cell. Immunol. 100:57-65.

Katz, IR, Thorbecke, GJ, Bell, MK, Yin, J-Z, Clarke, D, Zucker, MB (1986b). Protease-induced immunoregulatory activity of platelet factor 4. Proc Nat Acad Sci USA 83:3491-3495.

Maione, TE, Gray, GS, Petro, J, Hunt, AJ, Donner, AL, Bauer, SI, Carson, HF, Sharpe, RJ (1990). Inhibition of angiogenesis by recombinant human platelet factor-4 and related peptides. Science 247:77-79.

Matsushima, K, et al (1988) Molecular cloning of a human monocyte-derived neutrophil chemotactic factor (MDNCF) and the induction of MDNCF mRNA by interleukin-1 and tumor necrosis factor. J. Exp. Med. 167:1883-1893.

Niewiarowski, S, Paul, P (1981). Platelet granule proteins with mitogenic and antiheparin activity. In: Gordon, JL, (ed.), "Platelets in Biology and Pathology-2." Elsevier, Amsterdam, pp 91-106.
Park, KS, Rifat, S, Eck, H, Adachi, K, Surrey, S, Poncz, M (1990). Biologic and biochemic properties of recombinant platelet factor 4 demonstrate identity with the native protein. Blood 75:1290-1295.
Sharpe, RJ, Byers HR, Scott, CF, Bauer, SI, Maione, TE. (1990). Growth inhibition of murine melanoma and human colon carcinoma by recombinant human platelet factor 4. J Nat Cancer Inst 82:848-653.
Yin, J-Z, Zucker, MB, Clarke, D, Bell, MK, Thorbecke, GJ (1988). Prevention by a platelet-derived factòr (platelet factor 4) of induction of low dose tolerance to pneumococcal polysaccharides. Cell. Immunol. 115:221-227.
Zucker, MB, Katz, IR, Thorbecke, GJ, Milot, DC, Holt, J (1989). Immunoregulatory activity of peptides related to platelet factor 4. Proc Nat Acad Sci USA 86:7571-7574.

Cellular and Cytokine Networks in
Tissue Immunity, pages 125-130

NEUTROPHIL-ACTIVATING PROTEINS IN INFLAMMATORY SKIN-DISEASES

Jens - M. Schröder

Department of Dermatology,
University of Kiel,
D-2300 Kiel, FRG

In several skin diseases neutrophil-rich tissue infiltrates are observable. Whereas some of these diseases are of infectious nature several other dermatoses including psoriasis, which are termed neutrophilic dermatosis (Christophers, 1987) histologically are characterized by the formation of sterile pustules and/or neutrophil-rich tissue infiltrates without any signs of infection. Reasons for neutrophil accumulation in such diseased tissues are largely unknown. It has been discussed that PMN-chemotactic factors like the complement split product C5a or Leukotriene B_4 could be responsible for PMN-infiltration. These chemotaxins, however, don't show a leukocyte specificity and therefore do not explain preferential neutrophil tissue infiltration.

We addressed the question which is the major chemotactic signal compound present in lesional psoriatic epidermis, which could be responsible for PMN-infiltration of the epidermis.

The availability of large amounts of lesional psoriatic scale material offered a chance to biochemically characterize PMN-chemotactic factors present in inflammatory disease material. We therefore extracted psoriatic scales (50 - 500 grams) and investigated both, lipid-like PMN-chemotaxins as well as proteinaceous attractants. Initial experiments showed that both lipid-like and proteinaceous PMN-chemotactic factors are present in psoriatic scales. Serial dilution experiments however revealed that proteinaceous attractants were the most abundant chemotaxins in lesional psoriatic scale material (Schröder and Christophers, 1986, Camp et al., 1986).

When these proteinaceous chemotactic factors were analyzed for molecular size by G-75-gel chromatography it became clear that at least two attractants of similar M_r are present (Schröder and Christophers, 1986). The compound with higher M_r (~ 15 kDa), which is a minor compound, could be identified as $C5a_{des\ arg}$. The second one, which reproducibly was detected in psoriatic scales and was present in large amounts tentatively was termed "anionic neutrophil activating protein, ANAP" and appeared to be a new PMN-chemotactic protein (Schröder and Christophers, 1986). Cross desensitization experiments using PMN, which were preincubated with 10^{-8} M NAP-1/IL-8, revealed that biological responses to fractions containing ANAP were markedly decreased, whereas - as expected - $C5a_{des\ arg}$ depedent enzyme-release was not affected (Schröder and Christophers, 1986). These data indicated that ANAP apparently binds to the same PMN-receptor as NAP-1/IL-8 does and therefore could be structurally similar or identical to NAP-1/IL-8.

We were able to purify ANAP obtained from pooled lesional psoriatic scales by cation-exchange HPLC followed by different reversed phase HPLC-steps as well as size exclusion HPLC (Schröder et al., submitted for publication).

As a result three major neutrophil-activating proteins could be purified to homogeneity which tentatively were termed β_1-ANAP, β_2-ANAP and α_2-ANAP (Schröder et al. submitted). Fig. 1 shows a typical final RP-HPLC run for purification of two of these ANAP-factors. SDS-PAGE-analysis of these three polypeptides revealed major lines corresponding to a M_r of 7.8, 8.2 and 7.7. kDa for β_1-ANAP, β_2-ANAP and α_2-ANAP (Schröder et al. submitted). All three ANAPs could be obtained in sufficient amounts for aminoterminal amino acid sequencing. Whereas β_1-ANAP and β_2-ANAP were identical in its amino acid sequence, ß$_1$-ANAP is an aminoterminally truncated form of ß$_2$-ANAP. The sequence of both, ß$_1$-ANAP and ß$_2$-ANAP is identical to that found for neutrophil-activating protein 1 (Tab. 1 and Schröder et al., submitted). By sequence analysis as well as M_r determination (SDS-PAGE as well as size exclusion HPLC) ß$_2$-ANAP is identical with NAP-1/IL-8.

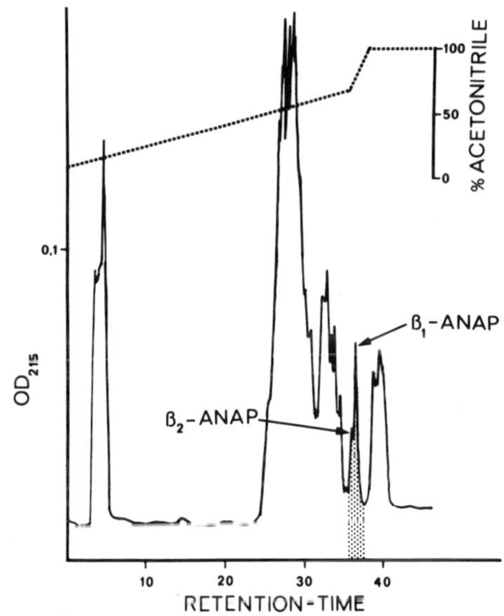

Figure 1. RP-18-HPLC of ß-ANAP. The chromatogram shows the final purification step of ß$_1$- and ß$_2$-ANAP. Arrows indicate elution-position of both ANAPs. Biological activity is shown by

---

α_2-ANAP revealed similarities in its aminoterminal sequence with NAP-1/IL-8 and is identical with the 16 kDa-moiety of melanoma growth stimulatory activity, MGSA (Richmond et al., 1988). Both aminoterminal amino acids of α_2-ANAP could not be identified. It is possible that α_2-ANAP is O-glycolysated as recently supposed for the 16 kDa-moiety of MGSA (Richmond et al., 1988). Molecular size estimation of all three ANAPs by size exclusion HPLC as well as SDS-PAGE analysis revealed relative molecular masses between 8 and 10 kDa indicating that intact cytokines, not however, carboxy-terminal truncation products were isolated. This suggestion was supported by evaluation of specific activities of these three ANAPs.

Stimulation of half maximal chemotactic migration of PMN by β_1-ANAP, β_2-ANAP as well as α_2-ANAP preparations has been found to be similar to that found for authentic NAP-1/IL-8, its 69 residue form as well as the neutrophil activating protein 3 (NAP-3), which is identical with MGSA (data not shown and [Schröder et al., 1990]). Therefore there is ample evidence now that biologically intact cytokines like NAP-1/IL-8 as well as MGSA/gro are present in lesional skin material of psoriasis.

It is interesting to speculate that the presence of NAP-1/IL-8 and gro/MGSA-related proteins may be responsible for accumulation of predominantly neutrophils and to a less degree also T-lymphocytes in the psoriatic lesion, because NAP-1/IL-8 is known to be a potent and highly efficient chemotactic factor for PMN in vitro (Schröder et al., 1987). Although NAP-1/IL-8 is also a potent chemotaxin for T-lymphocytes in vitro (Gronhoj-Larsen et al., 1989) it appears to be of low efficacy (Leonard et al., 1990). In contrast to other chemotaxins like LTB_4, C5a, FMLP or PAF NAP-1/IL-8 is neither a chemotactic factor for monocytes or eosinophils (Schröder et al., 1987).

Table 1. NH_2-terminal amino acid sequences of some ANAPs*

α_2-ANAP :	XXVATELRXQXLQTLYG...
16 kD-MGSA:	XXVATELRXQX...
β_1-ANAP :	ELRXQXIKTYSKPFHPK...
β_2-ANAP :	SAKELRXQXIKTYSKPFHPK...
NAP-1/IL-8:	SAKELRXQXIKTYSKPFHPK...

* The single letter code of amino acids was used.

X: amino acid could not be detected

Apparent specificity of NAP-1/IL-8 for neutrophils in inducing chemotactic responses led to the hypothesis that this cytokine could be of importance in (non-infectious) inflammatory reactions where histologically neutrophils are detectable. Investigations of scale material of different origin revealed that in psoriasis, eczema as well as ichthyosis congenita high amounts of both IL-8 and gro/MGSA-related neutrophil attractants are detectable. On the other hand we did not detect any NAP-1/IL-8-related cytokines in the stratum corneum of patients with UV-burns, Lyell-syndrome or drug reactions (unpublished observation). Moreover neither heel callus or normal epidermis did contain significant amounts of either NAP-1/IL-8 or MGSA/gro (data not shown and M. Sticherling, unpublished observation). The finding of excessively elevated amounts of both, NAP-1/IL-8 and MGSA/gro-related cytokines in the scale material obtained from patients with ichthyosis is unexpected and reveals that elevated tissue levels of NAP-1/IL-8-related cytokines apparently do not necessarily result in PMN-accumulation, because in skin lesions of patients with ichthyosis histologically no signs of a PMN-infiltrate are observable. It appears, that NAP-1/IL-8-related cytokines are detectable when epidermal scaling is observable (produced by epidermal hyperproliferation). Therefore it is intriguing to speculate about a direct or indirect role of NAP-1/IL-8-related cytokines as epidermal growth stimulators. Interestingly recent findings of in vitro epidermal cell growth stimulation supports this concept (Krueger et al., 1990).

REFERENCES

Camp RDR, Fincham NJ, Cunningham EM, Greaves MW, Morris J, Chu A (1986). Psoriatic skin lesions contain biologically active amounts of an interleukin 1-like compound. J Immunol 137: 3469-3474.

Christophers E (1987). Neutrophile Dermatosen. In: Braun-Falco O, Schill WB (eds.) Fortschritte der praktischen Dermatologie und Venerologie. Springer Verlag, Berlin, New

York, London, Paris, Tokyo, 195-202.

Gronhoj-Larsen C, Anderson AO, Appella E, Oppenheim JJ, Matsushima K (1989). The Neutrophil Activating Protein (NAP-1) Is Also Chemotactic for T-Lymphocytes. Science 243: 1464-1466.

Krueger G, Jörgensen C, Miller C, Schröder J-M, Sticherling M, Christophers E (1990). Effects of IL-8 on epidermal proliferation. J Invest Dermatol 94: 545 (abstract).

Leonard EJ, Skeel A, Yoshimura T, Noer K, Kutvirt S, Van Epps D (1990). Leukocyte specificity and binding of human neutrophil attractant/activation protein-1 (NAP-1). J Immunol 144: 1323-1330.

Richmond A, Balentien E, Thomas HG, Flaggs G, Barton DE, Spiess J, Bardoni R, Francke U, Derynck R (1988). Molecular characterization and chromosomal mapping of melanoma growth stimulatory activity, a growth factor structurally related to ß-thromboglobulin. EMBO J 7: 2025-2033.

Schröder J-M, Christophers E (1986). Identification of $C5a_{des\ arg}$ and an Anionic Neutrophil-Activating Peptide (ANAP) in Psoriatic Scales. J Invest Dermatol 87: 53-58.

Schröder J-M, Mrowietz U, Morita E, Christophers E (1987). Purification and partial biochemical characterization of human monocyte-derived neutrophil-activating peptide that lacks Interleukin 1 activity. J Immunol 139: 3474-3483.

Schröder J-M, Perssoon NLM, Christophers E (1990). Lipopolysaccharide-stimulated human monocytes secrete, apart from neutrophil-activating peptide 1/Interleukin 8, a second neutrophil-activating protein. NH_2-terminal amino acid sequence identity with Melanoma Growth Stimulatory Activity. J Exp Med 171: 1091-1100.

Schröder J-M, Gregory H, Young J, Christophers E (1990). Neutrophil activating proteins in psoriasis. Submitted for publication.

Cellular and Cytokine Networks in
Tissue Immunity, pages 131-136

HUMAN AND MOUSE MONOCYTE CHEMOTACTIC PROTEINS (MCP) : PRODUCTION AND IDENTIFICATION

Benny Decock, Riccardo Bertini, Jean-Pierre Lenaerts, René Conings, Alfons Billiau, Alberto Mantovani and Jo Van Damme

Laboratory of Immunobiology, Rega Institute for Medical Research, University of Leuven, B-3000 Leuven, Belgium (B.D., J.-P.L., R.C., A.B., J.V.D.) and Istituto di Ricerche Farmacologiche "Mario Negri", 20157 Milano, Italy (R.B., A.M.)

INTRODUCTION

Progress in leukocyt chemotaxis research has been accelerated by the identification of cytokines with chemotactic activity. First, a protein with chemotactic activity specific for granulocytes could be isolated from cultures of a variety of normal and transformed human cells. The factor has also been shown to be chemotactic for T-lymphocytes and is now known as interleukin 8 (IL-8; Matsushima and Oppenheim, 1989). This molecule has been found to induce granulocytosis and skin reaction, respectively, upon systemic and local injection in experimental animals (Van Damme et al, 1988). More recently, a monocyte chemotactic protein (MCP) has been purified from cultures of human glioma (Yoshimura et al, 1989a), myelomonocytic (Matsushima et al, 1989) and sarcoma (Van Damme et al, 1989) cell lines and from cultures of normal human blood mononuclear leukocytes (Yoshimura et al, 1989b; Decock et al, 1990) and fibroblasts (Van Damme et al, 1989). The amino acid sequence of this protein (Robinson et al, 1989; Yoshimura et al, 1989c; Furutani et al, 1989; Van Damme et al, 1989; Decock et al, 1990), named monocyte chemoattractant protein-1 (MCP-1) and monocyte chemotactic and activating factor (MCAF), showed low but significant similarity with the IL-8 sequence. MCP and IL-8 have been demonstrated to belong to 2 different but related protein families (Matsushima and Oppenheim, 1989; Leonard and Yoshimura, 1990; Van Damme, 1991). In this report we describe the production and isolation of MCP of both human and mouse origin.

MATERIALS AND METHODS

Leukocytes were isolated from human buffy coats by treatment with Plasmasteril (Fresenius, Bad Homburg, Germany). Mononuclear cells were obtained by centrifugation of leukocyte suspensions on Ficoll-sodium metrizoate (Lymphoprep; Nyegaard, Oslo, Norway). Preparations of adherent mononuclear leukocytes, consisting of 80 % monocytes, were obtained by incubating mononuclear cells in plastic culture flasks to adhere and by washing away the non-adherent cells. Granulocytes were isolated from total leukocyte preparations by lysis of remaining erythrocytes in water and by centrifugation in a Percoll gradient (1.054 g/ml; Pharmacia, Uppsala, Sweden).

Induction experiments were performed by incubating confluent fibroblast and tumor cell monolayers and mononuclear leukocytes (5×10^6 cells/well) in 24-well (1.9 cm^2) dishes for 48 h at 37°C in culture medium supplemented with 2 % serum containing one of the following inducer substances : lipopolysaccharide (LPS) from *E. coli* (Difco, Detroit, MI), concanavalin A (ConA; Calbiochem, San Diego, CA), double-stranded RNA polyriboinosinic:polyribocytidylic acid (poly rI:rC; P-L Biochemicals, Milwaukee, WI), measles virus (Attenuvax strain), natural human IL-1ß and IL-6 purified to homogeneity (Van Damme et al, 1988), recombinant murine tumor necrosis factor α (mTNF-α; Innogenetics, Antwerp, Belgium), murine IL-1α (mIL-1α; kindly provided by P. Lomedico, Hoffmann La Roche, Nutley, NJ), Newcastle disease virus (NDV; strain Komarov) and Sendai virus. Virus in culture supernatants was inactivated at pH 2 after the induction period.

Chemotactic activity for monocytes and granulocytes was measured under agarose according to the method of Nelson et al (1975) as described previously (Van Damme et al, 1989). Mononuclear cells (10^6 cells/well) and granulocytes (2×10^5 cells/well) from a single blood donor were exposed for 2 h at 37°C to test samples. Chemotactic activity in cell supernatants was expressed as percentage of maximal migration distance obtained with pure natural human MCP and IL-8.

The production and purification procedures for human and murine MCP were as described previously (Van Damme et al, 1989). Conditioned supernatants were processed by batch adsorption to controlled pore glass beads (CPG-10-350; Serva, Heidelberg, Germany). Adsorbed protein was applied to a heparin-Sepharose CL-6B (Pharmacia) column and subsequently eluted with a NaCl gradient. Fractions containing chemotactic activity were subjected to cation-exchange FPLC at pH 4 in formate buffer using a Mono S column (Pharmacia). MCP eluted with a NaCl gradient from the FPLC column was further purified by reverse-phase HPLC on a C8 Aquapore RP-300 column (Applied Biosystems, Foster City, CA), equilibrated with 0.05 % trifluoroacetic acid and eluted with an acetonitrile gradient.

The amino acid sequence of purified proteins and protein fragments was determined with an Applied Biosystems 477A/120A sequencing system.

RESULTS

Production of monocyte chemotactic activity by human fibroblasts and mononuclear leukocytes

The culture supernatants of confluent monolayers of normal human embryonic fibroblasts and of human mononuclear leukocytes stimulated with LPS, ConA, poly rI:rC, measles virus, IL-1ß and IL-6 were collected and tested for the presence of monocyte chemotactic activity (MCP). Chemotactic activity for granulocytes (IL-8) was also measured in the test samples. The results of 4 induction experiments are summarized in Table 1. Unstimulated cells did not produce detectable amounts of chemotactic activity. Production of MCP was accompagnied with IL-8 production in all combinations. Double-stranded RNA, measles virus and IL-1 induced chemotactic activity in cultures of both fibroblasts and mononuclear leukocytes. Stimulation of mononuclear cells with ConA and LPS also resulted in the production of chemotactic activity. Both fibroblasts and mononuclear cells treated with IL-6 failed to produce chemotactic activity.

TABLE 1. Production of MCP and IL-8 (% of maximal migration distance) by human fibroblasts and mononuclear leukocytes in response to different inducer substances

Inducer	Fibroblasts		Leukocytes	
	MCP	IL-8	MCP	IL-8
Control	<10	<10	<10	<10
LPS (50 μg/ml)	<10	<10	43	84
ConA (10 μg/ml)	ND	ND	43	72
polyrI:rC (100 μg/ml)	66	53	17	39
measles v.($10^{4.6}$ $TCID_{50}$/ml)	52	85	17	52
IL-1β (100 U/ml)	59	69	30	26
IL-6 (1000 U/ml)	<10	<10	<10	<10

Production of monocyt chemotactic activity by human tumor cells

Confluent monolayers of MG-63 osteosarcoma, HEp-2 epidermal carcinoma, Bowes melanoma and Malavu hepatoma cells were tested for MCP and IL-8 production in the presence of the inducer substances IL-1ß, poly rI:rC and measles virus. MG-63 sarcoma cells showed an induction profile resembling that of the normal fibroblasts. HEp-2 carcinoma cells were poor producers of chemotactic activity irrespective of the inducer substance. Bowes melanoma cells only responded to double-stranded RNA by producing exclusively IL-8 activity. IL-1 stimulated Malavu hepatoma cells to produce high amounts of both MCP and IL-8. Measles virus was a moderate and good inducer of MCP and IL-8, respectively, in hepatoma cells.

Production of monocyte chemotactic activity by mouse fibroblasts and L929 cells

Confluent monolayers of mouse embryonic fibroblasts and L929 cells were stimulated with mTNF-α, mIL-1α, IL-1β, poly rI:rC, NDV or Sendai virus. The results of 2 induction experiments are summarized in Table 2. Supernatants of unstimulated cells did not contained detectable amounts of chemotactic activity. Although cytokines stimulated both embryonic fibroblasts and L929 cells to produce MCP, the 2 viruses seemed to be the most potent stimulators. Remarkably no measureable granulocyte chemotactic activity was detected in culture supernatant of stimulated mouse cells (data not shown).

TABLE 2. Production of MCP (% of maximal migration distance) by mouse embryonic fibroblasts and L929 cells in response to different inducer substances

Inducer	Fibroblasts MCP	L929 cells MCP
Control	< 5	< 5
mTNF-α (0.3 ng)	15	5
mIL-1α (100 U/ml)	26	12
IL-1β (100 U/ml)	35	18
polyrI:rC (100 μg/ml)	23	24
NDV (20 HAU/ml)	45	40
Sendai v.(640 HAU/ml)	42	42

Isolation of human MCP produced by normal fibroblasts, MG-63 osteosarcoma cells and adherent mononuclear leukocytes

Chemotactic activity produced by confluent monolayers of normal embryonic fibroblasts and MG-63 osteosarcoma cells stimulated with poly rI:rC or IL-1 was concentrated and partially purified by adsorption to controlled pore glass beads. MCP and IL-8 showed comparable affinity for heparin. Cation-exchange FPLC of the chemotactic activity eluted from the heparin column resulted in the separation of MCP and IL-8. MCP eluted at about 0.5 M NaCl and IL-8 was found in the FPLC fractions containing 0.9 M salt. SDS-PAGE analysis of the FPLC-purified MCP produced by embryonic fibroblasts revealed a 15 kDa protein, whereas the MG-63 MCP migrated as a 10 and 15 kDa proteindoublet. Both MCP molecules, however, were N-terminally blocked, since no amino acid sequence was obtained when the proteins were subjected to Edman degradation. MCP-1/MCAF had also a blocked N-terminus which was found to be the result of the presence of a pyroglutamic acid residue (Robinson et al, 1989). In order to obtain amino acid sequence information, the purified MCP from MG-63 cells was digested with trypsin and the resulting protein fragments were, after separation by reverse-phase HPLC, subjected to amino acid sequence analysis. The amino acid sequences of 3 tryptic fragments, in total 22 residues, were identical with parts of the MCP-1/MCAF sequence.

MCP was also isolated from culture medium conditioned by LPS-stimulated adherent mononuclear leukocytes, consisting of 80 % monocytes. Although this MCP was subjected to the same purification procedure as fibroblast MCP, FPLC-purified MCP preparations were shown to contain considerable amounts of contaminating proteins which had to be removed by reverse-phase HPLC. SDS-PAGE analysis of homogeneous MCP produced by adherent mononuclear cells revealed protein bands of 10 and 15 kDa. After subjection to amino acid sequence analysis most of the isolated MCP was shown to have a blocked N-terminus, but also minor amounts of a molecule with a sequence starting at amino acid residue 6 of the MCP-1/MCAF sequence were detectable.

Isolation of murine MCP produced by L929 cells

Murine MCP produced by NDV-infected L929 cells was purified to homogeneity with the procedure used to isolate human MCP, including adsorption to controlled pore glass beads, heparin affinity chromatography, cation-exchange FPLC and reverse-phase HPLC. Homogeneous murine MCP occured as a 8 kDa protein upon SDS-PAGE analysis. In analogy with its human counterpart, this protein was also shown to have a blocked N-terminus and was therefore cleaved with the Asp-N endoproteinase. The 17 amino acid residue sequence obtained from a purified protein fragment was found to be identical with part (residues 3-19) of the cDNA-derived sequence of murine JE, identified as the mouse counterpart of human MCP (Rollins et al, 1988).

CONCLUSIONS

We could isolate human MCP from cultures of double-stranded RNA- or IL-1-stimulated embryonic fibroblasts and osteosarcoma cells and from LPS-stimulated adherent mononuclear leukocytes. MCP was purified by adsorption to controlled pore glass beads, heparin affinity chromatography, cation-exchange FPLC and reverse-phase HPLC. Irrespective of the cellular source, MCP was shown to have a blocked N-terminus. Amino acid sequence analysis of protein fragments revealed a unique MCP sequence. The difference at the molecular level between the 10 and 15 kDa MCP molecules observed upon SDS-PAGE is at present unknown.

Mouse MCP was induced, purified and identified under similar conditions as its human counterpart. The absence of measurable chemotactic activity for granulocytes in the supernatants of stimulated mouse cells could be explained by the insensibility for mouse IL-8 of the human granulocytes used in the assay. A discrepancy was noticed when the mouse MCP molecular weight determined by SDS-PAGE of purified protein (8 kDa) was compared to that predicted from the JE cDNA sequence (> 12 kDa; Rollins et al, 1988).

Recently another protein belonging to the MCP protein family, RANTES, was also found to be chemotactic for monocytes and T-lymphocytes (Schall et al,1990).

REFERENCES

Decock B, Conings R, Lenaerts J-P, Billiau A, Van Damme J (1990). Identification of the monocyte chemotactic protein from human osteosarcoma cells and monocytes : detection of a novel N-terminally processed form. Biochem Biophys Res Comm 167:904-909.

Furutani Y, Nomura H, Notake M, Oyamada Y, Fukui T, Yamada M, Larsen CG, Oppenheim JJ, Matsushima K (1989). Cloning and sequencing of the cDNA for human monocyte chemotactic and activating factor (MCAF). Biochem Biophys Res Comm 159:249-255.

Leonard EJ, Yoshimura T (1990). Human monocyte chemoattractant protein-1 (MCP-1). Immunology Today 11:97-101.

Matsushima K, Oppenheim JJ (1989). Interleukin 8 and MCAF : novel inflammatory cytokines inducible by IL1 and TNF. Cytokine 1:2-13.

Matsushima K, Larsen C, DuBois G, Oppenheim JJ (1989). Purification and characterization of a novel monocyte chemotactic and activating factor produced by a human myelomonocytic cell line. J Exp Med 169:1485-1490.

Nelson RD, Quie PG, Simmons RL (1975). Chemotaxis under agarose : a new and simple method for measuring chemotaxis and spontaneous migration of human polymorphonuclear leukocytes and monocytes. J Immunol 115:1650-1656.

Robinson EA, Yoshimura T, Leonard E, Tanaka S, Griffin PR, Shabanowitz J, Hunt DF, Appella E (1989). Complete amino acid sequence of a human monocyte chemoattractant, a putative mediator of cellular immune reactions. Proc Natl Acad Sci USA 86:1850-1854.

Rollins BJ, Morrison E, Stiles CD (1988). Cloning and expression of JE, a gene inducible by platelet-derived growth factor and whose product has cytokine-like properties. Proc Natl Acad Sci USA 85:3738-3742.

Schall TJ, Bacon K, Toy KJ, Goeddel DV (1990). Selective attraction of monocytes and T lymphocytes of the memory phenotype by cytokine RANTES. Nature 347:669-671.

Van Damme J, Van Beeumen J, Opdenakker G, Billiau (1988). A novel, NH_2-terminal sequence-characterized human monokine possessing neutrophil chemotactic, skin-reactive, and granulocytosis-promoting activity. J Exp Med 167:1364-1376.

Van Damme J, Van Beeumen J, Decock B, Van Snick J, De Ley M, Billiau A (1988). Separation and comparison of two monokines with lymphocyte-activating factor activity: IL-1ß and hybridoma growth factor (HGF). J Immunol 140:1534-1541.

Van Damme J, Decock B, Lenaerts J-P, Conings R, Bertini R, Mantovani A, Billiau A (1989). Identification by sequence analysis of chemotactic factors for monocytes produced by normal and transformed cells stimulated with virus, double-stranded RNA and cytokine. Eur J Immunol 19:2367-2373.

Van Damme J (1991). Interleukin-8 and related molecules. In: Thomson AW (ed), "Immunology and Molecular Biology of Cytokines", London: Academic Press, in press.

Yoshimura T, Robinson EA, Tanaka S, Appella E, Kuratsu J-I, Leonard EJ (1989a). Purification and amino acid analysis of two human glioma-derived monocyte chemoattractants. J Exp Med 169:1449-1459.

Yoshimura T, Robinson EA, Tanaka S, Appella E, Leonard EJ (1989b). Purification and amino acid analysis of two human monocyte chemoattractants produced by phytohemagglutinin-stimulated human blood mononuclear leukocytes. J Immunol 142:1956-1962.

Yoshimura T, Yuhki N, Moore SK, Appella E, Lerman MI, Leonard EJ (1989c). Human monocyte chemoattractant protein-1 (MCP-1). Full-length cDNA cloning, expression in mitogen-stimulated blood mononuclear leukocytes, and sequence similarity to mouse competence gene JE. FEBS Letters 244:487-493.

Cellular and Cytokine Networks in
Tissue Immunity, pages 137-142

Molecular Basis of Leukocyte Chemotactic Responses

John Didsbury and Ralph Snyderman

Department of Medicine, Duke University Medical Center, Box 3680, Durham, NC 27710, USA.

SUMMARY: Cloning of cDNA encoding the human formylpeptide chemoattractant receptor indicates it to be a member of the class of seven membrane spanning domain receptors which couple to G proteins. Indeed, chemoattractant receptors on leukocytes initiate migratory and cytotoxic activities via GTP-binding proteins. Leukocyte activation by chemoattractants stimulate sequential metabolic pathways involving phospholipase C then phospholipase D. The formylpeptide receptor physically associates with both a heterotrimeric G protein and a low molecular mass GTP-binding protein. These multiple GTP-binding proteins may regulate the function of chemoattractant receptors.

Phagocytes migrate along gradients of chemoattractants including C5a, a complement fragment, leukotriene B_4 (LTB_4), platelet-activating factor (PAF), interleukin 8-like cytokines and certain products of bacterial protein synthesis (i.e. formylmethionyl peptides). N-formylated synthetic oligopeptides [e.g. N-formyl-methionyl-leucyl phenyalanine, (fMet-Leu-Phe or fMLP)] are useful probes to study leukocyte activation (Snyderman et al.,1990).

The response of leukocytes to chemoattractants is initiated by activation of cell surface receptors. Specific receptors for chemotactic factors on phagocytic leukocytes when ligated initiate metabolic events which lead to their accumulation at sites of inflammation and activation of their cytotoxic potential. The best characterized chemotactic factor receptor is the one which binds formylpeptides. Neutrophil receptors for both lipid (LTB_4, PAF) and peptide (C5a, fMLP) chemoattractants all possess a single ligand binding subunit and appear to be monomeric (for review see Snyderman et al.,1990). The molecular mass of fMLP, C5a and LTB_4 receptors is similar with kDas of ~50-70. The total number of receptors for each chemoattractant is in the same moderately abundant range with 0.5-2.8 x 10^5 receptors per cell. Two classes of binding sites, one high affinity (Kd 0.2-0.5nM) and one low affinity (Kd 20-500nM) are found for each receptor. Guanine nucleotides modulate the interconvertibility of high affinity to low affinity sites for each of these receptors suggesting that each chemoattractant receptor is associated with a G protein. Based on these similarities it is likely that all of these receptors will be structurally homologous to one another and like other G protein-coupled receptors will contain a seven membrane spanning domain structure with extracellular and cytoplasmic tails.

Recent advances now make it possible to identify the structure-function relationships of chemoattractant receptors for their activation of disparate cellular functions. Boulay et al. have recently cloned the formylpeptide chemoattractant and have shown it to have the characteristic seven membrane spanning domains of G protein-coupled receptors (Boulay et al. 1990). We have used the nucleotide sequence of this receptor and cloned it from differentiated HL-60 cell mRNA by reverse transcription PCR. The cDNA was put into the transient eukaryotic expression vector pRK5 under control of a CMV enhancer/promoter. We have transfected human embryonic kidney cells using calcium phosphate mediated transfection such that 40-45% of the cells express formylpeptide receptor, with an average of 500,000 receptors per cell. In calcium flux experiments measured by Indo-1 fluorescence, the formylpeptide receptors undergo homologous desensitization.

Chemoattractants stimulate the directed migration of leukocytes, but at higher concentrations, also may induce them to secrete lysosomal enzymes and produce superoxide anions. Motility-related functions occur at low doses of chemoattractants (ca. 10^{-9}M fMLP) whereas secretory functions require 20-50-fold higher concentrations (Snyderman et al.,1988). Both of these responses are initiated by binding of chemoattractants to specific cell surface receptors.

Neutrophil responses to chemoattractants fall into two broad categories which govern the migratory versus cytotoxic (microbicidal/secretory) activities of the cells (Snyderman et al.,1988,1990). The evidence for discrete regulation of the two types of responses are based on dose-response relationships, activity of different chemoattractants, kinetics and pharmacological manipulations. Migratory or chemotactic responses occur at doses of chemoattractant which are at least 20-fold lower than those needed to stimulate cytotoxic processes such as the respiratory burst or exocytosis. Based on our biochemical studies phagocyte activation by fMet-Leu-Phe we have delineated two sequential phases. The first correlates with activation of chemotaxis, is called the rapid phase, and is activated by both the peptide chemoattractants (fMLP, C5a) and lipid chemoattractants (PAF, LTB_4). This phase involves ligand binding to its receptor which activates the coupled G protein ($Gi\alpha2$) by stimulating its binding of GTP. Pertussis toxin which ADP-ribosylates certain G proteins blocks the action of all chemoattractants at this step. The activated G protein causes a phospholipase C-mediated phosphodiesteric cleavage of phosphatidylinositol 4,5-bisphosphate (PIP_2) to form inositol 1,4,5-triphosphate (IP_3) and diacylglycerol (DAG)(Smith et al.,1985,1986). A phospholipase C is implicated in this step based on analysis of the inositol phosphates produced [i.e. formation of IP_3 coincident with a loss of PIP_2]. Activation of a phosphoinositide-specific phospholipase C has also been demonstrated for other chemoattractant receptors [C5a, LTB_4,PAF and NAF(IL-8)](Clancy et al.,1983, Lapetina,1982, Braquet et al.,1987, Peveri et al.,1988). The IP_3 formed from PIP_2 causes the release of calcium from intracellular stores and the DAG activates protein kinase C. Chelation of intracellular calcium with EGTA attenuates the responses invoked by fMLP implicating a role for calcium in this phase.

The products of the first phase (IP_3, its metabolites and DAG) may initiate the second sustained phase in the presence of high doses of chemoattractant ($>10^{-8}$M fMLP or C5a)(Truett et al. 1988). Activation of this phase correlates with stimulation of the respiratory burst and exocytosis. The peptide chemoattractants (fMLP, C5a) are strong activators of the second phase while lipid chemoattractants (LTB_4, PAF) are poor activators. These discrepences amongst chemoattractants should prove extremely useful in defining the structure-function relationships of their cloned receptors. The second phase is characterized by: (a) an influx of extracellular calcium presumably by activation of a calcium channel via an isomer of IP_3 and subsequently (b) a second, larger and more sustained production of phosphatidic acid and DAG. Protein kinase C involvement is indicated by the fact that fMLP stimulation of this phase results in translocation of protein kinase C activity to the membrane and phorbol esters can mimic certain fMLP generated responses. Fatty acid analysis of DAG produced during the second phase indicates that it arises from hydrolysis of phosphatidylcholine potentially via activation of phospholipase D or a phosphatidylcholine selective-phospholipase C. Involvement of extracellular calcium in initiating this process is supported by the observations that calcium ionophores increase cytosolic calcium levels in leukocytes and stimulate superoxide production, degranulation and DAG production (Truett et al.,1988). Moreover, the second phase is diminished by chelation of extracellular calcium.

In addition to previously mentioned data, several other lines of evidence demonstrate the association of the formylpeptide receptor with G proteins (Snyderman et al.,1988). Prebound formylpeptide receptor-ligand complexes on intact permeabilized neutrophils undergo an increased rate of dissociation in response to GTPγS and a partially purified formylpeptide receptor-radioligand complex exhibited a similar response to GTPγS. The formylpeptide receptor-radioligand complex elutes in three distinct peaks when chromatographed on DEAE-Fractogel. One peak is free receptor, a second co-elutes with a 40kDa pertussis toxin substrate which we have identified as Giα2. Interestingly, a third peak of receptor is associated with a ca. 28kDa GTP-binding protein (Polakis et al.,1989) tentatively identified as *ral* (unpublished observation). Both the 40kDa G protein and the low molecular mass GTP-binding protein are physically associated with the receptor since GTPγS enhances ligand dissociation from the complex and dissociation of the receptor from the GTP-binding proteins. Furthermore, fMLP stimulates both GTPase activity and the rate of GTPγS binding to leukocyte membranes.

These results imply association of the formylpeptide receptor with multiple G proteins and a potential novel role for low molecular mass G proteins in signal transduction or transport of the receptor to the cell surface. The low molecular mass G proteins appear to be involved in a broad array of cell functions including differentiation, growth, cytoskeletal organization and vesicular transport and secretion (Hall, 1990).

Association of the formylpeptide receptor with multiple G proteins (i.e. Giα2 and low molecular weight GTP-binding proteins) may be a mechanism by which the receptor governs multiple functions (e.g. chemotaxis and secretion). This possibility represents a potentially novel and intriguing mechanism of signal transduction.

Alternatively, the low molecular weight GTP-binding protein associated with the receptor could mediate receptor trafficking. Cloning and genetic manipulation of chemoattractant receptors will allow us to explore the structure-function relationships of this interesting association with G proteins and should provide new insight into receptor-mediated signal transduction processes.

The inflammatory process, while generally protective, can lead to severe tissue destruction. Understanding the precise regulation of the locomotive versus cytotoxic potential of leukocytes could lead to more rational designs of anti-inflammatory agents. For example, we have already shown that a hexadecapeptide (mastoporan) can directly activate leukocyte G proteins and biologic activities of neutrophils (Perianin and Snyderman,1989). Precise definition of the sites of receptor-G protein interactions could lead to a more rational design of pharmacological agents which activate or inhibit the inflammatory processes.

REFERENCES:

Boulay F, Tardif M, Brouchon L, Vignais P (1990). Synthesis and use of a novel N-formyl peptide derivative to isolate a human N-formyl peptide receptor cDNA. Bioch.Biophys.Res. Commun. 168:1103-1109.

Braquet PL, Torqui L, Shen TY, Vargaftig BB (1987). Perspectives in platelet-activating factor research. Pharmacol. Rev. 39:97-145.

Clancy RM, Dahinden CA, Hugli TE (1983). Arachidonate metabolism by human polymorphonuclear leukocytes stimulated by N-formyl-Met-Leu-Phe or complement component C5a is independent of phospholpiase activation. Proc. Natl. Acad. Sci. USA 80:7200-7204.

Hall A (1990). The cellular functions of small GTP-binding proteins. Science. 249:635-640.

Jesaitis AJ, Naemura JR, Painter RG, Sklar LA, Cochrane C.(1982). Intracellular localization of N-formyl chemotactic receptor and Mg2+ dependent ATPase in huaman granulocytes. Biophys. Biochem. Acta 719:556-568.

Lapetina EG (1982). Regulation of arachidonic acid production: role of phospholipases C and A2. Trends Pharmacol. Sci. 3:115-118.

Polakis PG, Evans T, Snyderman R (1989). Multiple chromatographic forms of the formylpeptide chemoattractant receptor and their relationship to GTP-binding proteins. Biochem. Biophys. Res. Commun. 161:276-283.

Perianin A, Snyderman R (1989). Mastoporan, a wasp venom

peptide, identifies two discrete mechanisms for elevating cytosolic calcium and inositol trisphosphates in human neutrophils. J. Immunol. 143:1669-1673.

Peveri P, Walz A, Dewald B, Baggiolini (1988). A novel neutrophil-activating factor produced by human mononuclear phagocytes. J. Exp. Med. 167:1547-1559.

Smith CD, Lane BC, Kusaka I, Verghese MW, Snyderman R (1985). Chemoattractant-receptor induced hydrolysis of phosphatidylinositol 4,5-biphosphate in human polymorphonuclear leukocyte membranes: requirement of a guanine nucleotide regulatory protein. J. Biol. Chem. 260:5875-5878.

Smith CD, Cox CC, Snyderman R (1986). Receptor-coupled activation of phosphoinositide-specific phospholipase C by an N protein. Science 232:97-100.

Snyderman R, Uhing RJ (1988). Phagocytic cells: stimulus-response coupling mechanisms. In: Gallin JI, Snyderman R, Goldstein IM (eds.), "Inflammation: Basic Principles and Clinical Correlates," New York: Raven Press Ltd., pp 303-323.

Snyderman R, Perianin A, Evans T, Polakis P, Didsbury, JR (1990). G Proteins and Neutrophil Function. In: Moss J, (ed.), "ADP-Ribosylating Toxins and G Proteins: Insights into Signal Transduction," Washington, D.C.:American Society for Microbiology, pp 295-323.

Truett AP, Verghese M, Dillon SB, Snyderman R (1988). Calcium influx stimulates a second pathway for sustained diacylglycerol production in leukocytes activated by chemoattractants. Proc. Natl.Acad. Sci. USA 85:1549-1553.

Cellular and Cytokine Networks in
Tissue Immunity, pages 143-149

INOSITOL PHOSPHATES IN NEUTROPHIL ACTIVATION

Didier Pittet, Christian Van Delden and Daniel P. Lew

Division of Infectious Diseases
University Hospital of Geneva, 1211 Geneva 4, Switzerland

Neutrophils are highly motile, phagocytic cells, vital for human host defenses. They are capable of sensing and killing microbes through the sequential activation of specific cell surface receptors, leading to a variety of biological responses. Optimal neutrophil function include adherence, chemotaxis, phagocytosis, exocytosis, as well as production of highly reactive oxygen metabolites. Several types of receptors in neutrophils, are coupled to a plasma membrane phospholipase (PLC) via nucleotide (GTP) binding proteins. PLC cleaves PtdIns(4,5)P_2 into inositol trisphosphate, Ins(1,4,5)P_3, and diacylglycerol. The two latter compounds act as intracellular messengers, mobilizing intracellular calcium from intracellular stores and activating protein kinase C, respectively.

We recently reviewed different aspects of the regulation and role of calcium signal in phagocyte activation [1, 2]. In this review, we will focus on recent aspects of phosphoinositide turnover in neutrophil activation.

Complexity of phosphatidylinositol turnover

Two types of plasma membrane-associated kinases phosphorylate phosphatidylinositol (PtdIns) into several isomeric forms of the polyphosphatidylinositol lipids (PtdInsP, PtdInsP_2, PtdInsP_3). PtdIns can be sequentially phosphorylated by specific kinases (type II) leading to the production of PtdIns(4)P and PtdIns(4,5)P_2. Together, these two species make up only 10% of the total inositol lipids pool. The cleavage of the membrane phospholipid PtdIns(4,5)P_2 leads to the generation of Ins(1,4,5)P_3. Ins(1,4,5)P_3 generation is a central event of signaling mechanisms coupling extracellular stimuli to the activation of cells of different species ranging from algae to man. In neutrophils, PtdIns-linked receptor activation is associated with chemoattractant stimulation, adherence, FcRIII-mediated phagocytosis, and has been reported to be involved in different cellular processes such as actin-polymerization, and possibly exocytosis.

The type I kinase, PtdIns-3-kinase, phosphorylates phosphoinositides on position 3 of the inositol ring, generating PtdIns(3)P, PtdIns(3,4)P_2 and PtdIns(3,4,5)P_3. Auger et al. reported that the type I kinase products only appeared after cell stimulation with growth factors-like substances in parallel with the activation of protein-tyrosine kinases [3]. Tyrosine kinase activity associated with retinoic acid stimulation has been identified in HL-60 cells [4]. Interestingly, a transient elevation in both PtdIns(3,4)P_2 and PtdIns(3,4,5)P_3 has been described in chemoattractant stimulated neutrophils [5]. The type I kinase may thus be present also in human neutrophils where its activity appears independent of $[Ca^{2+}]_i$. The real significance of this pathway of PtdIns$P_{(s)}$ generation remains to be further defined.

Ins(1,4,5)P_3 metabolism is regulated by a series of specific phosphomonoesterases and kinases. The two key enzymes in this metabolism are the Ins(1,4,5)P_3 5-phosphatase and the Ins(1,4,5)P_3 3-kinase. The Ins(1,4,5)P_3 3-kinase specifically converts Ins(1,4,5)P_3 into Ins(1,3,4,5)P_4. As described in other cellular systems, we have found in HL-60 cells, that the affinity of the 3-kinase for Ins(1,4,5)P_3 is higher than that of the 5-phosphatase (0.4 μM and 16 μM, respectively; unpublished results). Moreover, whereas the 5-phosphatase is Ca^{2+} independent, the 3-kinase is regulated by Ca^{2+}/calmodulin and its activity increases markedly with increases in $[Ca^{2+}]_i$. In addition, the 5-phosphatase also degrades Ins(1,3,4,5)P_4 into Ins(1,3,4)P_3, the ratio of its two substrates probably determining their relative rate of hydrolysis. Thus, following cell surface receptor occupancy, the activity of the Ins(1,4,5)P_3 3-kinase and 5-phosphatase drives the metabolism into the tris/tetrakisphosphate pathway. In HL-60 cells, several highly phosphorylated $InsP_{(s)}$ result from Ins(1,3,4,5)P_4 metabolism, highlighting the importance of the initial drive through this pathway (see figure).

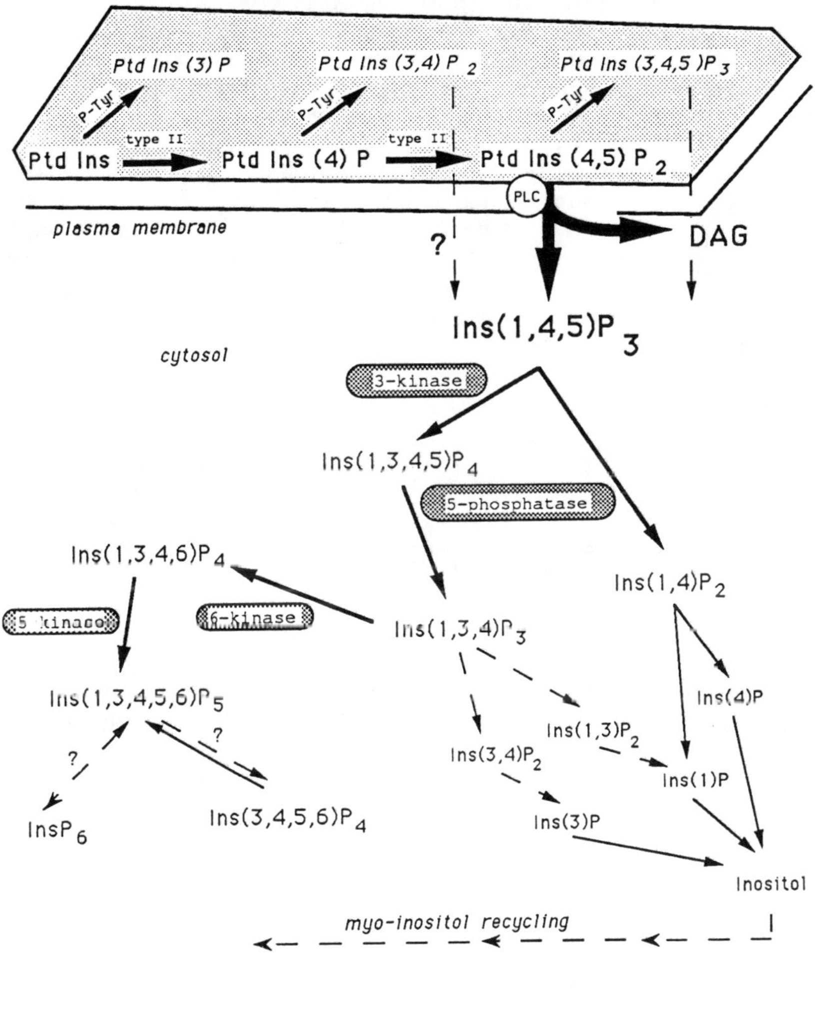

Metabolism of inositol phosphates

Figure 1.

Measuring inositol phosphates

Studies of inositol phosphate metabolism are generally performed using steady state radioactive labeling of the $PtdInsP_{(s)}$ and $InsP_{(s)}$, attempting to approach isotopic equilibrium. Because of the short viability of neutrophils once isolated from blood and the need of labeling periods longer than 24 h, it is difficult to measure $InsP_{(s)}$ production from $[^3H]$*myo*-inositol-labeled neutrophils. Two ways to overcome this problem are to use HL-60 cells or to perform metal dye-detecting (MDD) analysis, which does not require radiotracer labeling. We recently used this technique to quantify the absolute intracellular concentrations of $InsP_{(s)}$ both in HL-60 cells [6] and human neutrophils. This analysis revealed high intracellular levels of $Ins(1,4,5)P_3$ in resting neutrophils, the existence of several not yet described $InsP_{(s)}$, as well as unexpected changes in highly phosphorylated $InsP_{(s)}$ (in preparation).

A role for inositol phosphates, other than $Ins(1,4,5)P_3$

The reasons for the complex metabolic pathway leading to the generation of multiple $InsP_{(s)}$ are still unclear. Experimental evidences suggest a function in the regulation of $[Ca^{2+}]_i$ for certain isomers, such as $Ins(1,3,4,5)P_4$, but the contribution of inositol phosphates other than $Ins(1,4,5)P_3$ remains to be defined. $Ins(1,3,4,5)P_4$ may modulate $[Ca^{2+}]_i$ through several mechanisms: 1) the reuptake of Ca^{2+} into intracellular stores; 2) the control of the Ca^{2+} transfer process between $Ins(1,4,5)P_3$-sensitive and -insensitive pools; 3) the modulation of Ca^{2+} influx through the plasma membrane or 4) the potentiation of $Ins(1,4,5)P_3$-induced Ca^{2+} mobilization. However, this later effect could not be observed in subcellular fractions of HL-60 cells. Different aspects of the metabolism of $Ins(1,3,4,5)P_4$ in HL-60 cells [7] and human neutrophils, suggest its potential role as an intracellular messenger. Detailed analysis of $Ins(1,3,4,5)P_4$ generation reveals 1) rapid kinetics following agonist stimulation, 2) high sensitivity to minute dose of agonists, 3) higher amounts following increased agonist concentrations, and 4) $[Ca^{2+}]_i$-dependent accumulation. We characterized Ca^{2+} influx in parallel to the analysis of InsP accumulation in intact HL-60 cells. Only

$Ins(1,3,4,5)P_4$ generated upon fMLP stimulation correlated temporally with Ca^{2+} influx [7]. In contrast to fMLP, LTB_4 only weakly stimulates Ca^{2+} influx in human neutrophils [8]. LTB_4 also stimulates $PtdIns(4,5)P_2$ hydrolysis. Although the amounts of $Ins(1,4,5)P_3$ produced upon maximal concentrations of LTB_4 and fMLP are similar, the levels of $Ins(1,3,4,5)P_4$ are lower with the former agonist [9]. Although these results do not allow definitive conclusion, they strongly support a role for $Ins(1,3,4,5)P_4$ and $[Ca^{2+}]_i$ in the modulation of agonist-induced Ca^{2+} influx in myeloid cells.

Using MDD analysis, we observed unexpected changes in absolute intracellular concentration of several highly phosphorylated $InsP_{(s)}$, other than $Ins(1,3,4,5)P_4$, upon agonist stimulation in HL-60 cells. Importantly, $Ins(1,3,4,5,6)P_5$ levels were 36 μM in resting cells (100 fold higher than the levels of $Ins(1,4,5)P_3$) and increased to more than 50 μM 1 min after agonist stimulation; in absolute terms, this rise is larger than that of any other InsP. Preliminary results in human neutrophils confirm these observations. Their physiological significance remains to be studied.

Some studies have suggested cellular functions for highly phosphorylated $InsP_{(s)}$. Their potential involvement in the control of short-term (i.e secretion) or long-term (i.e growth) functions is consistent with their kinetics of accumulation: rapid, high and sustained levels, persisting for prolonged period of time. Another possible role for highly phosphorylated $InsP_{(s)}$ could be the interaction between intracellular messenger systems. In HL-60 cells, the levels of the highly phosphorylated $InsP_{(s)}$ change during cell differentiation, suggesting a role in trophic regulation and/or in cell adaptation (R. Michell, personal communication). Clearly, the role of highly phosphorylated $InsP_{(s)}$ in gene regulation deserves further investigation. Finally, it has been suggested that $InsP_5$ and $InsP_6$ are extracellular signals [10]. In human neutrophils, using MDD analysis, we could not show any secretion of $InsP_{(s)}$ by chemoattractant stimulated cells or any accumulation of $InsP_{(s)}$ in a subcellular compartment.

Distinct pools and metabolic pathways

The study of InsP metabolism is complicated by the existence of metabolically distinct pools of precursor phospholipids, as well as by the unexpected variety of inositol phosphate isomers. In neutrophils, both Ins(1,3,4)P_3 and Ins(1,3,4,5)P_4 could potentially originate from a PtdInsP other than PtdIns(4,5)P_2. However, even a single receptor-controlled event, such as PtdIns(4,5)P_2 hydrolysis, can lead to the generation of a large number of potential second messenger compounds, which regulate $[Ca^{2+}]_i$ and possibly other cellular processes. In addition, MDD analysis using radiolabelled HL-60 cells strongly support the existence of different pools of $InsP_{(s)}$ and thus multiple pathways are stimulated during cell activation.

The reasons for such labyrintic pathways are still unclear. The role of Ins(1,4,5)P_3 as a second messenger is unequivocal. The possible modulating function of Ins(1,3,4,5)P_4 on $[Ca^{2+}]_i$ needs further investigations. The formation of Ins(1,3,4,5)P_4, as well as other highly phosphorylated $InsP_{(s)}$, is an energy-consuming process which utilizes ATP. It seems unlikely that cells would employ this energetically-unfavorable metabolic pathway unless it is useful to support cellular function(s). Individual cells may preferentially utilize certain isomers or combination of InsP isomers to regulate particular functions.

We can only predict an exciting future in this research area over the next following years.

Acknowledgements: the work presented in this review has been performed in collaboration with A Monod, E Huggler, J Gil, W Schlegel, KH Krause, GW Mayr, C Wollheim. Supported by a grant of the Swiss National Research Foundation (No 3.829.0.87).

REFERENCES

1. Di Virgilio F, Stendahl O, Pittet D, Lew PD, Pozzan T (1990). Cytoplasmic calcium in phagocyte activation. In: Grinstein S, Rotstein OD (eds), "Mechanisms of Leukocyte Activation" Academic Press, pp 179-205.
2. Lew PD (1989). *Eur J Clin Invest* **19**:338-346.
3. Auger KR, Serunian LA, Soltoff SP, Libby P, Cantley LC (1989). *Cell* **57**:167-75.
4. Chapekar MS, Hartman KD, Knode MC, Glazer RI (1987). *Mol Pharmacol* **31**:140-145.
5. Traynor-Kaplan AE, Thompson B, Harris A, Taylor P, Omann GM, Sklar LA (1989). *J Biol Chem* **264**:15668-78.

6. Pittet D, Schlegel W, Lew PD, Monod A, Mayr GW (1989). *J Biol Chem* **264**:18489-18493.
7. Pittet D, Lew PD, Mayr GW, Monod A, Schlegel W (1989). *J Biol Chem* **264**:7251-7261.
8. Merrit JE, Jacob R, Hallam (1989). *J Biol Chem* **264**:1522-1527.
9. Dillon SB, Murray JJ, Verghese MW, Snyderman R (1987). *J Biol Chem* **262**:11546-11552.
10. Vallejo M, Jackson T, Lightman S, Hanley MR (1987). *Nature* **330**:656-658.

Cellular and Cytokine Networks in
Tissue Immunity, pages 151-156

THE MECHANISM OF PHAGOSOMAL ACIDIFICATION IN PHAGOCYTIC CELLS

Gergely L. Lukacs*¶, Ori D. Rotstein¶ and Sergio Grinstein*

*Division of Cell Biology, Research Institute, Hospital for Sick Children, 555 University Ave., M5G 1X8 and ¶Department of Surgery Toronto General Hospital, 200 Elizabeth St., M5G 2C4 and The Institute of Medical Science, University of Toronto

INTRODUCTION

Despite the well-documented occurrence of phagosomal acidification, the mechanism underlying this process remains unclear (1). Proposed mechanisms of phagosomal acidification include increased lactic acid production during phagocytosis, proton generation during superoxide formation, carbonic anhydrase-coupled proton transport, Na^+/H^+ exchange, proton pumping via a H^+-ATPase and phagosome-lysosome fusion. Available evidence supporting each of these potential mechanisms is mostly indirect (see ref. in 1,2).

In the present study phagosomal pH was measured by monitoring the fluorescence of fluorescein isothiocyanate (FITC)-labelled, opsonized *Staphylococcus aureus* that were ingested by thioglycolate-elicited murine peritoneal macrophages. Using this technique, the putative role of H^+-pumping ATPases in phagosomal acidification was investigated.

RESULTS

Phagosomal acidification. To measure phagosomal acidification, macrophages were allowed to phagocytose FITC-labelled bacteria, washed and stored at 4°C to prevent further acidification and phagosome-lysosome fusion as described in ref. 3. When cells were allowed to carry out phagocytosis for only 2 min, the initial intraphagosomal pH (pH_p) recorded upon rewarming the cells to 37°C was 7.4

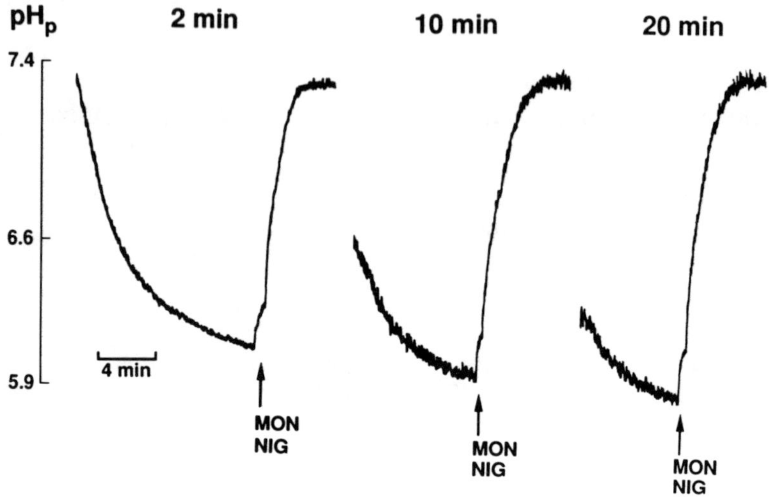

Fig.1.Phagosomal acidification in macrophages. Macrophages were allowed to ingest FITC-labelled *S. aureus* for the period of time indicated on the figure, washed and resuspended in Na^+ medium at 37°C for fluorescence determination. Monensin (MON):4 μM and nigericin (NIG):20 μM were added at the arrow.

(similar to the extracellular pH). In contrast, when cells 10 min or 20 min prior to the measurement the initial initial pH_p recorded was 6.74 ± 0.15 (n=28) and 6.47 ± 0.11 (n=8) , respectively, indicating that phagosomal acidification had already taken place and was (at least partially) preserved during the subsequent washes and incubation in the cold (Fig.1.). Unless otherwise specified, a phagocytosis period of 10 min was chosen for the experiments described hereafter. Upon rewarming to 37°C, pH_p decreased further at an initial rate of 0.20 ± 0.04 pH unit/min (n=20) and reached a steady state at 5.89 ± 0.18 (n=28) in 6-8 min.

ATP-dependence of phagosomal acidification. Based on the well defined role of vacuolar-type H^+-ATPases in the acidification of intracellular organelles (1,4), it was hypothesized that phagosomal acidification was mediated via a H^+-ATPase, likely of the vacuolar type. This was tested by analyzing the ATP-dependence of phagosomal acidification. To attain an efficient and reversible ATP depletion, the plasma membrane of macrophages was permeabilized by electrical discharges. With an optimal electric field (2.3 kV/cm), ca. 80% of the cells lost their ability to exclude trypan blue from the cytoplasm, meanwhile preserving their content of plasma membrane was confirmed examining the loss of the impermeant, fluorescent indicator BCECF from the cytosol (3). In contrast to intact cells, the pH_p of porated cells remained near neutrality (7.01 ± 0.06; n=8) after resuspension at 37 °C, presumably due to depletion of ATP and/or Mg^{2+} through leakage. Reintroduction of ATP and Mg^{2+} initiated a rapid drop in pH_p. Phagosomal acidification was not observed when either ATP or Mg^{2+} alone were added, suggesting that the simultaneous presence of the nucleotide and the divalent cation is required. The rate of Mg-ATP-stimulated acidification in permeabilized cells averaged 0.16 ± 0.04 pH/min (n=8) and the final pH_p attained was 6.16 ± 0.14 (n=8).

The hydrolysis of the high energy gamma-phosphate bond of ATP appeared to be required for H^+ (equivalent) translocation, since the non-hydrolyzable ATP analog AMP-PNP failed to support the acidification (3). Substitution of Mg^{2+} by Ca^{2+} greatly diminished the rate of acidification. These data are consistent with the notion that a H^+-pumping ATPase is involved in acidification of the phagosome. To further define the nature of this ATP-dependent mechanism, the inhibitor sensitivity profile of phagosomal acidification was examined.

<u>Inhibitor sensitivity of phagosomal acidification in intact and electroporated macrophages.</u> There are three types of proton pumping ATPases, which differ in their pharmacological properties (see 1,4 for reviews): phosphorylated or E_1E_2-type ATPases, F_1F_0-ATPases and vacuolar type H^+-ATPases. Similarly vanadate, an inhibitor of phosphorylated ATPases, did not alter the rate of Mg-ATP induced phagosomal acidification at concentrations of 100-200 µM in permeabilized cells.The membrane permeant inhibitors of the F_1F_0 -ATPase, oligomycin and azide, which were tested in intact cells, also did not affect the rate of phagosomal acidification. These results suggest that the phagosomal pump is neither of the E_1E_2 type nor of the mitochondrial type, but is possibly a vacuolar H^+-ATPase. This notion was

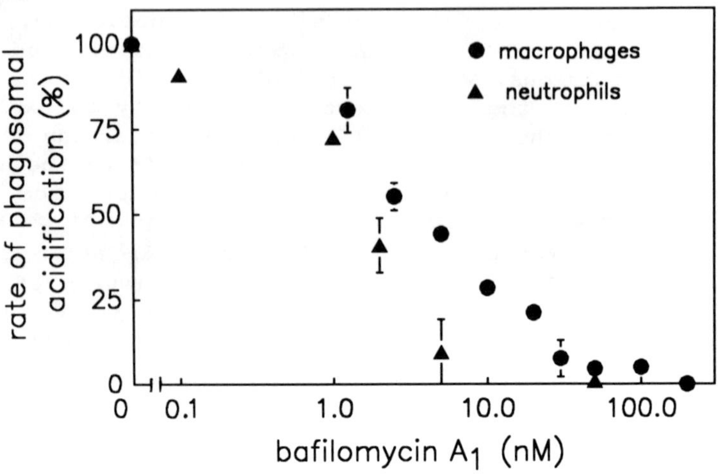

Fig.2. Concentration dependence of bafilomycin A_1 inhibition of phagosomal acidification in murine macrophages and human neutrophils. Data are means ± SE of 3-8 experiments. Where absent, error bars were smaller than the symbol.

further supported by results obtained with several vacuolar-type H^+-ATPase inhibitors. Dicyclohexylcarbodiimide (DCCD) inhibited phagosomal acidification in both intact and electroporated cells with comparable potency (app. $K_i \approx 20$ µM). N-ethylmaleimide (NEM), which has been reported to inhibit vacuolar H^+-ATPases at µM concentrations (1,4), blocked the Mg-ATP induced acidification of permeabilized macrophages with an apparent K_i of 30 µM. The Mg-ATP induced acidification of electroporated cells was also inhibited in the presence of nitrate, a selective inhibitor of the vacuolar-type H^+-ATPase. Half-maximal inhibition was obtained at 25 mM (3).

Bafilomycin A_1 is the most potent and specific inhibitor of the vacuolar-type H^+-ATPases available. In the nM range, this antibiotic blocks the activity of vacuolar, but not of E_1E_2 or F_1F_0-ATPases (5). Dose response curves examining the effect of bafilomycin A_1 on the rate of phagosomal acidification in intact murine macrophages and human neutrophils yielded an apparent K_i of 1-3 nM (Fig.2.), a value that is similar to the K_i reported for inhibition of the vacuolar H^+ pump in isolated chromaffin granules,

Neurospora crassa vacuoles, and Golgi vesicles (5,6). The phagosomal acidification in permeabilized cells was also found to be sensitive to bafilomycin A_1 and the apparent K_i was 5 nM.

DISCUSSION

The present study provides evidence supporting the concept that phagosomal acidification is mediated via a vacuolar-type H^+-ATPase. This conclusion was based on two major approaches. First, the Mg-ATP dependence of the process was demonstrated in electroporated cells. That acidification required ATP hydrolysis was indicated by the failure of AMP-NPN or ATPγS to support acidification. The second line of evidence indicating involvement of proton pumps was mainly pharmacological. In addition, this approach revealed that the phagosomal pumps are of the vacuolar type. Briefly, the acidification was insensitive to oligomycin and azide, ruling out the involvement of mitochondrial type (F_1F_0) H^+-ATPases. Similarly, phagosomal acidification in electroporated cells was insensitive to vanadate, implying that proton transport is not mediated by E_1E_2 type H^+-ATPases. In contrast, a variety of well known inhibitors of the vacuolar-type H^+-ATPase diminished or prevented phagosomal acidification. NEM in permeabilized, and DCCD in both intact and permeabilized cells substantially inhibited phagosomal acidification, at concentrations reported to inhibit other vacuolar pumps (1,4). Moreover, the acidification in permeabilized cells was blocked by nitrate. Perhaps the most convincing evidence was obtained with bafilomycin A_1, a highly selective blocker of vacuolar-type H^+-ATPases (5), which completely inhibited phagosomal acidification at submicromolar concentrations both in intact and permeabilized cells.

The phagosomal pumps might be an intrinsic component of the plasma membrane (7). On the other hand, proton pumps might be incorporated into the phagosomal membrane upon fusion of lysosomes or other intracellular organelles (1,2). However, in our experimental system phagosomal acidification persisted under conditions where increases in cytoplasmic $[Ca^{2+}]_i$ were prevented in BAPTA loaded cells (3), thereby precluding phagosome to lysosome fusion (8). Moreover, little (<5%) phagosome-lysosome fusion was observed in electron micrographs 10 min after initiation of phagocytosis.

Furthermore, bafilomycin A_1-sensitive acidification was noted in our system as early as 2 min after phagocytosis had been initiated. This time period is considered to be too short for the occurrence of phagosome-lysosome fusion. It would therefore appear that acidification is initiated *prior* to lysosomal fusion. This conclusion is in keeping with earlier results demonstrating that phagosomal acidification is detectable before the appearance of lysosomal enzyme activity in the phagosomes (9).

REFERENCES

1. Mellman, I., Fuchs, R., and Helenius, A. (1986). Acidification of the endocytic and exocytic pathways. Ann. Rev. Biochem. 55, 663-700

2. Mollinedo, F., Manara, F. S., and Schneider, D.L. (1986). Acidification activity of human neutrophils. J. Biol. Chem. 261, 1077-1082

3. Lukacs, G.L., Rotstein, O., and Grinstein, S.(1990). Phagosomal acidification is mediated by a vacuolar-type H^+-ATPase in murine macrophages. J. Biol. Chem. in press.

4. Forgac, M. (1989). Structure and function of vacuolar class of ATP-driven proton pumps. Physiol. Rev. 69, 765-796

5. Bowman, E. J., and Siebers, A., and Altendorf, K. (1988). Bafilomycins: A class of inhibitors of membrane ATPases from microorganisms, animal cells, and plant cells. Proc. Natl. Acad. Sci. 85, 7972-7976

6. Moriyama, Y., and Nelson, N. (1989). H^+-translocating ATP-ase in Golgi apparatus. J. Biol. Chem. 264, 18445-18450

7. Swallow, C. J., Grinstein, S., and Rotstein, O. D. (1990). A vacuolar type H^+-ATPase regulates cytoplasmic pH in macrophages. J. Biol. Chem. 265, 7645-7654

8. Jaconi, M. E. E., Lew, D.E., Carpentier, J.-L., Magnusson, K. E., Sjogren, M., and Stendhal, O. (1990). Cytosolic free calcium elevation mediate the phago-lysosome fusion during phagocytosis in human neutrophils. J. Cell Biol. 110, 1555-1564

9. McNeil, P. L., Tanasugarn, L., Meigs, J. B., and Taylor, D. L. (1983). Acidification of phagosomae is initiated before lysosomal enzyme activity is detected. J. Cell Biol. 97, 692-702

Cellular and Cytokine Networks in Tissue Immunity, pages 157-162

Lipid Second Messengers: Protein Kinase C Dependent and Independent Pathways

Robert M. Bell, Toshiro Okazaki and Yusuf A. Hannun
Departments of Biochemistry (R.M.B., T.O.) and Medicine (Y.A.H.), Duke University Medical Center, Durham, North Carolina 27710

Increasingly, the breakdown products of the cellular lipids are being implicated as second messengers or as lipid mediators within a complex network of signal transduction pathways. The function of membrane lipids was once thought to be limited to forming the permeability barrier of the cell and internal vesicular and organellar systems. The diversity of these lipids, however, suggested additional cellular functions.

The glycerolipids serve as reservoirs for bioactive molecules that are produced when cells are acted upon by growth factors, hormones or neurotransmitters (Figure 1) (Exton, 1990; Bishop and Bell, 1988). Platelet activating factor (PAF) and arachidonic acid and its metabolites have been recognized for some time to be critically involved in cell regulation. The role of phosphoinositide breakdown products in cell regulation has recently come into sharp focus through a series of discoveries: IP_3 functions to mobilize intracellular calcium (itself a second messenger); sn-1,2-diacylglycerol (DAG) is a second messenger that binds to and activates members of the protein kinase C family (Nishizuka, 1984); and finally, phosphatidic acid produced by action of phospholipase D or by DAG kinase is emerging as a bioregulator (Exton, 1990; Moolenaar, 1986; Murayama and Ui, 1987). One of its potential sites of action is on GAP (GTPase Activity Protein), a protein which modulates ras (Tsai et al., 1989).

Recent discoveries suggest that the cellular sphingolipids also serve as reservoirs from which bioactive

Fig.1 Glycerolipids: Reservoirs for Bioactive Lipids (●)

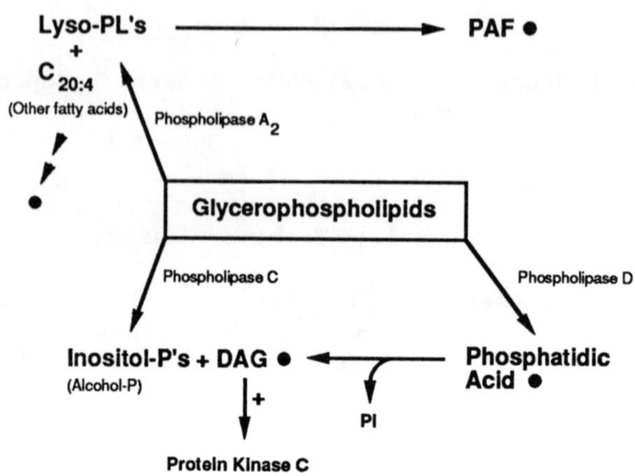

lipid second messengers or lipid mediators are produced (Hannun and Bell, 1989). A series of pathways analogous to those known to function on the cellular glycerolipids are emerging (Figure 2). At least three groups of bioactive molecules are known: sphingosine, lysosphingolipids and ceramide (Hannun and Bell, 1987; Hannun and Bell, 1989; Okazaki et al., 1989). A sphingomyelin cycle functioning in human promyelocytic cells may turn out to be the first of a number of cycles functioning to transiently produce sphingolipid derived second messengers and lipid mediators (Okazaki et al., 1989). These discoveries and hypothesis emerged from the observation that sphingosine, the basic building block of the cellular sphingolipids, inhibited protein kinase C (Hannun et al., 1986).

Fig.2 Sphingolipids: Potential Reservoirs for Bioactive Lipid Breakdown Products (●)

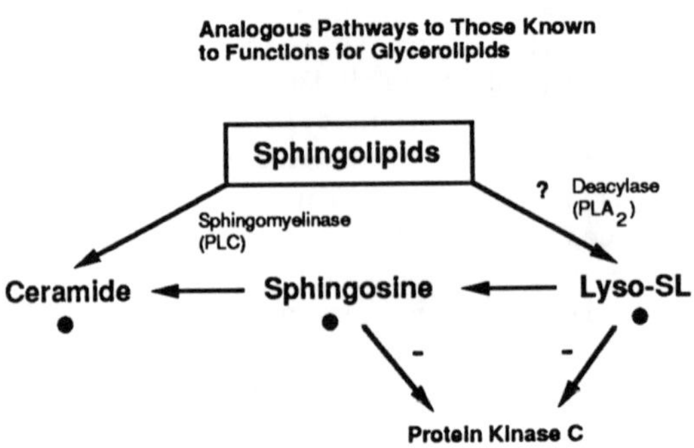

Protein kinase C denotes a family of closely related ser/thr protein kinases that are regulated by DAG, phospholipid and calcium. The isozymes of protein kinase C are differentially expressed in cells and tissues. Each of them binds and is activated by phorbol esters, potent tumor promoters. Protein kinase C isoforms appear to possess distinct functional domains that can be separated from one another. The catalytic domains resemble those of other ser/thr protein kinases. The regulatory domains possess the high affinity phorbol ester binding sites; since phorbol ester binding is dependent on calcium and phospholipid, these domains also possess these high specificity sites. Finally, each isozyme contains a pseudosubstrate site near its amino terminus. The biochemical properties of these kinases are somewhat different (Burns et al., 1990; Schaap and Parker, 1990); later members of the family appear to be calcium independent (Ono et al., 1988; Ono et al., 1989). Notably, recent studies suggest that each regulatory domain may possess two phorbol binding sites (Burns & Bell, unpublished).

Sphingosine was found to inhibit protein kinase C <u>in vitro</u>; it is a competitive inhibitor with respect to DAG and it inhibits phorbol ester binding <u>in vitro</u> and in cells including platelets, neutrophils and HL60 cells. In platelets, sphingosine inhibits phosphorylation of the 40 kDa protein, aggregation and secretion (Hannun et al., 1986). The inhibitory actions of sphingosine are overridden with cell permeable DAGs or phorbol esters. Sphingosine does not inhibit PI turnover, DAG production, or calcium transients. A similar set of observations were made in human neutrophils where sphingosine inhibits the oxidative burst in response to phorbol esters, F-Met-Leu-Phe, opsonized zymosan, or arachidonic acid (Wilson et al., 1986; Lambeth et al., 1988). Further, sphingosine inhibits the production of PAF, arachidonic acid and LTB_4 (McIntyre et al., 1987) without interfering with DAG generation, normal calcium transients or other events. Addition of cell permeable DAGs or phorbol esters overcomes the inhibitory actions of sphingosine. In the hairless mouse, sphingosine blocks phorbol ester induced inflammatory response (Gupta et al., 1988); it blocks the invasion of monocytes and neutrophils into phorbol ester treated epidermis.

These and other findings led to the hypothesis that sphingolipid breakdown products may function physiologically in cell regulation or in pathobiology. The involvement of lysosphingolipids in the pathogenesis of the sphingolipidosis was hypothesized (Hannun and Bell, 1987). Finally, the existence of sphingolipid cycles was proposed.

A sphingomyelin cycle was discovered in HL60 cells treated with physiological levels of vitamin D_3 (Okazaki et al., 1989). Such treatment led to the breakdown of 25% of the cellular sphingomyelin in 1.5 to 2 hr. By 4-6 hrs., sphingomyelin levels normalized. The products of the breakdown were ceramide and phosphocholine indicating the involvement of a sphingomyelinase of the C type fully analogous to the phospholipase Cs known to breakdown glycerolipids (Compare Figs 1&2). Increased sphingomyelinase activity preceded sphingomyelin turnover in HL60 cells (Okazaki et al., 1989). Importantly, the addition of exogenous sphingomyelinase to HL60 cells at subthreshold levels of vitamin D_3 caused differentiation, thus demonstrating that vitamin D_3 dependent sphingomyelin degradation was not an epiphenomenon. Cell permeable ceramides have been developed which can replace vitamin D_3 (Okazaki et al., 1990). The mechanism by which these agents affect cell differentiation is not known. Ceramides do not affect protein kinase C, and the cell permeable ceramides are not metabolized to sphingosine. Clearly, protein kinase C is not the target.

These studies provide a new conceptual and experimental field of research. Many studies are now possible because cell permeable sphingolipid metabolites are available and appropriate analytical methods have been developed. The sites of action and the mechanisms for signal generation and attenuation need to be described. Such studies will likely lead to new fundamental insight into cellular regulation and the roles of lipid breakdown products in those processes.

REFERENCES

Bishop B, Bell R (1988). Functions of diacylglycerol in glycerolipid metabolism, signal transduction and cellular transformation. Oncogene Res. 2:205-218.

Burns D, Bloomenthal J, Lee M-H, Bell R (1990). Expression of the α, ßII, and γ protein kinase C isozymes in the baculovirus-insect cell expression system. J. Biol. Chem. 265: 12044-12051.

Exton J (1990). Signaling through phosphatidylcholine. J. Biol. Chem. 265:1-4.

Gupta A, Fisher G, Elder J, Nickolff B, Voorhees J (1988). Sphingosine inhibits phorbol ester-induced inflammation, ormithine decarboxylase activity, and activation of protein kinase C in mouse skin. J. Invest. Dermatol. 91:486-491.

Hannun Y, Bell R (1987). Lysosphingolipids inhibit protein kinase C: Implications for sphingolipidoses. Science 235:670-674.

Hannun Y, Bell R (1989). Functions of sphingolipids and sphingolipid breakdown products in cellular regulation. Science 243: 500-507.

Hannun Y, Loomis C, Merrill, Jr. A, Bell R (1986). Sphingosine inhibition of protein kinase C activity and of phorbol dibutyrate binding in vitro and in human platelets. J. Biol. Chem. 261:12604-12609.

Lambeth J, Burnham D, Tyagi S (1988). Sphinganine effects on chemoattract anti-induced diacylglycerol generation, calcium fluxes, superoxide production, and on cell viability in the human neutrophil. J. Biol. Chem. 263:3818-3822.

McIntyre T, Reinhold S, Prescott S, Zimmerman G (1987). Protein kinase C activity appears to be required for the synthesis of platelet-activating fact of and leukotriene B_4 by human neutrophils. J. Biol. Chem. 262:15370-15376.

Moolenaar W, Kruijer W, Tilly B, Verlaan I, Bierman A, de Laat S (1986). Growth factor-like action of phosphatidic acid. Nature 323:171-173.

Murayama T, and Ui M (1987). Phosphatidic may stimulate membrane receptors mediating adenylate cyclase inhibition and phospholipid breakdown in 3T3 fibroblasts. J.Biol.Chem. 262:5522-5529.

Nishizuka Y (1984). Turnover of inositol phospholipids and signal transduction. Science 225: 1365-1370.

Okazaki T, Bell R, Hannun Y (1989). Sphingomyelin turnover induced by vitamin D_3 in HL-60 cells. J. Biol. Chem. 264:19076-19080.

Okazaki T, Bizlawaska A, Bell R, Hannun Y (1990). Role of ceramide as a lipid mediator of 1α, 25-dihydroxyvitamin D_3-induced HL-60 cell differentiation. J. Biol. Chem. (in press).

Ono Y, Fujii T, Ogita K, Kikkawa U, Igarashi K, Nishizuka Y (1988). The structure expression and properties of additional members of the protein kinase C family. J. Biol. Chem. 263: 6927-6932.

Ono Y, Fujii T, Ogita K. Kikkawa U, Igarashi K, Nishizuka Y (1989). Protein kinase C subspecies from rat brain: Its structure, expression, and properties. Proc. Natl. Acad. Sci, USA 86:3099-3103.

Schaap D, Parker P (1990). Expression, purification and characterization of protein kinase C-ϵ. J. Biol. Chem. 265:7301-7307.

Tsai M-H, Yu C-L, Wei F-S, Stacey D (1989). The effect of GTPase activating protein upon Ras is inhibited by mitogenically responsive lipids. Science 243:522-526.

Wilson E, Olcott M, Bell R, Merrill,Jr. A, Lambeth J, (1986). Inhibition of the oxidative burst in human neutrophils by sphingoid long-chain bases. J. Biol. Chem. 261:12616-12623.

Cellular and Cytokine Networks in Tissue Immunity, pages 163-168

Mechanisms of macrophage pH regulation and their functional significance in the inflammatory microenvironment.

Ori D. Rotstein, Carol J. Swallow, Sergio Grinstein, Gergely Lukacs.

Department of Cell Biology, Hospital for Sick Children Research Institute (S.G., G.L.) and Department of Surgery, University of Toronto (C.J.S., G.L. and O.D.R) Toronto, Ontario, Canada.

INTRODUCTION

Cells of the monocyte/macrophage system play an important role in the coordination of the host response against infection. Within the inflammatory microenvironment, maintenance of cytoplasmic pH (pH_i) within the physiological range, by these cells, is threatened by the production of metabolic acid following cell activation, as well as by diffusion of protons from the acidic extracellular milieu. If left unopposed by pH_i regulatory mechanisms, these stresses will result in cytoplasmic acidification, suboptimal enzyme activity and thus, cell dysfunction. The purpose of this discussion is to review recent studies investigating the mechanisms of pH_i regulation in macrophages and the role of these mechanisms in maintaining optimal antimicrobial function.

MECHANISMS of pH_i REGULATION IN MONOCYTES AND MACROPHAGES

Monocytes and macrophages regulate their pH_i through three predominant ion transport systems (Swallow et al, (1990a). These are: 1) the Na^+/H^+ antiport;
2) the Na^+-dependent $HC)_3^-/Cl^-$ exchanger; and
3) a vacuolar-type H^+ ATPase.

<u>The Na^+/ H^+ Antiport:</u>
The Na^+/H^+ antiport exchanges extracellular Na^+ for intracellular H^+, thus counteracting the tendency of cells to become acidic. The properties of the Na^+/H^+ antiport

are similar to those described for most mammalian cells. The stoichiometry of the exchange reaction is one Na^+ for one H^+, so that the process is electroneutral and insensitive to changes in membrane potential. Under physiological conditions, the markedly inward gradient for Na^+ drives the net extrusion of protons. The rate of proton extrusion is increased by cytoplasmic acidification, yet inhibited by external acid. These effects of extracellular protons make the Na^+/H^+ antiport relatively ineffective in regulating pH_i when the cells are suspended in acidic media.

The Na^+ -Dependent HCO_3^-/Cl^- Exchanger:
While macrophages derived from a variety of sites and species have been tested for Na^+/H^+ exchange activity, only the monocyte-like cells of the U937 line have been examined for Na^+ -dependent HCO_3^-/Cl^- exchange (Ladoux et al, 1987). This plasma membrane transporter mediates the uptake of extracellular Na^+ and HCO_3^- in exchange for cytoplasmic Cl^- and possibly H^+. Two acid equivalents are extruded by the cell per cycle. As with the Na^+/H^+ antiport, Na^+ -dependent HCO_3^-/Cl^- exchange is driven by the inward Na^+ gradient. Thus, Na^+-dependent HCO_3^-/Cl^- exchange can also counteract cytosolic acidification.

The Vacuolar-type H^+-ATPASE:
Recent work in our laboratory has revealed the existence of an additional, novel pH_i regulatory pathway in phagocytic cells. We initially observed that, unlike most other cell types reported, macrophages can recover to their physiological pH_i following an acid pulse even in the nominal absence of Na^+ and HCO_3^-. Under these conditions, Na^+/H^+ exchange and the HCO_3^--dependent systems are inoperative and cannot account for the observed recovery. Accordingly, the pH_i recovery from acidification was unaffected by amiloride and its analogs or by disulfonic stilbenes (Swallow et al, 1988). The intracellular alkalinization was accompanied by an increased rate of extracellular acidification, indicating translocation of acid equivalents across the plasma membrane. Thus, the data suggested the presence of a Na^+- and HCO_3^--independent proton extrusion process.

Further analysis indicated that this proton transport process was inhibited by N-ethylmaleimide and by N,N'-dicyclohexylcarbodiimide. These agents are effective blockers of proton-transporting ATPases in mitochondria and other intracellular membranes (Forgac, 1989), raising the possibility that a proton-pumping ATPase also existed in the membrane of phagocytes. Consistent with this notion, ATP depletion of the cells prior to acid loading precluded the Na^+ and HCO_3^--independent pH_i recovery. Various classes of proton pumps have been described in other cells types which are readily distinguishable on the basis of their pharmacological properties. Mitochondrial or F_1F_0 type proton pumps are exquisitely sensitive to oligomycin and to azide, while these drugs do not affect other types of pumps. A second type of pump (E_1E_2 type), such as the gastric H^+/K^+ ATPase, forms a stable phosphorylated intermediate and is inhibited by vanadate. Finally, a third type of pump present in lysosomes, secretory granules, Golgi vesicles and vacuoles (hence called "vacuolar type" H^+-ATPases) is resistant to both oligomycin and vanadate, yet is inhibited by 7-chloro-4- nitrobenz-2-oxa-1,3-diazole, by nitrate and by p-chloro- mercuribenzenesulfonate. The mechanism mediating proton extrusion from macrophages was found to be sensitive to the latter group of inhibitors, while it was resistant to both vanadate and oligomycin. These findings enabled us to tentatively assign the macrophage pump to the vacuolar class of proton ATPases.

A more conclusive identification of the type of ATPase involved in pH_i regulation in macrophages was accomplished using bafilomycin A_1. This macrolide antibiotic was recently reported to be an effective means of differentiating the three major types of proton pumps (Bowman et al, 1988). Vacuolar H^+-ATPases are exquisitely sensitive to bafilomycin, whereas E_1E_2 and F_1F_0 ATPases are only moderately sensitive or completely insensitive, respectively. We found bafilomycin to be a very potent (apparent K_i = 3 nM) blocker of the Na^+ and HCO_3^--independent pH_i recovery of acid-loaded macrophages, confirming that this process is mediated by a vacuolar-type of proton ATPase. The pH_i recovery of macrophages was accompanied by a hyperpolarization of the membrane potential, as would be expected for an outwardly oriented electrogenic proton pump of the vacuolar type. Recent studies have reported a similar type of pump activity in alveolar macrophages (Bidani et al, 1989).

ACTIVATION OF THE PLASMALEMMAL VACUOLAR H^+ ATPASE IN MACROPHAGES.

In urinary epithelial cells, plasmalemmal vacuolar H^+ ATPase are asymmetrically localized to the luminal border of the cell and serve to extrude H^+ into the urine. These pumps are not present constitutively in the plasma membrane but rather reside in vesicles immediately beneath the brush border membrane. In response to cellular acidification, these vesicles are exocytically translocated into the plasma membrane. This process has been shown to be mediated via a rise in cytoplasmic calcium in response to intracellular acidification and to require the presence of an intact microtubular system (Schwartz and Al-Awqati, 1988). As in urinary epithelial cells, cytoplasmic acidification caused a marked increase in cytoplasmic calcium in peritoneal macrophages. However, cells preloaded with the cytoplasmic calcium chelator BAPTA and suspended in calcium-free medium to obviate the calcium rise in response to cytoplasmic acid-loading, demonstrated equivalent proton pump activity, thus showing that a calcium rise was not required for activation of the pump. Furthermore pH recovery proceeded normally in the presence of 0.1 mM colchicine, indicating that microtubular assembly was not critical to the activity of the proton pump (Swallow et al, 1990b). The data thus support the concept that a vacuolar type H^+ ATPase is constitutively present in the plasma membrane of macrophages and is activated in response to cytoplasmic acidification. Confirmation of this localization requires further study using antibodies directed against the pump.

FUNCTIONAL SIGNIFICANCE OF PLASMALEMMAL H^+ ATPASES IN MACROPHAGES

Maintenance of pH_i in an acidic microenvironment:

The pH of the inflammatory microenvironment has been reported to fall as low as 5.7 (Bryant et al, 1980). As noted above, function of the H^+-ATPase may be vitally important in the maintenance of near-physiological pH_i insofar as the Na^+/H^+ antiport and HCO_3^-/Cl^-- exchange are rendered ineffective under these conditions. We examined pH_i regulation in cells suspended in media of normal and acidic pH (Swallow et al, 1990c). At an extracellular pH of 7.35, the plasmalemmal proton pump contributed little to pH_i homeostasis. By contrast, when the medium pH was lowered to 6.7, inhibition of the proton pump with bafilomycin A_1 caused pH_i to fall significantly from 6.8 to 6.6. This reduction translated into a functional impairment of the cell as evidenced by the reduced superoxide generation in response to phorbol esters.

<u>The proton pump as a mediator of extracellular acidification:</u>

In addition to its role in regulating pH_i, the plasmalemmal H+ ATPase may serve to acidify the extracellular milieu. Such acidification may have functional consequences including direct microbicidal activity, activation of extracellular hydrolytic enzymes and enhancement of cytokine function. While the pH directly beneath adherent macrophages has been reported to be as low as 3.6, the mechanism underlying the acidification has not been defined (Silver et al, 1988). However, osteoclasts which are derived from cells of the monocyte/macrophage lineage are known to resorb bone in part by proton extrusion into the cleft between the cell and the bone substratum. In these cells, acidification appears to be mediated by a vacuolar-type H^+ ATPase asymmetrically localized on the cell surface (Blair et al, 1989).

<u>Vacuolar-type H^+ ATPases mediate phagosomal acidification:</u>

Acidification of the newly-formed phagosome following ingestion of a microorganism is an important microbicidal mechanism. Specifically, acidification is required for phagosome-lysosome fusion and subsequent activation of the acid hydrolases released into the phagosomal compartment. The mechanism of phagosomal acidificaiton was studied by monitoring changes in fluorescence of fluorescein isothiocyanate-labelled <u>Staphylococcus aureus</u> following their ingestion by macrophages (Lukacs et al, 1990). The pH of the phagosome spontaneously decreased to 5.8. In both intact and electroporated cells, this reduction was inhibited by ATP depletion and inhibitors of vacuolar-type H^+ ATPases, but not by inhibitors of F_0F_1-type or E_1-E_2 -type H^+ ATPases. When phagosome-lysosome fusion was prevented by cytoplasmic calcium depletion, acidification occurred normally indicating that the vacuolar H^+ ATPases were not derived from fusion with lysosomes. These findings are compatible with the concept that phagosomal acidification is mediated by a vacuolar-type H^+-ATPase. The origin of the pump is not clear but its constitutive presence in the plasma membrane of macrophages suggests an attractive hypothesis.

REFERENCES:

Bidani A, Brown SE, Heming TA, Guriel R, Dubose TO Jr (1989). Cytoplasmic pH in pulmonary macrophages: recovery from acid load is Na^+-independent and NEM sensitive. Amer J Physiol 257:C65-76.

Blair HC, Teitelbaum SL, Ghiselli R, Gluck S (1989). Osteoclastic bone resorption by a polarized vacuolar proton pump. Science 245: 855-857.

Bryant RE, Rashad AL, Mazza JA, Hammond D (1980). B-lactamase activity in human pus. J Infect Dis 142: 594- 601.

Forgac M (1989). Structure and function of vacuolar class of ATP-driven proton pumps. Physiol Rev 69:765-796.

Horwitz MA, Maxfield FR (1984). Legionella pneumophila inhibits acidification of its phagosome in human monocytes. J Cell Biol 99: 1936-43.

Ladoux A, Krawice I, Cragoe EJ Jr, Abita JP, Frelin C (1987). Properties of the Na^+-dependent $Cl^-/HC)_3^-$ exchange system in U937 human leukemic cells. Eur J Biochem 170:43-49.

Lukacs G, Rotstein OD, Grinstein S (1990). Phagosomal acidification is mediated by a vacuolar-type H^+-ATPase in murine macrophages. J Biol Chem, in press.

Schwartz CJ and Al-Awqati Q (1986). Regulation of transepithelial H^+ transport by exocytosis and endocytosis. Ann Rev Physiol 48: 153-161.

Silver IA, Murrills RJ, Etherington DJ (1988). Microelectrode studies on the acid microenvironment beneath adherent macrophages and osteoclasts. Exp Cell Res 175: 266-276.

Swallow CJ, Grinstein S, Rotstein OD (1988). Cytoplasmic pH regulation by an ATP dependent and N,N'-dicyclohexylcarbodiimide-sensitive mechanism. J Biol Chem 263: 19558-19563.

Swallow CJ, Grinstein S, Rotstein OD (1990a). Regulation and functional significance of cytoplasmic pH in phagocytic leukocytes. In: Grinstein S, Rotstein OD (eds), "Mechanisms of Leukocyte Activation", Academic Press pp 227-249.

Swallow CJ, Grinstein S, Rotstein OD (1990b). A vacuolar type H^+ ATPase regulates cytoplasmic pH in macrophages. J Biol Chem 265: 7645-7654.

Swallow CJ, Grinstein S, Sudsbury RA, Rotstein OD (1990c). Modulation of the macrophage respiratory burst by an acidic environment: the critical role of cytoplasmic pH regulation by proton extrusion pumps. Surgery 108:363-368.

Cellular and Cytokine Networks in
Tissue Immunity, pages 169-175

THE ROLE OF GTP-BINDING PROTEINS IN THE CONTROL OF MAST CELL EXOCYTOSIS

Meir Aridor and Ronit Sagi-Eisenberg

Department of Chemical Immunology
The Weizmann Institute of Science
Rehovot 76100, Israel

SUMMARY

Basic secretagogues of mast cells induce histamine secretion from ATP-permeabilized and resealed cells in a process that is dependent on the internal application of GTP; independent of phosphoinositide breakdown and inhibited by pertussis toxin (PtX) treatment. In addition, basic secretagogues of mast cells stimulate the GTPase activity G-proteins in a cell-free system and significantly reduce PtX-catalyzed ADP-ribosylation of G-proteins. Based on these findings, we conclude that basic secretagogues activate exocytosis in a receptor-independent manner by directly activating G-proteins that play a role in stimulus-secretion coupling. Basic secretagogues are capable of inducing secretion in a mechanism that bypasses phosphoinositide breakdown by directly activating a G-protein that is located downstream from phospholipase C, namely the putative G_E protein. G_E is a PtX-substrate and therefore most probably belongs to the heterotrimeric G-proteins of the Gi class.

INTRODUCTION

Mast cells play a central role in immediate hypersensitivity reactions. Physiologically, the secretory response of mast cells can be induced by aggregation of their cell surface specific receptors for immunoglobulin E (IgE) by the corresponding antigen (1). In addition, mast cell degranulation can also be elicited by a number of positively charged substances, collectively known as the basic secretagogues of mast cells (2). These include the synthetic compound 48/80, polymers of basic amino acids and biologically active peptides such as substance P.

The mechanisms by which mast cell secretagogues bring about secretion are not understood. A number of cellular events take place after stimulation of mast cells (3-8), nevertheless their mode of activation and contribution to secretion have not yet been resolved. We (9) and others (10) have previously shown that exocytosis can be induced by the combined presence of Ca^{2+} ionophores and phorbol esters, suggesting that Ca^{2+} rise and protein kinase C (PKC) activation interact synergistically to elicit exocytosis. This finding implicates phosphoinositide (PIP_2) hydrolysis as playing a major role in stimulus-secretion coupling. However, while both IgE-mediated and basic secretagogues induced exocytosis are accompanied by PIP_2 breakdown, there are a number of important differences in their mode of action implying that signals additional to those resulting from PIP_2 breakdown, must be involved in activation of exocytosis.

The exocytotic processes initiated by IgE or by basic secretagogues differ in their sensitivities to PtX (11). This observation implies that GTP-binding proteins (G-proteins) may, at least in part, mediate the additional signals leading to exocytosis. In fact, the involvement of at least two different G-proteins, one coupled to phospholipase C (PLC) activation (G_P) and the other directly regulating exocytosis (G_E) has been suggested (12). We have therefore undertaken studies aimed at evaluating the relative contributions of the putative G-proteins G_p and G_E to the overall process of exocytosis.

RESULTS AND DISCUSSION

To determine whether the PIP_2-PLC could be activated by a G-protein in intact mast cells, we have employed ATP to reversibly permeabilize the cells and introduce non-hydrolyzable analogues of GTP into them (13). Introduction of GTP-γ-S (100 μM) into the cytosol of mast cells stimulated both histamine secretion and diacylglycerol (DAG) formation measured by generation of its phosphorylation product phosphatidic acid (PA) (Fig. 1). GTP-γ-S-induced PA formation was inhibited when neomycin, an aminoglycoside antibiotic known to bind to and inhibit phosphoinositide breakdown, was introduced into the cells during their permeabilization (13). This observation indicated that the source of the PA formed in response to entrapment of GTP-γ-S was PIP_2 metabolism. The stimulatory effect of

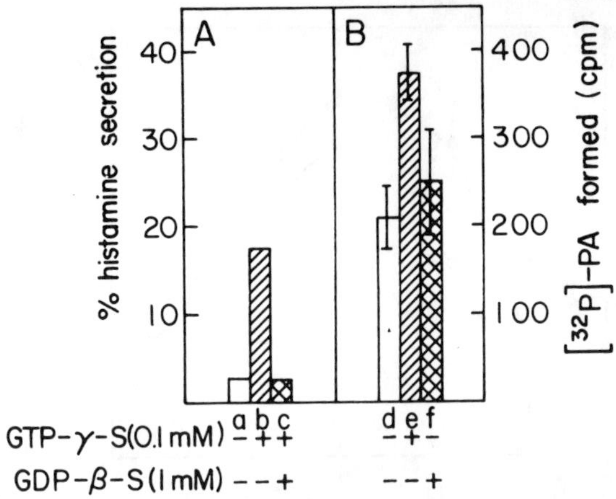

Figure 1. Effects of GTP-γ-S on histamine secretion and PA formation. Purified {^{32}P}-labeled mast cells were permeabilized in the absence (a,d) or presence of GTP-γ-S (0.1 mM) (b,e) or GTP-γ-S (0.1 mM) + GDP-β-S (1 mM) (c,f). After resealing, the cells were further incubated for 20 min at 30°C and histamine and {^{32}P}-labeled PA determined.

GTP-γ-S on both secretion and PA production could be inhibited by the simultaneous introduction of excess of GDP-β-S (1 mM) into the cells (Fig. 1). These results indicate that activation of a G-protein within intact cells leads to the concomitant activation of a PLC.

The effect of GTP-γ-S was biphasic and at high concentrations (> 100μM) it self inhibited PA formation (Fig. 2). This dual regulation of PLC activity by GTP-γ-S suggests that in analogy with the adenylate cyclase system, two G-proteins, a stimulatory and inhibitory G-protein, are involved in regulating PLC activity. Indeed, in other cellular systems, the existence of a PLC-inhibiting G-protein has been indicated (14,15).

The close correlation between GTP-γ-S-induced PA formation and histamine secretion implies that the continuous activation of a PIP_2-hydrolyzing PLC by a stimulatory G-protein suffices to trigger histamine secretion. Moreover, it may imply that G_E activation requires the generation of the second messengers DAG and IP_3 to raise internal Ca^{2+} concentrations and activate PKC. However, neither a rise in Ca^{2+} by means of Ca^{2+} ionophores nor activation of PKC by TPA were able to restore exocytosis in 1 mM GTP-γ-S-loaded cells. In contrast, treating the cells with a subdose of the basic secretagogue 48/80, that by itself

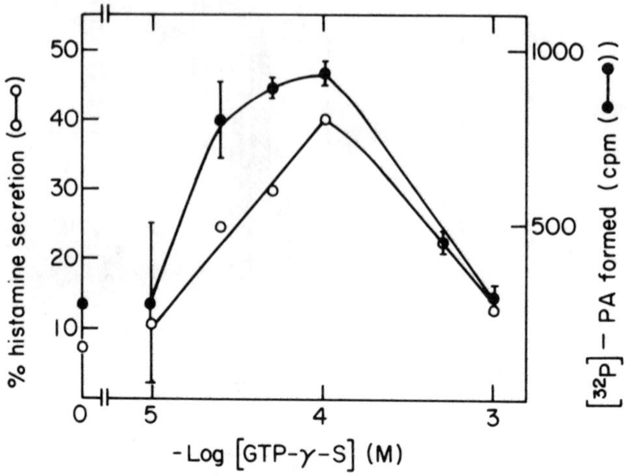

Figure 2. GTP-γ-S-induced histamine secretion and PA formation. Purified mast cells were {^{32}P}-labeled, permeabilized in the presence of the indicated GTP-γ-S concentrations and treated as described under Fig. 1.

failed to induce secretion, markedly potentiated histamine secretion. Moreover, secretion under these conditions was not accompanied by PA formation and was resistant to depletion of Ca^{2+} from internal stores (13). At higher concentrations, 48/80 could also reactivate PLC leading to PA formation (13). These findings demonstrate that activation of a G-protein, other than the PLC activating G-protein, is sufficient for inducing release. Moreover, this putative G-protein, which was previously designated G_E (12), can be activated directly by an external ligand, i.e. by compound 48/80. To validate this model, we extended our studies to examine whether neomycin, that is a positively charged molecule, may activate secretion from mast cells in a mechanism that is independent of phosphoinositide breakdown. Indeed, we could show (16) that when loaded alongside GTP-γ-S, into ATP-permeabilized cells, neomycin, at concentrations higher than 1 mM induces histamine secretion in a process that is dependent on the internal application of GTP but is independent of phosphoinositide breakdown (Fig. 3). Neomycin was also found to induce histamine secretion from intact mast cells by a mechanism that is similar to that utilized by other basic secretagogues of mast cells. The strict dependency of induced exocytosis on GTP together with the high sensitivity to PtX (11) suggest that activation of mast cells by basic reagents is highly

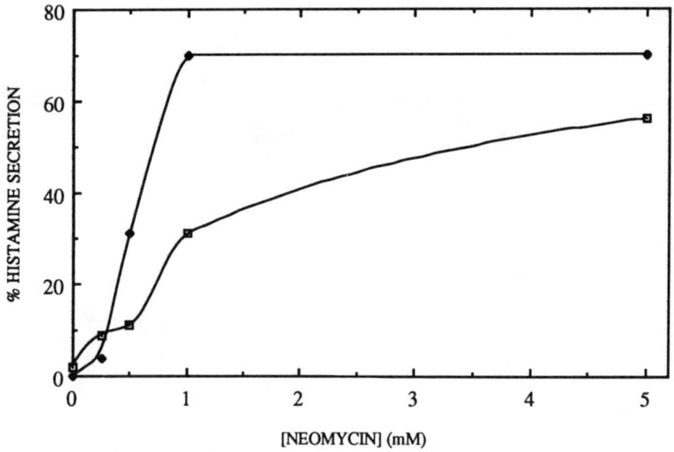

Figure 3. Effect of GTP on neomycin-induced histamine secretion from permeabilized mast cells. Purified mast cells were permeabilized in the presence of the indicated concentrations of neomycin and the presence (◆-◆) or absence (◘-◘) of GTP (1 mM). Cells were subsequently resealed and histamine secretion determined.

---

dependent on G-protein activation. It was reported that mastoparan, another basic secretagogue of mast cells, directly activates purified G-proteins (17). Since receptors for polybasic compounds on mast cells have not been identified (18,19), we examined whether compound 48/80 and neomycin, like mastoparan, may be capable of directly activating G-proteins. For this purpose, we measured the GTPase activity of brain membranes that are enriched in G_i/G_o proteins. Both 48/80 and mastoparan stimulated 2-fold the GTPase activity of cholate-solubilized membranes (13). This effect of 48/80 was dose-dependent, with the half-maximal effect obtained at 2.5 μg/ml and maximal effect at 10 μg/ml (Fig. 4). Similarly, neomycin stimulated 4-fold the GTPase activity of cholate-solubilized rat brain membranes in a PtX-inhibitable manner (16). In addition, neomycin, compound 48/80 and mastoparan significantly reduced (by approximately 80%) the ADP-ribosylation of PtX-substrates present in rat brain membranes (16).

Low Mr GTP-binding proteins of the ras family have been implicated as playing a role in secretion. The question, therefore, arises whether G_E, the G-protein associated with exocytosis, belongs to the ras family or whether it is a member of the heterotrimeric G-proteins. One way to address this question would be to examine the PtX sensi-

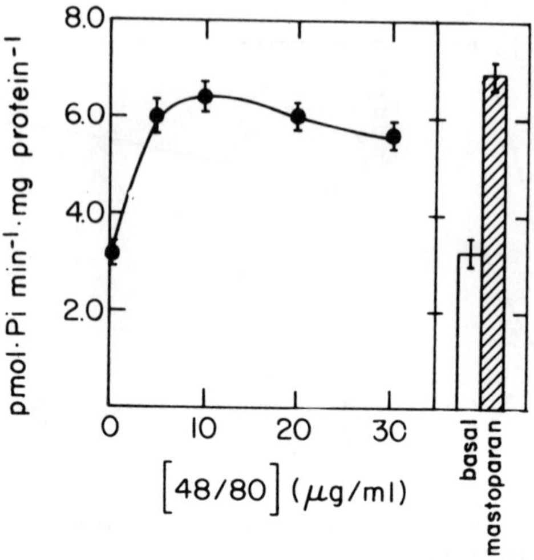

Figure 4. Activation of GTPase activity by 48/80 and mastoparan. Rat brain membranes (5 mg/ml) were solubilized with 1% cholate. Aliquots (20 μg) were incubated with the indicated concentrations of 48/80 or 150 μg/ml of mastoparan and GTPase activity determined.

tivity of G_E. However, in previous experiments G_E-dependent secretion could only be induced by introducing GTP-γ-S into the cells. Under such conditions, GTP-γ-S can dissociate ADP-ribosylated proteins and relieve their inhibition. The finding that internally applied neomycin, while blocking PLC activation, can still activate secretion from mast cells loaded with GTP provided us with a system where PtX-sensitivity of G_E-induced secretion could be tested. Using these conditions, we could demonstrate (16) that release induced by internally applied neomycin is inhibitable by PtX. Based on this finding we conclude that G_E is a PtX substrate and therefore, most probably, belongs to the heterotrimeric class of signal transducing G-proteins.

REFERENCES

1. Segal DM, Taurog J, Metzger H (1977). Proc Natl Acad Sci USA 74: 2993-2997.
2. Lagunof D, Martin TW, Read G (1983). Ann Rev Pharmacol Toxicol 23: 331-351.
3. Ali H, Cunha-Melo JR, Saul WF, Beaven MA (1990). J Biol Chem 265: 745-753.

4. Gruchalla RS, Dinh TT, Kennerly DA (1990). J Immunol 144: 2334-2342.
5. Yamada K, Okano Y, Miura K, Nozawa Y (1987). Biochem J 247: 95-99.
6. Corcia A, Schweitzer-Stenner R, Pecht I, Rivnay B (1986). EMBO J 5: 849-854.
7. Mohr FC, Fewtrell C (1987). J Biol Chem 262:10638-10643.
8. Holgate SJ, Lewis RA, Austen KF (1980). Proc Natl Acad Sci USA 77: 6800-6804.
9. Sagi-Eisenberg R, Pecht I (1984). Immunol Lett 8: 237-241.
10. Katakmi Y, Kaibuchi K, Sawamura Y, Takai Y, Nishizuka Y (1984). Biochem Biophys Res Commun 121: 573-578.
11. Saito H, Okajima F, Molski TFP, Shaafi RI, Ui M, Ishizaka T (1987). J Immunol 138: 3927-3934.
12. Cockcroft S, Howell TW, Gomperts BD (1987). J Cell Biol 105: 2745-2750.
13. Aridor M, Traub L, Sagi-Eisenberg R (1990). J Cell Biol 111: 909-917.
14. Oberdisse E, Lapetina EG (1987). Biochem Biophys Res Commun 144: 1188-1196.
15. Limor R, Schvartz I, Hazum E, Ayalon D, Naor Z. (1989). Biochem Biophys Res Commun 159: 209-215.
16. Aridor M, Sagi-Eisenberg R. (1990). J Cell Biol 111: In press.
17. Higashijima T, Uzu S, Nakajima TR, Ross E (1988). J Biol Chem 263: 6491-6494.
18. Repke H, Bienert M (1987). FEBS Lett 221: 236-240.
19. Repke H, Piotrowski W, Bienert M, Foreman JC (1987). J Pharmacol Exp Therap 243: 317-321.

Cellular and Cytokine Networks in
Tissue Immunity, pages 177-182

Modulation of endothelium and monocytes by tumor-derived factors

Matthias Clauss, Satoshi Ogawa, and David Stern

Department of Physiology, Columbia University, College of Physicians and Surgeons, New York City, New York 10032

Modulation of endothelial cell function in the tumor bed, with the induction of increased vascular permeability and activation of the hemostatic system, are of special importance for both tumor growth (1) and metastases (2). Increased permeability leads to the escape of plasma components, including fibrinogen, and procoagulant events which can promote formation of a fibrin gel, serving as a substrate for tumor and blood vessel growth. Although induction of clot formation would seem to favor only tumor growth, intravascular coagulation with formation of occlusive thrombi could also locally reduce blood flow, thereby depriving the tumor of oxygen and nutrients. In this context, when low doses of tumor necrosis factor/cachectin (TNF) were infused into mice bearing methylcholanthrene A (meth A)-induced fibrosarcomas, intravascular fibrin formation was observed, resulting in occlusive thrombi and a major drop in blood flow, all of which were localized in the tumor bed (3). An important potential mechanism through which TNF can initiate this localized thrombotic process involves induction of endothelial synthesis and expression of tissue factor, a cell surface procoagulant cofactor which is believed to be the major initiator of coagulation in vivo (4).

To understand mechanisms which could account local enhancement of procoagulant events in tumor vasculature, we analyzed conditioned medium of meth A tumor cells for the ability to enhance TNF-mediated induction of endothelial tissue factor in vitro. Such activity could be found in serum-free conditioned media which had been concentrated by ultrafiltration, batch adsorbed and eluted from a cation exchanger (thereby removing more than 90% of protein), and subsequently applied to a heparin column. Chromatography on heparin-ultragel separated the procoagulant inducing activity into two pools (Fig. 1): activity I eluted at ≈0.15 M NaCl, whereas activity II required ≈0.8 M NaCl for elution.

Further purification of activity I, which we termed Meth A factor, was achieved on the FPLC using the ion exchangers Mono Q and Mono S, and reversed phase with Pro RP as described (5). A single band resulted from preparative gel elution after SDS-PAGE containing all of the tissue factor inducing activity with Mr ≈ 44,000 Da under nonreduced and 56,000 Da under reduced conditions (see fig.1, inset for activity I). Although the activity was stable to heat, even in the presence of SDS, it could be destroyed by treatment with beta-mercaptoethanol at 98°C for 5 min. or by incubation with proteases at 37°C. Although purified Meth A factor revealed no intrinsic procoagulant activity, it induced procoagulant

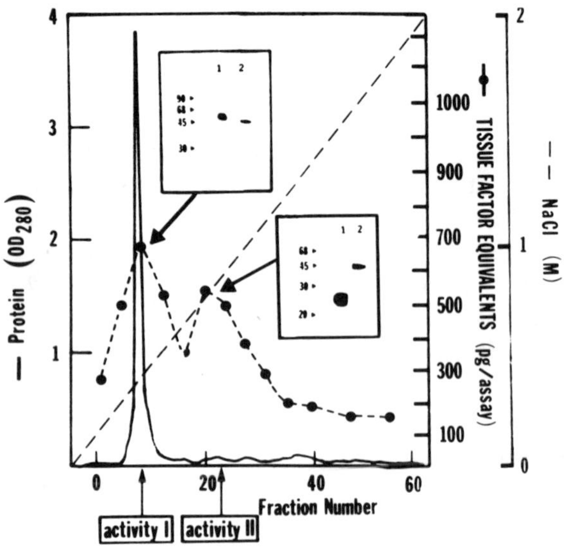

Figure 1. Chromatography of partially purified meth A-conditioned medium on heparin-ultragel. Meth A conditioned medium was subjected to batch adsorption on S Sepharose (after a 1:1 dilution in 50 mM MES-buffer (pH 5.5) and acidified to pH 5.5 with hydrochloric acid), step-eluted with 1 M NaCl, 100 mM MES (pH 6.8), dialyzed against phosphate (50 mM; pH 7.4), and then applied to heparin-ultragel. The heparin column was eluted with an ascending salt gradient (0 to 2 M NaCl), and fractions were assayed for their ability to induce tissue factor activity in endothelial cells as described elsewhere (4). The two separated peaks of activity (I and II, indicated with arrows) were further purified as described recently (4,6). The purified two factors corresponding to either activity I or II were then analyzed on SDS-polyacrylamide gel electrophoresis as shown in the two insets: 1, on reduced and 2, on non-reduced gels.

activity in endothelial cells, as assessed by means of a two stage coagulation assay. The induction was dose- dependent, being half-maximal at 6-8 pM and maximal at 15-20 pM. About 7-fold (maximal) enhancement of the procoagulant activity was be observed during coincubation with rTNF. The induced procoagulant activity was factor VII dependent, could be blocked by incubation with a monoclonal antibody to tissue factor and was be inhibited by cycloheximide, indicating that the observed activity was de novo synthesized tissue factor. Tissue factor activity was detectable by 2 hrs, reached a maximum by 6 hrs and thereafter declined to the baseline.

Meth A factor-mediated induction of tissue factor in the presence of TNF was not simply due to a change in cell surface expression: increased tissue factor activity of endothelial monolayers incubated with meth A factor/TNF was parallelled by an increase in total tissue factor antigen in the endothelium and is ≈3-times more than in the functional assay as determined by ELISA. The immunological data matched to the results of Northern blots, showing much stronger induction of tissue factor mRNA with both meth A factor and TNF together than was observed in the functional assay. Since the functional tissue factor assay only detects of tissue factor on the cell surface, this finding suggests that either not all the induced tissue factor is expressed on the cell surface (5) or nonfunctional tissue factor is present.

The material in the second activity peak with higher affinity for immobilized heparin was purified by batch adsorption on Fast S, followed by chromatography on FPLC Mono S and reversed phase HPLC (C_4), as described recently (6). When peak fractions from the reversed phase column were subjected to SDS-polyacrylamidgelelectrophoresis, a single major band was observed (see also Fig.1, inset for activity II), migrating with an apparent Mr corresponding to ≈23,000 Da under reducing conditions and 46,000 Da under non-reducing conditions. Endothelial tissue factor inducing activity could be eluted from the same position on the gel as the band, either from reducing or non-reducing conditions. N-terminal sequence analysis showed that five of the first seven residues of the murine ≈46 kDa polypeptide were identical to that reported for guinea pig Vascular Permeability Factor (VPF), which in turn was shown to be identical to Vascular Endothelium Growth Factor (VEGF)(7). The sequence of the murine ≈46 kDa factor was Ala-Pro-Thr-Thr-Glu-Gly-Glu, whereas the sequence of guinea pig VPF (7) is Ala-Pro-Met-Ala-Glu-Gly-Glu (in the case of bovine VPF/VEGF, four of the first seven residues are identical)(8).

The identity of the 46 kDa polypeptide with VPF was confirmed by blocking experiments with a monospecific, neutralizing antibody to guinea pig VPF, which inhibited most of the tissue factor inducing activity. Furthermore, purified guinea pig VPF also induced procoagulant activity in endothelium, which could be neutralized by monospecific antibody to tissue factor. Taken together, these data provided strong support for the conclusion that the murine ≈46 kDa polypeptide with high affinity for heparin, was the murine homologue of VPF.

VPF is a polypeptide mediator produced constitutively by certain tumor cells and other cell lines, which increases vascular permeability and stimulates endothelial proliferation (9,10). In addition to these properties, we have shown that VPF induces tissue factor in endothelial cells as well as in monocytes and macrophages. Although the time course of tissue factor induction by VPF was similar to that of meth A factor, the dose dependence was somewhat different: with VPF the maximal response occurred at ≈1 nM, and the half-maximal response occurred at ≈ 300 pM. Priming of endothelial cells with meth A factor resulted in further enhancement of VPF induced tissue factor activity in the presence of TNF.

Another new and striking function for VPF was the induction of monocyte chemotaxis, which was not simply due to enhanced chemokinesis, as shown by checkerboard analysis. VPF induced migration of monocytes through endothelial cell layers grown on collagen membranes. Neither polymorphonuclear leukocytes nor lymphocytes were attracted by VPF.

In terms of mechanisms through which meth A-factor, VPF and TNF bring about changes in cellular properties, we considered the possibility that the tumor-derived factors could enhance endothelial binding sites for TNF. Pilot radioligand binding studies with radioiodinated TNF have shown that meth A factor increases the affinity and number of endothelial binding sites, providing a possible basis for apparent enhancement of TNF-induced tissue factor production in the presence of meth A factor. However, no significant effect of VPF on the binding of TNF to the endothelial cell surface could be seen, suggesting that VPF and TNF may reinforce each others' actions at an intracellular site. In this context, VPF has recently been shown to induce a rise in endothelial cytosolic calcium (11), suggesting a possible common locus in intracellular signal transduction mechanisms at which TNF and VPF could act.

Although in vivo studies will be required to understand the biologic significance of these two tumor-derived factors, the spectrum of changes they can induce in the vasculature suggests that they participate in increasing vascular permeability and procoagulant response of monocytes/macrophages as well as of endothelial cells. In this sense they may have an important role in the accumulation of tumor stroma, thereby supporting tumor and vascular growth. Furthermore, the ability of these factors to enhance endothelial tissue factor induction in response to TNF suggests a possible role in the enhancement of TNF-induced tumor necrosis.

References:

1. Dvorak, H. 1986. Tumors: Wounds that do not heal. Similarities between tumor stroma generation and wound healing. New Eng. J. Med. 315:1650.
2. Rickles, F. R., Hancock, W. W., Edwards, R. L., and L. R. Zacharski. 1988. Antimetastatic agents. Role of cellular procoagulants in the pathogenesis of fibrin deposition in cancer and the use of anticoagulants and/or antiplatelet drugs in cancer treatment. Seminars in thrombosis and hemostasis. 14:88.
3. Nawroth, P., D. Handley, G. Matsueda, R. De Waal, H. Gerlach, D. Blohm, and D. Stern. 1988. Tumor necrosis factor/cachectin-induced intravascular fibrin formation in meth A fibrosarcomas. J. Exp. Med. 168:637.
4. Clauss, C., C. Murray, M. Vianna, R. De Waal, G. Thurston, P. Nawroth, H. Gerlach, M. Gerlach, R. Bach, P. Familletti, and D. Stern. 1990. A polypeptide factor produced by fibrosarcoma cells that induces endothelial tissue factor and enhances the procoagulant response to tumor necrosis factor/cachectin. J. Biol. Chem. 265:7078.
5. Ryan, J., Brett, J, Kisiel, W., and D. Stern. 1990. Tumor necrosis factor-induced endothelial cell tissue factor is principally associated with the subendothelial matrix. Blood, in press.
6. Clauss, M., Gerlach, M., Gerlach, H., Brett, J., Wang, F, Familletti, P. C., Pan, Y-C. E., Olander J. V., Connolly, D. T., and D. Stern. Vascular permeability factor: A tumor derived polypeptide which induces endothelial cell and monocyte procoagulant activity, and promotes monocyte migration. J. Exp. Med. 172, in press.
7. Keck, P., S. Hauser, G. Krivi, K. Sanzo, T. Warren, J. Feder, and D. Connolly. 1989. Vascular permeability factor, an endothelial cell mitogen related to PDGF. Science (Wash DC) 246:1309.
8. Leung, D., G. Cachianes, W-J. Kuang, D. Goeddel, N. Ferrara.

1989. Vascular endothelial growth factor is a secreted angiogenic mitogen. Science (Wash DC) 246:1306.

9. Senger, D. S. Galli, A. Dvorak, C. Perruzzi, V. Harvey, and H. Dvorak. 1983. Tumor cells secrete a vascular permeability factor that promotes accumulation of ascites fluid. Science (Wash DC) 219:983.

10. Connolly, D., D. Heuvelman, R. Nelson, J. Olander, B. Eppley, J. Delfino, N. Siegel, R. Leimbruber, and J. Feder. 1989. Tumor vascular permeability factor stimulates endothelial cell growth and angiogenesis. J. Clin. Invest. 84:1470.

11. Brock, T., H. Dvorak and D. Senger. 1990. Tumor-secreted vascular permeability factor (VPF) increase endothelial cell cytosolic calcium. Faseb J. 4:#2071

Cellular and Cytokine Networks in
Tissue Immunity, pages 183-188

Endothelial Cell-Lymphocyte Interactions

J.S. Pober, C.C.W. Hughes, C.O.S. Savage, F.J. Schoen and P. Libby

Departments of Pathology and Medicine, Brigham and Women's Hospital and Harvard Medical School, Boston, MA 02115

INTRODUCTION

Cell-mediated immune reactions, such as delayed-type hypersensitivity (DTH), may be elicited in the peripheral tissues of an individual sensitized to a specific foreign protein antigen by rechallenge with the specific antigen. A critical early event in this process is the presentation of the foreign protein to circulating antigen-specific memory T cells. Antigen presentation, performed by an immune accessory cell, involves processing of the antigen, often by limited proteolysis, and display of the processed antigen in a complex with a self class I or class II MHC molecule on the surface of the accessory cell. To produce T cell activation, the accessory cell must also provide antigen-independent costimulator signals to the T cell (Weaver and Unanue, 1990). In this report, we will review recent work demonstrating that human endothelial cells (EC) possess the potential to effectively present antigens to T cells because they can express MHC molecules and costimulator activities, implying that EC may serve to initiate cell mediated immune reactions. We propose that antigen presentation by EC to T lymphocytes is physiological in that it contributes to host defense against foreign organisms. In addition, we suggest that in the setting of transplantation, foreign EC in the arteries of allografts, will present allogeneic MHC molecules and costimulator activities to host T cells, leading to an anti-graft chronic DTH reaction. Such a reaction to graft EC may underlie the syndrome of transplant-associated arteriosclerosis (TxAA).

MHC MOLECULE EXPRESSION BY ENDOTHELIAL CELLS

Vascular EC cultured from a variety of human vessels, including umbilical vein, dermal microvessels or saphenous vein, express low levels of class I MHC molecules (restriction elements used to present antigen to $CD8^+$ T cells) but do not express detectable levels of class II molecules (restriction elements used to present antigen to $CD4^+$ T cells). Early studies with cultured EC revealed that human IFN-γ both increased the level of synthesis and expression of class I molecules and caused *de novo* synthesis and expression of class II molecules (HLA-DR>HLA-DP>>HLA-DQ) (Pober et al., 1983; Collins et al., 1984). Other cytokines, notably IFN-α/β and TNF/LT, further increased class I expression but suppressed the induction of class II expression (Collins et al., 1986; Lapierre et al., 1988). EC could also be induced to express class II molecules when incubated with allogeneic $CD8^+$ T cells. In contrast, co-culture with allogeneic $CD4^+$ T cells failed to cause class II molecule synthesis in EC (Pardi et al., 1987; Doukas and Pober, 1990). This is because $CD4^+$ T cells cultured with EC are induced to secrete an as yet uncharacterized inhibitor of class II molecule expression (Doukas and Pober, 1990). These data suggest that, *in vivo*, resting (class I^+, class II^-) EC may present class I associated antigens to $CD8^+$ T cells, and that this interaction causes expression of class II molecules so that activated EC may then present antigen to $CD4^+$ T cells. Upon antigen-triggered activation, both types of T cells will secrete cytokines, such as TNF and IFN-γ, that initiate inflammatory reactions. $CD4^+$ T cells are more traditionally associated with development of intense DTH reactions, and induced expression of class II molecules may be necessary for this to occur. Class II molecules are indeed induced during the course of experimental DTH in baboon (Munro et al., 1989).

COSTIMULATOR ACTIVITIES OF ENDOTHELIAL CELLS

Comparative studies of EC with other cell types revealed that many different cells in culture, including fibroblasts and smooth muscle cells, could express comparable levels of class II MHC molecules upon IFN-γ treatment (Pober et al., 1983; Collins et al., 1984) [although EC did appear more responsive in organ culture (Messadi et al., 1988) or *in vivo* (Munro et al., 1989)]. However, experiments with cultured dermal fibroblasts revealed that although class II-expressing cells of this type could be lysed by class II-specific cytolytic T lymphocytes (Pober et al., 1983) and could present protein antigens to T cell clones (Umetsu et al., 1985), fibroblasts could not fully activate resting T cells in either primary allogeneic responses (Pober et al., 1983; Geppart and Lipsky, 1985) or secondary responses to protein antigens such as tetanus toxoid (Umetsu et al., 1986). Antigen presentation by fibroblasts, although incapable of causing T cell proliferation, did cause T cells to become responsive to exogenous IL-2 (Umetsu et al., 1986). We reasoned, therefore, that since IFN-γ-treated EC can fully activate resting lymphocytes to proliferate in both primary allogeneic responses (Pober et al., 1983; Pober et al., 1986) and secondary responses to protein antigens (Wagner et al., 1985), EC must express costimulator activities that function to enhance IL-2 secretion by antigen-activated T cells.

In support of this hypothesis, we demonstrated that EC markedly augment (typically by 3-8 fold) IL-2 synthesis by T cells activated suboptimally or even supraoptimally by a polyclonal stimulator (Guinan et al., 1989; Hughes et al., 1990). Costimulator activity depends upon cell contact and is partly mediated by EC LFA-3 interacting with T cell CD2. More recent experiments have established that costimulator activity is present in lightly paraformaldehyde-fixed EC and can be partly mimicked by micelles of phosphatidyl inositol (PI)-linked LFA-3. PI-LFA-3 cannot fully replace EC and combinations of PI-LFA-3 and EC are more effective than either costimulator alone. Moreover, since many cells, including fibroblasts, express comparable levels of LFA-3 as EC, either LFA-3 on EC must be structurally different from that on fibroblasts to account for EC efficiency or the other signal(s) provided by EC must be relatively EC specific. The LFA-3-independent signal has not yet been identified. Antibody blocking studies have not supported a role for an LFA-1:ICAM-1 interaction, a VLA-4:VCAM-1 interaction, a CD44 interaction or a CD28:B7 interaction.

Ongoing studies suggest that EC costimulation, measured as increases in T cell IL-2 transcripts or IL-2 secretion in the presence of the polyclonal T cell mitogen phytohemagglutinin (PHA), may be mediated, in part, by superinduction of c-fos mRNA (and presumably Fos protein) in the activated T cell. Fos is one of two subunits of the AP-1 transcription factor (the other being Jun) that enhances IL-2 transcription. Specifically, we have found that isolated peripheral blood T cells constitutively express c-jun transcripts and that PHA acts to induce IL-2, in part by causing a low level, transient burst of c-fos transcripts (peak 30 min). In the presence of EC, the steady state level of c-jun is unaffected, but the level of the PHA-induced burst of c-fos transcripts may increase up to ten fold. This EC effect does not appear to involve stabilization of c-fos mRNA and probably results from increased c-fos transcription.

ENDOTHELIAL CELLS IN TRANSPLANT-ASSOCIATED ARTERIOSCLEROSIS

Our cell culture studies, summarized above, have identified properties of EC that may allow them to function as antigen presenting cells *in vivo*. Under normal circumstances, we propose that this activity will occur primarily in postcapillary venules, the site of leukocyte extravasation and accumulation in protective reactions such as DTH to foreign protein antigens. However, we believe our findings also have relevance to pathologic reactions. In allogeneic transplantation, graft EC may play a role as a stimulator of rejection. Recent support for this hypothesis has come from histologic examination of human coronary arteries following cardiac transplantation. These vessels are prone to undergo an accelerated occlusive obliteration of the lumen, caused by progressive smooth muscle cell accumulation in the arterial intima. This process, which we call TxAA, can occur in 6 months to a few years and is a major cause of late graft loss. Its pathogenesis is unknown. Immunocytochemical examination of early arterial lesions reveals a subendothelial band-like infiltrate of $CD4^+$ and $CD8^+$ T cells and macrophages, abutting upon $HLA\text{-}DR^+$ luminal EC (Salomon et al.). Such EC are clearly activated because arterial EC are normally $HLA\text{-}DR^-$. Since cultured arterial EC, like venous EC, can stimulate primary allogeneic responses and display costimulator activities, the observed *in situ* relationships imply that there is T cell recognition and activation of graft EC. We believe the histological appearance of these early lesions is most consistent with that of a DTH reaction to the foreign endothelium. In later, more stenotic lesions, smooth muscle cells accumulate in the deeper layers of the intima, accounting for the progressive luminal obliteration. It seems likely that the smooth muscle cells, which do not express HLA-DR, have been recruited and stimulated to proliferate by cytokines released as a consequence of the anti-endothelial reaction. Experiments to characterize the function and specificities of the T cells in the arterial wall, and thereby test our interpretation, are currently underway.

ACKNOWLEDGEMENTS

We thank our many colleagues whose work is discussed in this review. Supported by NIH grants HL-36003, HL-43364 and HL-36028.

REFERENCES

Collins T, Korman AJ, Wake CT, Boss JM, Kappes DJ, Fiers W, Ault KA, Gimbrone MA Jr, Strominger JL, Pober JS (1984). Immune interferon activates multiple class II major histocompatibility complex genes and the associated invariant chain gene in human endothelial cells and dermal fibroblasts. Proc Natl Acad Sci (USA) 81:4917-4921.

Collins T, Lapierre LA, Fiers W, Strominger JL, Pober JS (1986). Recombinant human tumor necrosis factor increases mRNA levels and surface expression of HLA-A,B antigens in vascular endothelial cells and dermal fibroblasts *in vitro*. Proc Natl Acad Sci (USA) 83:446-450.

Doukas J, Pober JS (1990). Lymphocyte-mediated activation of cultured endothelial cells (EC): $CD4^+$ T cells inhibit EC class II MHC antigen expression despite secreting IFN-γ and increasing EC class I MHC and ICAM-1 antigen expression. J Immunol 145:1088-1098.

Geppart TD, Lipsky PE (1985). Antigen presentation by interferon-γ-treated endothelial cells and fibroblasts: differential ability to function as antigen presenting cells despite comparable Ia expression. J Immunol 1935:3750-3762.

Guinan EC, Smith BR, Doukas JT, Miller RA, Pober JS (1989). Vascular endothelial cells enhance T cell responses by markedly augmenting IL-2 concentrations. Cell Immunol 118:166-177.

Hughes CCW, Savage COS, Pober JS (1990). Endothelial cells augment T cell IL-2 production by a contact dependent mechanism involving CD2:LFA-3 interaction. J Exp Med 171:1453-1467.

Lapierre LA, Fiers W, Pober JS (1988). Three distinct classes of regulatory cytokines control endothelial cell MHC antigen expression: Interactions with immune (γ) interferon differentiate the effects of tumor necrosis factor and lymphotoxin from those of leukocyte (α) and fibroblast (β) interferons. J Exp Med 167:794-804.

Messadi DV, Pober JS, Murphy GF (1988). Effects of recombinant gamma interferon on HLA-DR and DQ expression by skin cells in short term organ culture. Lab Invest 58:61-67.

Munro JM, Pober JS, Cotran RS (1989). Tumor necrosis factor and interferon-γ induce distinct patterns of endothelial activation and associated leukocyte accumulation in skin of *Papio anubis*. Am J Pathol 135:121-133.

Pardi R, Bender JR, Engleman EG (1987). Lymphocyte subsets differentially induce class II human leukocyte antigens on allogeneic microvascular endothelial cells. J Immunol 139:2585-2592.

Pober JS, Collins T, Gimbrone MA Jr, Cotran RS, Gitlin JD, Fiers W, Clayberger C, Krensky AM, Burakoff SJ, Reiss CS (1983). Lymphocytes recognize human vascular endothelial and dermal fibroblast Ia antigens induced by recombinant human interferon. Nature 305:726-729.

Pober JS, Collins T, Gimbrone MA Jr, Libby P, Reiss CS (1986). Inducible expression of class II major histocompatibility complex antigen and the immunogenicity of vascular endothelium. Transplantation 41:141-146.

Salomon RN, Hughes CCW, Payne DD, Schoen FJ, Pober JS, Libby P. Human coronary transplant-associated arteriosclerosis: evidence for a chronic immune reaction to activated graft endothelial cells. Manuscript submitted.

Umetsu DT, Pober JS, Jabara HJ, Fiers W, Yunis E, Burakoff SJ, Reiss CS, Geha RS (1985). Human dermal fibroblasts present tetanus toxoid antigen to antigen specific T cell clones. J Clin Invest 76:254-260.

Umetsu DT, Katzen D, Jabara HJ, Geha RS (1986). Antigen presentation by human dermal fibroblasts: activation of resting T lymphocytes. J Immunol 136:440-445.

Wagner CR, Vetto RM, Burger DR (1985). Subcultured human endothelial cells can function independently as fully competent antigen presenting cells. Hum Immunol 13:33-47.

Weaver CT, Unanue ER (1990). The costimulatory function of antigen-presenting cells. Immunol Today 11:49-55.

Cellular and Cytokine Networks in
Tissue Immunity, pages 189-194

ENDOTHELIAL CELL - LEUKOCYTE INTERACTIONS IN IN VIVO MODELS OF INFLAMMATION

Malcolm L. Watson and Timothy J. Williams

Department of Applied Pharmacology, National Heart & Lung Institute, London SW3 6LY.

One of the key events in the acute inflammatory reaction is the interaction of leukocytes with the vascular endothelium. The importance of this interaction was proposed more than a century ago by Cohnheim (1889), based on *in vivo* microscopic examination of damaged tissue. In recent years *in vitro* studies have provided insight into the molecular mechanisms involved in cell activation and the adhesive process, and we have applied these findings to *in vivo* studies of inflammation.

Numerous mediators are known to cause leukocyte accumulation and extravasation *in vivo* following local application. These include lipid mediators such as leukotriene B_4 (LTB_4), the complement activation product C5a, the cytokines IL-1, IL-8/NAP-1 and TNF as well as bacterial products such as lipopolysaccharide and N-formylated peptides (eg fMLP). These mediators are also able to increase vascular permeability by a neutrophil-dependent mechanism (eg. Wedmore & Williams, 1981; Rampart *et al.*1989; Buckley *et al.*1990). The first event in leukocyte extravasation is leukocyte-endothelial cell adhesion, and it is not clear from the *in vitro* evidence whether this occurs following an action of chemotactic substances on the endothelium (Hoover *et al.*1984) or on the leukocyte (Tonnesen *et al.*1984). Based on *in vivo* experiments in which the accumulation of radiolabelled leukocytes in response to intradermal injection of fMLP or PAF could be selectively reduced by preinjection of skin sites with the same mediator, Colditz & Movat (1984) proposed that chemoattractant receptors regulating neutrophil accumulation exist on postcapillary venular endothelial cells.

In order to determine the role of receptors on the leukocyte in the process of emigration *in vivo* our laboratories have examined the effect of uncoupling neutrophil chemoattractant receptors from cellular responses using pertussis toxin (Nourshargh & Williams, 1990). Pretreatment of neutrophils with pertussis toxin (PT) abolished *in vitro* adhesion and degranulation responses to C5a and fMLP, but the cells remained responsive to phorbol esters, which bypass chemoattractant receptors coupled to PT-sensitive G proteins. Radiolabelled rabbit neutrophils were pretreated with PT before injecting into a recipient. Thus, the neutrophils were treated leaving the endothelium unaffected. Although PT pretreatment did not affect the circulation of neutrophils over the 4 hour experimental period, the local accumulation of PT-pretreated neutrophils in response to intradermally-injected C5a, fMLP and zymosan was virtually abolished when compared with the pronounced accumulation of control (non-pretreated) neutrophils to these stimuli. In this model therefore there is a requirement for neutrophil stimulation via a PT sensitive mechanism in order for neutrophil accumulation to occur in response to extravascular chemotactic stimuli. It is not clear how a mediator generated, or injected, extravascularly affects the neutrophil in the moving blood stream within the microvessel lumen. There is evidence that the mediator signal may be picked up as the neutrophil passes through the capillary and that the affected neutrophil then adheres downstream in the venule (Nagai & Katori, 1988).

The neutrophil CD11/CD18 complex has been demonstrated to be important in stimulated neutrophil adhesion to endothelial cells *in vitro* (Harlan *et al.* 1985) and patients with a genetic deficiency in these molecules suffer from recurrent infection without pus formation (Anderson *et al.* 1985). An inducible ligand, intercellular adhesion molecule-1 (ICAM-1), has been identified for at least one member of the CD11/CD18 complex. ICAM-1 expression on endothelial cells is induced by IL-1, TNF and lipopolysaccharide *in vitro* (Smith *et al.* 1988), and in a primate model ICAM-1 expression was detected following intradermal injection of TNF *in vivo* (Munro *et al.* 1989). Blocking antibodies which recognise either the CD11/CD18 complex or ICAM-1 can be used to examine the role of these molecules in mediating *in vivo* accumulation of leukocytes in response to inflammatory mediators or stimuli.

We have used a monoclonal antibody that recognises CD18, designated 60.3, to determine the role of the neutrophil CD18 complex in neutrophil accumulation in response to chemoattractants *in vivo* (Nourshargh *et al.* 1989). A similar protocol was used to that described for the pertussis toxin treated cells. Radiolabelled rabbit neutrophils were incubated *in vitro* with 60.3 before intravenous injection into a recipient animal and the ability of these cells to accumulate at dermal sites injected with chemoattractants was measured. 60.3 pretreatment caused a marked reduction of neutrophil accumulation in response to intradermal injection of C5a, LTB_4 and fMLP. Although these mediators may cause an increased expression of CD18 *in vitro*, these findings indicate that basally expressed CD18 is important for the accumulation of neutrophils in response to chemoattractants *in vivo*. Systemic treatment of rabbits with 60.3 also reduces cutaneous neutrophil accumulation in response to intradermal injection of chemoattractants as well as the plasma leakage caused by these agents (Arfors *et al.* 1987). Intravital microscopic examination of the rabbit tenuissimus muscle showed that 60.3 reduced leukocyte-endothelial adhesion in response to extravascular chemoattractant, but not the rolling of leukocytes along the vessel wall (Arfors *et al.* 1987), indicating that these two phenomena may involve different molecular mechanisms.

Increased adhesion *in vitro* may be mediated by changes in leukocyte CD11/CD18 complex or in endothelial ICAM-1 as well as other adhesion molecules (Springer, 1990). IL-1 induces leukocyte adhesion in vitro via an endothelium and protein synthesis -dependent mechanism (Bevilacqua *et al.* 1985), and most laboratories do not find IL-1 to stimulate neutrophils *in vitro*. *In vivo* accumulation of neutrophils in response to IL-1 (but not fMLP) is also dependent on protein synthesis (Rampart & Williams, 1988; Cybulsky *et al.* 1989). However, in common with chemoattractants such as C5a and fMLP, neutrophil accumulation in response to IL-1 is blocked by both pertussis toxin and 60.3 (Nourshargh *et al.* 1989; Nourshargh & Williams, 1990), raising the possibility that IL-1 may act via the local generation of chemoattractants. A likely candidate is IL-8, which is synthesised *de novo* in response to IL-1 by monocytes, fibroblasts and endothelial cells (Baggiolini *et al.* 1989). The ability of IL-1 to both increase endothelial adhesivity (via ICAM-1 and other molecules) and also to cause the production of IL-8 could account for its remarkable *in vivo* chemoattractant potency.

Other studies have examined the effect of anti-ICAM-1 antibodies on leukocyte recruitment in *in vivo* models of inflammation. Barton *et al* (1989) were able to inhibit phorbol ester induced neutrophil accumulation in rabbit lungs by pretreatment with anti-ICAM-1 antibody. In a primate model Wegner *et al* (1990) reduced lung eosinophil accumulation following aerosol antigen challenge by pretreatment with anti-ICAM-1, and this decrease was associated with a fall in airway responsiveness to methacholine.

While there has been considerable progress in understanding the adhesive interaction between the leukocyte and endothelium, little is known about subsequent events which lead to neutrophil dependent increased vascular permeability and the passage of leukocytes across the basement membrane. Neutrophil granule enzymes might appear to be likely candidates as common mediators of increased permeability at sites of vessel wall-neutrophil interaction, but using an *in vitro* vessel wall construct, Huber & Weiss (1989) were unable to demonstrate inhibition of neutrophil-mediated increased permeability with a variety of enzyme inhibitors. Neutrophil cationic proteins have been implicated *in vitro* and *in vivo* (Needham *et al.* 1988) and using an intravital system Rosengren *et al* (1989) reported that the polyanion dextran sulphate inhibits increased vascular permeability but not leukocyte extravasation in the hamster cheek pouch.

The interaction of leukocytes with the vascular endothelium and the increased vascular permeability associated with it are important early events in inflammatory reactions. These responses may be elicited by the action of chemical mediators on the leukocyte or the endothelium or on both cell types. The understanding of how this process occurs *in vivo* are essential for the rational treatment of inflammatory disease.

REFERENCES

Anderson D.C., Schmalsteig F.C., Finegold M.J., Hughes B.J., Rothlein R., Miller L.J., Kohl S., Tosi M.F., Jacobs R.L., Waldrop T.C., Goldman A.S., Shearer W.T. & Springer T.A. (1985). The severe and moderate phenotypes of heritable Mac-1, LFA-1 deficiency: their quantiative definition and relation to leukocyte dysfunction and clinical features. *J. Infect. Dis.*, **152**, 668-689.

Arfors K.E., Lundberg C., Lindbom L., Lundberg K., Beatty P.G. & Harlan J.M. (1987). A monoclonal antibody to the membrane glycoprotein complex CD18 inhibits polymorphonuclear leukocyte accumulation and plasma leakage in vivo. *Blood*, **69**, 338-340.

Baggiolini M., Walz A. & Kunkel S.L. (1989). Neutrophil-activating peptide-1/interleukin 8, a novel cytokine that activates neutrophils. *J. Clin. Invest.*, **84**, 1045-1049.

Barton R.W., Rothlein R., Ksiazek J. & Kennedy C. (1989). The effect of anti-intercellular adhesion molecule-1 on phorbol-ester-induced rabbit lung inflammation. *J. Immunol.*, **143**, 1278-1282.

Bevilacqua M.P., Pober J.S., Wheeler M.E., Cotran R.S. & Gimbrone M.A. (1985). Interleukin 1 acts on cultured human vascular endothelium to increase the adhesion of polymorphonuclear leucocytes, monocytes, and related cell lines. *J. Clin. Invest.*, **76**, 2003-2011.

Buckley T.L., Brain S.D. & Williams T.J. (1990). Oedema formation induced by IL-1 in vivo: interactions with the neuropeptide, calcitonin gene-related peptide (CGRP) in rabbit skin. *Br. J. Pharmacol.*, **99**, 94P.

Cohnheim J. (1889). Inflammation. In *Lectures on General Pathology. Section 1. The pathology of the circulation*. pp. 242-382. London: New Sydenham Society.

Colditz I.G. & Movat H.Z. (1984). Desensitization of acute inflammatory lesions to chemotaxins and endotoxin. *J. Immunol.*, **133**, 2163-2168.

Cybulsky M.I., McComb D.J. & Movat H.Z. (1989). Protein synthesis dependent and independent mechanisms of neutrophil emigration. *Am. J. Pathol.*, **135**, 227-237.

Harlan J.M., Killen P.D., Senecal F., Schwartz B.R., Yee E.K., Taylor R.F., Beatty P.G., Price T. & Ochs H.D. (1985). The role of neutrophil membrane glycoprotein GP-150 in neutrophil adherence to endothelium in vitro. *Blood*, **66**, 167-178.

Hoover R.L., Karnofsky M.J., Austen K.F., Corey E.J. & Lewis R.A. (1984). Leukotriene B_4 action on endothelium mediates augmented neutrophil/endothelial adhesion. *Proc. Natl. Acad. Sci. USA*, **81**, 2191-2193.

Huber A.R. & Weiss S.J. (1989). Disruption of the subendothelial basement membrane during neutrophil diapedesis in an in vitro construct of a blood vessel wall. *J. Clin. Invest.*, **83**, 1122-1136.

Munro J.M., Pober J.S. & Cotran R.S. (1989). Tumor necrosis factor and interferon-gamma induce distinct patterns of endothelial activation and associated leukocyte accumulation in skin of papio anubis. *Am. J. Pathol.*, **135**, 121-133.

Nagai K. & Katori M. (1988). Possible changes in the leukocyte membrane as a mechanism of leukocyte adhesion to the venular walls induced by leukotriene B_4 and fMLP in the microvasculature of the hamster cheek pouch. *Int. J. Microcirc.*, **7**, 305-314.

Needham L., Hellewell P.G., Williams T.J. & Gordon J.L. (1988). Endothelial functional responses and increased vascular permeability induced by polycations. *Lab. Invest.*, **59**, 538-548.

Nourshargh S., Rampart M., Hellewell P.G., Jose P.J., Harlan J.M., Edwards A.J. & Williams T.J. (1989). Accumulation of ^{111}In-neutrophils in rabbit skin in allergic and non-allergic inflammatory reactions in vivo: inhibition by neutrophil pretreatment in vitro with a monoclonal antibody recognising the CD18 antigen. *J. Immunol.*, **142**, 3193-3198.

Nourshargh S. & Williams T.J. (1990). Evidence that a receptor operated event on the neutrophil mediates neutrophil accumulation in vivo: pretreatment of ^{111}In-neutrophils with pertussis toxin in vitro inhibits their accumulation in vivo. *J. Immunol.*, in press.

Rampart M. & Williams T.J. (1988). Evidence that neutrophil accumulation induced by interleukin-1 requires both local protein biosynthesis and neutrophil CD18 antigen expression in vivo. *Br. J. Pharmacol.*, **94**, 1143-1148.

Rampart M., Van Damme J., Zonnekyn L. & Herman A.G. (1989). Granulocyte chemotactic protein/interleukin-8 induces plasma leakage and neutrophil accumulation in rabbit skin. *Am. J. Pathol.*, **135**, 1-5.

Rosengren S., Ley K. & Arfors K.-E. (1989). Dextran sulphate prevents LTB_4-induced permeability increase but not neutrophil emigration in the hamster cheek pouch. *Microvasc. Res.*, **38**, 243-254.

Smith C.W., Rothlein R., Hughes B.J., Mariscalco M.M., Rudloff H.E., Schmalstieg F.C. & Anderson D.C. (1988). Recognition of an endothelial determinant for CD18-dependent human neutrophil adherence and transendothelial migration. *J. Clin. Invest.*, **82**, 1746-1756.

Springer T.A. (1990). Adhesion receptors of the immune system. *Nature*, **346**, 425-434.

Tonnesen M.G., Smedley L.A. & Henson P.M. (1984). Neutrophil-endothelial cell interactions. Modulation of neutrophil adhesiveness induced by complement fragments C5a and C5a des arg and formyl-methionyl-leucyl-phenylalanine in vitro. *J. Clin. Invest.*, **74**, 1581-1592.

Wedmore C.V. & Williams T.J. (1981). Control of vascular permeability by polymorphonuclear leukocytes in inflammation. *Nature*, **289**, 646-650.

Wegner C.D., Gundel R.H., Reilly P., Haynes N., Letts L.G. & Rothlein R. (1990). Intercellular adhesion molecule-1 (ICAM-1) in the pathogenesis of asthma. *Science*, **247**, 456.

Cellular and Cytokine Networks in
Tissue Immunity, pages 195-203

COMMUNICATION BETWEEN ENDOTHELIUM AND LEUKOCYTES MEDIATED BY CYTOKINES

Elisabetta Dejana, Gianfranco Bazzoni, Inés Martìn-Padura, and Alberto Mantovani.

Istituto di Ricerche Farmacologiche "Mario Negri"
Via Eritrea 62, 20157 Milan, Italy

1. Introduction

Endothelial cells (EC) have long been defined as a "passive" lining of vessels, endowed with negative properties, the most important one being that of representing a non-thrombogenic substrate for blood. As such, EC were viewed to participate in tissue reactions essentially as target for injurious agents. The possibility to isolate and culture endothelial cells from various districts gave the tools for studying their complex reactions to a variety of activating stimuli. EC have, in this way, emerged as active participants in many physiological and pathological processes. It is now evident that hemostasis, inflammatory reactions and immunity involve close interactions between immunocompetent cells and vascular endothelium. In particular, the ontogeny and function of white blood cells require an intimate relationship with vascular EC. Cytokines are mediators of these complex bidirectional interactions between leukocytes and vascular elements (for review see Mantovani and Dejana, 1989).

2. Endothelial cells as targets for the action of cytokines

Cytokines are mediators of the complex bidirectional interactions between leukocytes and vascular elements. Cytokines produced by activated lymphoid and mononuclear phagocytes elicit a complex spectrum of responses in vascular cells. The responses elicited seem to follow discrete, essentially non overlapping, patterns (for review see Mantovani and Dejana, 1989).

IL-1 and TNF are the prototypes of cytokines which induce proinflammatory-prothrombotic changes in EC (Table 1). The antithrombotic properties of EC are profoundly altered by exposure to these inflammatory cytokines. IL-1 and TNF induce thromboplastin (PCA), which promotes activation of the coagulation system, and decrease the cell surface anticoagulant activity mediated by the thrombomodulin (TM)-protein C pathway. They induce production of "platelet activating factor" (PAF) and augment production of a plasminogen activator inhibitor (PAI) thus impairing the ability of the cells to dissolve a fibrin clot.

Table 1 - The proinflammatory/prothrombotic set of functions induced in endothelial cells by IL-1 and TNF.

EC function	Significance
PGI2; ↓ responsiveness to noradrenaline	Vasodilation Hypotension
↑ PCA, PAF, ↓ TM; ↑ PAI	Thrombosis
Adhesion molecules (ICAM-1, ELAM-1, VCAM-1); Chemotactic cytokines (IL-8, MCP, CSFs)	Extravasation of circulating cells (leukocytes,tumor cells)

For abbreviations, see text.

The only activity that is apparently in contrast with the "prothrombotic" pattern elicited by IL-1 and TNF is the production of prostacyclin (PGI_2) by activated EC (Rossi et al., 1985). PGI_2 is involved in vasodilation at sites of inflammation and cell-mediated immunity and in the hypotension associated with systemic administration of these mediators. Furthermore the ability of the cells to produce increased amounts of PGI_2 lasts for several hours and is probably important as a defense mechanism in inhibiting platelet aggregation and thrombus formation.

At variance with IL-1 and TNF, <u>interferon gamma (γIFN)</u> induces a series of EC responses that do not essentially overlap with those induced by these inflammatory mediators. In general γIFN induces EC to act as accessory cells. It augments the expression of MHC class I antigens and induces class II antigens and the invariant chain (Pober et al., 1983). In contrast to IL-1 and TNF, γIFN does not change EC properties in regulating coagulation and fibrinolysis.

Granulocyte- and granulocyte-macrophage-colony stimulating factors (G-CSF and GM-CSF, respectively) and fibroblast growth factors (FGF) all induce patterns of responses in EC that differ from those induced by IL-1 and TNF or γIFN. It is in particular noteworthy that these cytokines that regulate growth and differentiation of hematopoietic cells (G and GM-CSFs) (FGFs) induce proliferation and migration of EC (Bussolino et al., 1989 a,b). These phenomena are frequently accompanied by induction of lytic enzymes (as urokinase or collagenase) that facilitate cell migration and extracellular matrix digestion.

3. Endothelial cells as producers of cytokines

EC produce cytokines that regulate the hematopoietic system, the proliferation and differentiation of T and B cells and the recruitment of leukocytes at sites of inflammation (Table 2). As mentioned above, EC produce copious ampunts of classical CSFs (G, M and GM). Two of these molecules (G and GM-CSF) in turn act on endothelial cells inducing migration and proliferation. Thus EC are an important constituent of the hematopoietic microenvironment. Upon exposure to inflammatory stimuli (as endotoxin, IL-1 or TNF), EC produce IL-1 and interleukin-6 (IL-6) (Sironi et al., 1989; review Mantovani and Dejana, 1989). These are pleiotropic cytokines which affect activation and proliferation of different cell types as T and B lymphocytes and hemopoietic precursors. IL-1 also induces proliferation of arterial smooth muscle cells of the media and in this way possibly contributes to the vascular thickening during the atherosclerotic process (Libby et al., 1988; Raines et al., 1989). IL-1 and IL-6 also induce the release of acute phase proteins and, in this way, producing these peptides, EC take part in the regulation of specific immunity and acute phase responses. Finally EC have the capacity to produce CSFs and other cytokines (MCP and interleukin-8) which can activate and induce chemotactic migration of leukocytes as discussed in detail in the following section.

4. Leukocyte recruitment

EC express a series of adhesive structures on their membrane that are a substratum for monocyte, lymphocyte and polymorphonuclear cell adhesion. In resting conditions EC express two integral membrane proteins denominated "intercellular adhesion melecule" (ICAM-1 and ICAM-2) (Dustin and Springer, 1988). These proteins belong to the large superfamily of immunoglobulins and are homologous in their aminoacid sequences. They are expressed even without activation of EC and are probably responsible for the basal adhesion of leukocytes to the endothelial cell surface. The receptor of ICAM-1 and ICAM-2 is a member of the leukocyte integrin family, it has been denominated LFA-1 (or CD11a/18 or alß2) and is present on monocytes, polymorphonuclear leukocytes, lymphoid cells and related leukemic lines (Marlin and Springer, 1987; Staunton et al., 1989).

Table 2 - Cytokines produced by endothelial cells.

Cytokine	Stimulus	Function
IL-1	LPS IL-1 TNF IFN-γ	Lymphocyte activation; local and systemic inflammation; acute phase responses; hematopoiesis
IL-6	"spontaneous" LPS IL-1 TNF	Lymphocyte activation; acute phase response, hematopoiesis
CSFs	LPS IL-1 TNF modified LDL	Leukocyte recruitment and activation; hematopoiesis; EC proliferation and migration
Chemotactic factors (IL-8 and MCP)$^+$	LPS IL-1 TNF	Leukocyte recruitment and activation
PDGF	IL-1	Smooth muscle cell proliferation (atherosclerosis)

$^+$See Table 1

When EC are activated by the inflammatory mediators interleukin-1 (IL-1) and tumor necrosis factor (TNF) (and also to a minor extent by interferon γ) the expression of ICAM-1 is augmented (Dustin and Springer, 1988). In addition to increasing ICAM-1, IL-1 and TNF induce *de novo* expression of two novel adhesion structures denominated "endothelial leukocyte adhesion molecule 1" (ELAM-1) (Bevilacqua et al., 1989) and "vascular cell adhesion molecule" (VCAM) (Osborn et al., 1989).

The cDNA encoding ELAM-1 has recently been cloned (Bevilacqua et al., 1989) and shows it to be a member of an emerging family of cell adhesion molecules denominated "selectins". Other members defined so far are the MEL 14 homing receptor in lymphocytes (Gallatin et al., 1983) and the platelet and endothelial cell GMP140 (McEver and Martin, 1984). These molecules have a relatively high homology and share the common characteristic of containing a lectin domain, an epithelial growth factor domain and a complement binding domain. The lectin domain is probably the most important in determining the adhesive properties of these antigens through the binding to specific carbohydrate regions in the ligand cell or matrix proteins. VCAM, at variance, belongs to the immunoglobulin superfamily (Osborn et al., 1989) and is therefore unrelated to ELAM-1. Its receptor has been identified as the integrin molecule VLA-4 (or a_4b_1) (Elices et al., 1990).

As a consequence of expression of leukocyte adhesion structures, EC exposed to inflammatory stimuli provide a better substratum for the adhesion of polymorphonuclear cells, monocytes and lymphocytes. This structural change on EC membrane lasts several hours. Thus, at sites of inflammation and cell-mediated immune reactions, EC participate in white blood cell recruitment by changing their adhesive properties.

In addition to expressing molecules that act as substratum for adhesion, EC participate in the regulation of leukocyte extravasation by producing cytokines which are chemotactic for leukocytes. These include CSFs (see above) and members of a novel, emerging superfamily of chemotactic polypeptides (see Table 2; reviewed in Baggiolini et al., 1989; Mantovani, 1990; Wolpe and Cerami, 1989). We and others have shown that, upon stimulation with inflammatory signals (e.g. IL-I), EC produce IL-8 and monocyte chemotactic protein (MCP) (Strieter et al., 1989; Schroder and Christophers, 1989; Sica et al., 1990 a,b). The superfamily to which IL-8 and MCP belong is characterized by a structural hallmark represented by 4 conserved cysteins, the first two in tandem, which are probably important for the three dimensional structure of these molecules. The same 4 Cys motif is shared by cytokines belonging to the platelet factor 4 (PF4) family, except that the first 2 Cys tandem is interrupted by an intervening aminoacid. The pF4 family includes IL-8 and gro which are chemotactic for neutrophils. IL-8 (also referred to as neutrophil activating proteins, NAP-I) is a cytokine active on neutrophils, basophils, and lymphocytes (Baggiolini et al., 1989). IL-8 also induces migration of melanoma (Wang et al., 1990) and this together with augmented binding to EC may contribute to augmented metastasis after IL-I administration mice (Giavazzi et al., 1990). MCP is a cytokine selectively acti monocytes (Yoshimura et al., 1989; Matsushima et al., 1989; Bo al., 1990; Van Damme et al., 1989).

It was originally identified in supernatants of tumor cells and is probably one important determinant of macrophage infiltration in tumors (Bottazzi et al., 1983; Mantovani, 1990). By producing MCP and IL-8 (Strieter et al., 1989; Schroder and Christophers, 1989; Sica et al., 1990 a., b.), EC participate in chemotaxis of different leukocyte populations at sites of inflammation and cell-mediated immunity. Production of MCP by vessel wall elements (EC and smooth muscle cells) may in particular be relevant in the pathogenesis of atherosclerosis, in which monocyte extravasation is an early event, and vasculitis, where monocyte accumulate in and around vessel walls.

5. Overview

EC are strategically located at the very interface between circulating blood elements and tissues. It is therefore not surprising that these cells play an important active role in immunity, inflammation and hemostasis. Cytokine molecules are used as communication signals in the complex bidirectional interaction between leukocytes and EC. EC represent a source of cytokines and, at the same time, a target for the action of various of these polipeptide mediators. Cytokine-induced EC responses follow discrete patterns: a program related to inflammation and thrombosis is activated by IL-1 and TNF, while IFN-γ activates accessory cell function, and FGFs and G and GM-CSF elicit functions related to angiogenesis.

In the complexity of the activation patterns they can express, EC are reminiscent of mononuclear phagocytes: the long utilized term of "reticuloendothelial system", though now largely abandoned, reflected the recognition of this similarity and interrelationship.

References

Baggiolini M., Walz A. and Kunkel S.L.: Neutrophil-activating protein-1/interleukin 8, a novel cytokine that activates neutrophils. J. Clin. Invest. 84, 1045, 1989.

Bevilacqua M.P., Stengelin S., Gimbrone M.A.jr. and Seed B.: Endothelial-leukocyte adhesion molecule 1: An inducible receptor for neutrophils related to complement regulatory proteins and lectins. Science 243, 1160, 1989.

Bottazzi B., Colotta F., Sica A., Nobili N. and Mantovani A.: A chemoattractant expressed in human sarcoma cells (tumor-derived chemotactic factor, TDCF) is identical to monocyte chemoattractant protein-1/monocyte chemotactic and activating factor (MCP-1/MCAF). Int. J. Cancer. 45, 795, 1990.

Bottazzi B., Polentarutti N., Acero R., Balsari A., Boraschi D., Ghezzi P., Salmona M. and Mantovani A.: Regulation of the macrophage content of neoplasms by chemoattractants. Science 220, 210, 1983.

Bussolino F., Wang J.M., Defilippi P., Turrini F., Sanavio F., Edgell C.J., Aglietta M., Arese P. and Mantovani A.: Granulocyte- and granulocyte-macrophage-colony stimulating factors induce human endothelial cells to migrate and proliferate. Nature 337, 471, 1989a.

Bussolino F., Wang J.M., Turrini F., Alessi D., Ghigo D., Costamagna C., Pescarmona G., Mantovani A. and Bosia A.: Stimulation of the Na+/H+ exchanger in human endothelial cells activated by granulocyte- and granulocyte-macrophage- colony stimulating factor. Evidence for a role in proliferation and migration. J. Biol. Chem. 264, 18284, 1989b.

Dustin M.L. and Springer T.A.: Lymphocyte function-associated antigen-1 (LFA-1) interaction with intercellular adhesion molecule-1 (ICAM-1) is one of at least three mechanisms for lymphocyte adhesion to cultured endothelial cells. J. Cell Biol. 107, 321, 1988.

Elices M.L., Osborn L., Takada Y., Crouse C., Luhowskyj S., Hemler M.E. and Lobb R.R.: VCAM-1 on activated endothelium interacts with the leukocyte integrin VLA-4 at a site distinct from the VLA-4/fibronectin binding site. Cell 60, 577, 1990.

Gallatin W.M., Weissman I.L. and Butcher E.C. A cell-surface molecule involved in horgan specific homing of lymphocytes. Nature 304, 30, 1983.

Giavazzi R., Garofalo A., Bani M.R., Ghezzi P., Boraschi D., Mantovani A. and Dejana E.: Interleukin-l-induced augmentation of experimental metastases from a human melanoma in nude mice. Cancer Res. 50, 4771, 1990.

Libby P., Warner S.J.C. and Friedman G.B.: Interleukin 1: A mitogen for human vascular smooth muscle cells that induces the release of growth-inhibitory prostanoids. J. Clin. Invest. 81, 487, 1988.

Mantovani A.: Tumor-associated macrophages. Current Opinions Immunology 2, 699, 1990.

Mantovani A. and Dejana E.: Cytokines as communication signals between leukocytes and endothelial cells. Immunol. Today 10, 370, 1989.

Marlin S.D. and Springer T.A.: Purified intercellular adhesion molecule-1 (ICAM-1) is a ligand for lymphocyte function-associated antigen 1 (LFA-1). Cell 51, 813, 1987.

Matsushima K., Larsen C.G, DuBois G.C. and Oppenheim J.J.: Purification and characterization of a novel monocyte chemotactic and activating factor produced by a human myelomonocytic cell line. J. Exp. Med. 169, 1485, 1989.

McEver R.P. and Martin M.N.: A monoclonal antibody to a membrane glycoprotein binds only to activated platelets. J. Biol. Chem. 259, 9799, 1984.

Osborn L., Hession C., Tizard R., Vassallo C., Luhowskyi S., Chi-Rosso G. and Lobb R.: Direct expression cloning of vascular cell adhesion molecule 1, a cytokine-induced endothelial protein that binds to lymphocytes. Cell 59, 1203, 1989.

Pober J.S., Gimbrone M.A. Jr., Cotran R.S., Reiss C.S., Burakoff S.J., Fiers W. and Ault K.A.: Ia expression by vascular endothelium is inducible by activated T cells and by human γ-interferon. J. Exp. Med. 157, 1339, 1983.

Raines E.W., Dower S.K. and Ross R. Interleukin-1 mitogenic activity for fibroblasts and smooth muscle cells is due to PDGF-AA. Science 243, 393, 1989.

Rossi V., Breviario F., Ghezzi P., Dejana E. and Mantovani A.: Prostacyclin synthesis induced in vascular cells by interleukin-1. Science. 229: 174-176, 1985.

Schroder J.M. and Christophers E.: Secretion of novel and homologous neutrophil-activating peptides by LPS-stimulated human endothelial cells. J. Immunol. 142, 244, 1989.

Sica A., Matsushima K., Van Damme J., Wang J.M., Polentarutti N., Dejana E., Colotta F. and Mantovani A.: IL-1 transcriptionally activates the monocyte-derived neutrophil chemotactic factor/IL-8 gene in endothelial cells. Immunology. 69: 548-553, 1990a.

Sica A., Wang J.M., Colotta F., Dejana E., Mantovani A., Oppenheim J.J., Larsen C.G., Zachariae C.O.C. and Matsushima K.: Monocyte chemotactic and activating factor gene expression induced in endothelial cells by IL-1 and TNF. J. Immunol. 144, 3034, 1990b.

Sironi M., Breviario F., Proserpio P., Biondi A., Vecchi A., Van Damme J., Dejana E. and Mantovani A.: IL-1 stimulates IL-6 production in endothelial cells. J. Immunol. 142, 549, 1989.

Staunton D.E., Dustin M.L. and Springer T.A.: Functional cloning of ICAM-2, a cell adhesion ligand for LFA-l homologous to ICAM-1. Nature 339, 61, 1989.

Strieter R.M., Kunkel S.L., Showell H.J., Remick D.G., Phan S.H., Ward P.A. and Marks R.M.: Endothelial cell gene expression of a neutrophil chemotactic factor by TNF-α, LPS, and IL-ß. Science 243, 1467, 1989.

Van Damme J., Decock B., Lenaerts J.P., Conings R., Bertini R., Mantovani A. and Billiau A.: Identification by sequence analysis of chemotactic factors for monocytes produced by normal and transformed cells stimulated with virus, double-stranted RNA or cytokine. Eur. J. Immunol. 19, 2367, 1989.

Wang J.M., Taraboletti G., Matsushima K., Van Damme J. and Mantovani A.: Induction of haptotactic migration of melanoma cells by neutrophil activating protein/interleukin-8. Biochem. Biophys. Res. Commun. 169, 165, 1990.

Wolpe S.D. and Cerami A.: Macrophage inflammatory protein 1 and 2: Members of a novel superfamily of cytokines. FASEB J. 3, 2565, 1989.

Yoshimura T., Robinson E.A., Tanaka S., Appella E., Kuratsu J.I. and Leonard E.J.: Purification and amino acid analysis of two human glioma-derived monocyte chemoattractants. J. Exp. Med. 169, 1449, 1989.

Cellular and Cytokine Networks in Tissue Immunity, pages 205-212

SUBVERSION OF THE CYTOKINE NETWORK OF T CELL-MACROPHAGE INTERACTION BY THE HUMAN IMMUNODEFICIENCY VIRUS

Monte S. Meltzer, Lisa M. Baca, Jim A. Turpin, D. Chester Kalter, Carl Dieffenbach, Robert M. Friedman, and Howard E. Gendelman

H. M. Jackson Foundation, Rockville, MD 20850 (D.C.K., H.E.G.); Dept. Path., Uniformed Services Univ. Health Sciences, Bethesda, MD 20814 (C.D., R.M.F.); and Dept. Cell. Immunol., Walter Reed Army Inst. Res., Rockville, MD 20850 (M.S.M., L.M.B., J.A.T.)

Disease is the net result of interactions between pathogenic reactions induced by infectious agents and defensive maneuvers brought to bear by the infected host. In most instances, initial scavenger responses and subsequent induction of immunologically specific and nonspecific effector reactions resolve or contain the infection. The balance between parasite and host is weighed heavily on the side of the host, even in those infections where there is no sterile immunity (tuberculosis, epidemic typhus, leishmaniasis). Certain microorganisms have evolved mechanisms to shift this balance. Host immune reactions are evaded or directly subverted by infectious pathogens in several diseases. In African trypanosomiasis (sleeping sickness), the protozoan parasite induces a vigorous antibody response: opsinized trypomastigotes are rapidly cleared from blood. However, just as rapidly these parasites change surface antigens and evade this host defence mechanism. As a consequence of antigenic variation, successive waves of parasitemia occur, each inducing a different and temporarily effective antibody response until death of the host. Antigenic variation in response to selective pressures induced by circulating antibody is a relatively common evasion mechanism used by many microorganisms including the human immunodeficiency virus (HIV). But in addition to the evasion of neutralizing antibody through antigenic variation, HIV directly subverts the immune response. Such subversion of host defence by HIV is manifest in at least three arenas. First and best characterized is the pathognomonic depletion of CD4+ helper T cells throughout the disease. This T cell subpopulation initiates either directly or indirectly virtually all other immune phenomenon. HIV is tropic for and lytic to this vital T cell subset. Second, antibodies produced by the infected patient against HIV enhance virus uptake in CD4+ target cells and also expand the total pool of susceptible cells through FcR-mediated infection of CD4- target cells. Third, HIV subverts the cytokine network of T cell-macrophage interactions to enhance viral gene expression (IL-1, IL-2, IL-6, TNFα, MCSF, GMCSF) and incapacitate the major antiviral defence of the body, interferon (IFN) (1). This latter HIV-associated immune subversion is the subject of this report.

There is well established precedent for IFN as dominant regulatory molecules in host defence reactions against such retroviral infections as murine and avian leukemia and several lentiviral diseases. In visna-maedi virus infection virus replication in ovine macrophages is reduced ≥1000-fold by IFN released from T cells (2). The role of IFN in human retroviral disease is more complex. In HIV infection, IFN activity is paradoxically found in sera of patients with late stage HIV disease, and is an index of poor prognosis. But strong antiviral activity is reported with addition of IFNα, IFNβ, and IFNγ to HIV-infected T cells and macrophages (3). With PHA/IL-2 treated T cells, the time course for appearance and quantity of p24 antigen (Ag) in culture fluids of cells exposed to 500 IU/ml recombinant human IFNα at the time of HIV infection and continuously thereafter were indistinguishable from those of infected control cells through 3 wks (4). The frequency of cells that expressed HIV mRNA in control and IFN-treated cells (about 20% at 10 days by *in situ* hybridization) were also similar. In contrast, levels of virion-associated reverse transcriptase (RT) activity in culture fluids from these same IFN-treated cells were reduced 2 to 3-fold from those of infected control cells. Reduced levels of RT activity were matched by parallel reductions in infectious titer. In a series of 8 separate experiments with 3 different HIV isolates, maximal inhibition of RT activity in culture fluids of IFN-treated HIV-infected T cells was 50 to 70% that of infected control cells at 500 to 10,000 IU/ml IFN. No amount of IFN could prevent HIV infection or completely restrict virus replication. Coincident with this partial reduction in RT activity levels and infectious titer in the culture fluids of IFN-treated HIV-infected T cells, RT activity levels in cell lysates from the identical cultures were increased about 2-fold. Thus, the major effect of IFN on the replication of HIV in T cells is directed at virus assembly or release: the frequency of cells productively infected with virus and the levels of viral proteins produced by infected cells remain unchanged (or increased) by

IFN treatment; the number of virions released from these infected cells, however, is reduced about 2-fold.

In contrast to the relatively modest effect of IFN on the replication of HIV in T cells, the effect of this cytokine on monocytes was quite dramatic. Addition of 50 to 500 IU/ml IFN with the HIV inoculum and continuous exposure of monocytes to IFN thereafter completely abrogated productive virus infection. No p24 Ag or RT activity was detected in culture fluids of IFN-treated infected monocytes at any time after infection. Analysis of IFN-treated HIV-infected monocytes by *in situ* hybridization for HIV mRNA showed no evidence of productive infection 2 wks after virus challenge (20 to 30% of control infected monocytes expressed HIV mRNA at the same time point). Polymerase chain reaction amplification (PCR) of DNA in cell lysates of monocytes treated with IFN with LTR and *gag* primers showed no proviral DNA. Thus, monocytes treated with IFN at the time of virus challenge show no evidence of HIV infection: no viral protein, no viral mRNA, and no proviral DNA. IFN interrupts one or more early events in the virus replication cycle *before* the formation of proviral DNA: binding, uptake, uncoating, or reverse transcription. Despite obvious differences in response to IFN by T cells and monocytes, levels of IFN-induced antiviral enzyme activities in the two cell types were similar (Table 1). The exact mechanisms for IFN-induced anti-HIV activity in monocytes are not yet known but may include: (a) changes in virus receptor number or distribution (IFN-treated monocytes show marked changes in CD4, FcR, CD11a, and mannosylated protein receptors, each of which is implicated in the uptake of HIV into monocytes); (b) changes in the monocyte plasma membrane that interrupt fusion or uptake of the virion into the cell (IFN-treated cells show alterations in membrane fluidity, microfilament organization, and membrane proteases that damage bound virus); and (c) changes in subcellular compartments or cytosolic milieu that preclude reverse transcription (IFN-treated cells synthesize 2'-5'(A)oligonucleotides that induce RNases, and directly inhibit reverse transcription).

Addition of IFN to monocytes previously infected with HIV for 7 days induced a dramatic decrease in both p24 Ag and RT activity. Quantitation of the infectious virus released into culture fluids 2 days after IFN treatment showed a 1000-fold decrease in infectious titer, but only a 3-fold decrease in RT activity at the same time point. Such discordance suggests that most progeny virions produced after IFN-treatment are defective. However, analysis of these virions by transmission electron microscopy and by radioimmunoprecipitation with HIV-seropositive sera failed to document morphological-

Table 1. Effect of IFNα on HIV replication and induction of antiviral enzymatic activities in T cells and monocytes

	HIV REPLICATION			ANTIVIRAL ENZYMES		
	RT activity	HIV mRNA	proviral DNA	2'5'oligoA synthetase	RNase L	protein kinase (p68)
T cells						
	++	+++	+++	+++	+++	+++
monocytes						
before infection						
	0	0	0	+++	+++	+++
after infection						
	0	0	+++	+++	+++	+++

ly aberrant viral particles or abnormal proteins. Additionally, patterns of virus budding at the monocyte plasma membrane or within intracytoplasmic vacuoles were no different from those of control infected cultures. Ten to 14 days after IFN treatment, no p24 Ag or RT activity was detected in culture fluids or cell lysates of HIV-infected monocytes. IFN-treatment also induced a dramatic reversal of cytopathic changes associated with HIV-infection. Multinucleated giant cells were evident 7 days after infection with a frequency of about 20% of total cells. Addition of IFN to these cultures at 7 days was associated with a gradual decrease in the frequency of multinucleated giant cells and absence of cell lysis through 3 wks. In contrast, the frequency of multinucleated giant cells in control infected cultures increased to 30 to 50% of total cells and cell lysis was common.

In the absence of detectable levels of viral proteins (p24 Ag or RT activity), or of morphologic evidence for virus infection, proviral DNA was still detected 2 and 3 wks after virus challenge in monocytes treated with IFN 7 days after infection. PCR amplification of cell lysates with HIV DNA primers showed levels of proviral DNA in the IFN-treated infected monocytes equivalent to that of control infected cells. Southern blot analysis of DNA from IFN-treated and control infected cells showed similar results. Levels of HIV mRNA detected by Northern blot analysis in the IFN-treated HIV-infected monocytes were reduced >95% of those of control infected cells. Analysis of these same cell populations by *in situ* hybridization for HIV mRNA showed productive infection in 21 ± 3% untreated HIV-infected cells versus 1 ± 1% IFN-treated HIV-infected monocytes. The presence of high levels of proviral DNA in cells with little or no evidence for active transcription suggests true microbiological latency...and this in a nonreplicating cell with no direct evidence for integrated virus. Such transcriptional restriction of virus replication in the IFN-treated HIV-infected monocytes has no precedent in previously described retroviral systems.

The preceding data presents an apparent paradox. IFN shows potent antiviral activity in macrophages. IFN also has antiviral activity in HIV-infected patients: in a randomized, placebo-controlled trial, asymptomatic HIV-seropositive individuals given IFN daily for ≤12 wks remained free of AIDS-associated opportunistic infections (0 of 16 patients) for up to 3 years; 30% (5 of 16 patients) of the placebo-treated control patients developed such infections over the same time interval (5). Yet the major source of IFN during any infection is the macrophage. In HIV-infected patients, virtually all blood monocytes and most tissue macrophages (cells of the brain, lung, and lymph nodes excepted) are free of virus (1). If IFN is effective in HIV-infected patients, and most macrophages (the primary source of IFN) are free of virus infection, why is there HIV disease? The answer to this question may derive from from an HIV-induced defect in the immune system as significant for progression of disease as the well-known depletion of CD4+ T cells. Monocytes from HIV-infected patients and monocytes from HIV-seronegative donors infected *in vitro* with monocyto tropic HIV fail to produce IFN after any of numerous treatments with agents that induce high titers of IFN in cultures of control cells.

No IFN activity (inhibition of virus-induced cytopathic effects in human fibroblasts) was detected in culture fluids of uninfected or HIV-infected monocytes or T cells with any of 15 different HIV isolates at any time through 3 wks. Similarly, levels of TNFα, IL-1β, or IL-6 in these culture fluids are ≤1 pg/ml (6). Culture fluids from uninfected control monocytes treated with synthetic double-stranded RNA [poly(I).(C)] contain high levels of IFN activity: >1000 IU/ml 24 hr after treatment (Table 2). Antibody neutralization studies show >99% of antiviral activity is IFNα. In striking contrast, poly(I).(C)-treated monocytes infected with HIV 14 days previously produce little or no IFN activity at any time through 3 days. HIV-associated inhibition of poly(I).(C)-induced IFN activity in culture fluids of virus-infected monocytes increases with time after infection:<10% at 1, 50% at 3, 80% at 5, 90% at 7, and >99% at 14 days. It is important to note that at 14 days, <50% of monocytes in these cultures are positive for HIV mRNA by *in situ* hybridization. In replicate experiments with 3 different HIV isolates, no IFN activity (≤10 IU/ml) was detected in culture

Table 2. Cytokine activity (pg/ml by ELISA) and mRNA at 24 hr in HIV-infected monocytes treated with poly(I).(C)

IL-1β activity	IL-1β mRNA	IL-6 activity	IL-6 mRNA	TNFα activity	TNFα mRNA	IFNα activity	IFNα mRNA
Uninfected monocytes							
10	+++	900	+++	1100	+++	2400	+++
HIV-infected monocytes							
70	+++	300	+++	1650	+++	0	0

fluids of HIV-infected monocytes treated with poly(I).(C), New Castle disease virus or herpes simplex virus 10 to 30 days after HIV inoculation.

To further define the extent and specificity of the HIV-induced defect in IFN production in monocytes, we examined IFNα mRNA using coupled reverse transcription/PCR analysis. While IFNα mRNA was evident in cell lysates of uninfected monocytes 8 through 24 hrs after poly(I).(C) treatment, no IFNα mRNA was found in any cell lysate of HIV-infected monocytes treated with identical conditions and for identical time intervals. Replicate experiments with primer pairs specific for the mRNA transcripts of 3 different members of the IFNα family (IFNα1, IFNα2, IFNα13) showed significant levels of IFNα mRNA in cell lysates of uninfected poly(I).(C)-treated monocytes, but none in the HIV-infected cells. These results confirm the near absence of IFN activity in culture fluids of poly(I).(C)-treated, HIV-infected, monocytes and localize this HIV-associated defect to a transcriptional block.

The specificity of this HIV-associated transcriptional block in expression of IFNα genes was explored by quantitation of mRNA for several other cytokines induced in monocytes by poly(I).(C). Coupled reverse transcription/PCR analysis of mRNA for IL-1β, IL-6, and TNFα in cell lysates of uninfected and HIV-infected monocytes showed no cytokine mRNA. These results are consistent with the absence of these cytokines as detected by ELISA in monocyte culture fluids and with published reports (7). After poly(I).(C) treatment high and indistinguishable levels of mRNA of IL-1β, IL-6, and TNFα were identified in cell lysates from both uninfected and HIV-infected monocytes. High levels of mRNA were associated with similarly high concentrations of these same cytokines in culture fluids as detected by ELISA. The strong HIV-associated transcriptional block in the expression of IFNα genes was not evident in expression of several other cytokine genes. Moreover, while IFNα is the predominant IFN activity produced by monocytes, it is not the only IFN expressed by these cells. IFNβ and IFNω are minor species of IFN genetically distinct from the IFNa family of genes (8). Both uninfected and HIV-infected monocytes expressed IFNβ and IFNω mRNA after poly(I).(C) treatment: there was no differences in the amount or time course for appearance of these mRNA in cell lysates of uninfected or HIV-infected monocytes. These results, *in toto*, document a profound and highly specific transcriptional block in the expression of IFNα genes in monocytes infected with HIV. The inability of HIV-infected monocytes to express IFNα may represent an adaptive response by this virus to ensure its survival and unimpeded replication in monocytes. The inevitable result of this HIV-induced cytokine dysregulation is virus replication and persistence in mononuclear phagocytes.

In the HIV-infected patient, production of all IFN types is suppressed: production of IFNγ by PBMC of HIV infected patients is reduced; transcription of the IFNγ gene, but not the IL-2 gene, is impaired in HIV-infected T cells (9). Similarly, monocytes and PBMC from HIV-infected patients show a markedly reduced ability to secrete IFNα or express IFNα mRNA after exposure to vesicular stomatitis virus, influenza A virus, or herpes simplex virus-infected fibroblasts (10). The mechanism for the transcriptional block in IFNα gene expression is not yet known. Remarkably, HIV-infected monocyte cultures that exhibited this near absolute IFNα defect showed a frequency for productively infected cells of <50%. If the IFNα defect is a direct sequela of infection, then all cells must harbor the HIV provirus which in turn is expressed in only half of the monocytes. Alternatively, the IFNα defect may be mediated by a soluble factor released by HIV-infected cells that affects the entire cell population. This latter hypothesis is consistent with observations on PBMC of HIV-infected patients in which a cell population that is >99% virus-free shows a 1000-fold decrease in ability to produce IFNα (11).

REFERENCES

1. Meltzer MS, Skillman DS, Gomatos PJ, Kalter DC, Gendelman HE (1990). Role of mononuclear phagocytes inthe pathogenesis of human immunodeficiency virus infection. Ann Rev Immunol 8: 169-194.
2. Zinc MC and Narayan O (1989). Lentivirus-induced interferon inhibits maturation and proliferation of monocytes and restricts the replication of caprine arthritis encephalitis virus. J Virol 63: 2578-2584.

3. Kornbluth RS, Oh PS, Munis JR, Cleveland PH, Richman DD (1990). The role of interferons in the control of HIV replication in macrophages. Clin Immunol Immunopath 54: 200-219.
4. Gendelman HE, Baca L, Turpin J, Kalter DC, Hansen B, Orenstein JM, Dieffenbach C, Friedman RM, Meltzer, MS (1990). Regulation of HIV replication in infected monocytes by IFNα: mechanisms for viral restriction. J Immunol (in press).
5. Lane HC, Davey V, Kovacs JA, Feinberg J, Metcalf JA, Herpin B, Walker R, Deyton L, Davey RT Jr, Falloon J, Polis MA, Salzman NP, Baseler M, Masur H, Fauci, AS (1990). Interferon-α in patients with asymptomatic human immunodeficiency virus (HIV) infection A randomized, placebo-controlled trial. Ann Int Med 112: 805-812.
6. Gendelman HE, Friedman RM, Joe S, Baca LM, Turpin JA, Dveksler G, Meltzer MS, Dieffenbach C (1990). A selective defect of IFNα production in HIV-infected monocytes. J Exp Med (in press).
7. Molina J-F, Scadden DT, Amirault C, Woon A, Vannier E, Dinarello CA, Groopman JE (1990). Human immunodeficiency virus does not induce interleukin-1, interleukin-6, or tumor necrosis factor in mononuclear cells. J Virol 64: 2901-2906.
8. Adolf GR (1987). Antigenic structure of human interferon-ω^1(interferon $\alpha_{II}{}^1$): Comparison with other human interferons. J Gen Virol 68: 1669-1674.
9. Arya SK, Gallo RC (1985).: Human T cell growth factor (interleukin 2) and γ-interferon genes: expression in human T-lymphotropic virus type III-and type I-infected cells. Proc Natl Acad Sci USA 82:8691-8698.
10. Abb J, Piechowiak H, Zachoval R, Zachoval V, Deinhardt F (1986). Infection with human T-lymphotropic virus type III and leukocyte interferon production in homosexual men. Eur J Clin Microbiol 5: 365-368.
11. Voth R, Rossol S, Klein K, Hess G, Schutt KH, Schroder HC, Meyer Zum Buschenfelde K-H, Muller WEG (1990). Differential gene expression of IFN-α and tumor necrosis factor-α in peripheral blood mononuclear cells from patients with AIDS related complex and AIDS. J Immun 144: 970-975.

Cellular and Cytokine Networks in Tissue Immunity, pages 213-219

ROLE OF LEUKOCYTE ADHESINS IN THE INFECTION OF MONOCYTES AND T CELLS BY THE HUMAN IMMUNODEFICIENCY VIRUS-1 (HIV)

D. Chester Kalter, Howard E. Gendelman, and Monte S. Meltzer

H. M. Jackson Foundation (D.C.K.,H.E.G.) and Dept. Cell. Immunol.(M.S.M.), Walter Reed Army Inst. Res., Rockville, MD 20850

There are two major ways that HIV infection can spread between susceptible target cells. HIV virions released from an infected cell can infect other cells from the fluid phase at both local and distant sites. Infectious virus can also spread cell-to-cell without exposure to the extracellular milieu. Such cell-to-cell spread is described for herpes simplex, varicella-zoster, and rabies virus (1). HIV-induced syncytia in infected T cell and monocyte cultures (fusion between infected cells expressing gp120 and uninfected cells expressing CD4) enables cell-to-cell spread of virus. Zidovudine and neutralizing sera from patients infected with HIV prevent virus transmission from the fluid-phase, but have little or no effect on cell-to-cell spread of virus (2). On the other hand, monoclonal antibodies (mAb) against CD4 completely prevent both cell syncytia and cell-to-cell spread of virus (3). Despite this latter observation, there are several lines of evidence that suggest fusion of HIV-infected with uninfected cells requires membrane interactions in addition to those between gp120 and CD4: (a) the number of syncytia that form between HIV infected and uninfected cells does not correlate with CD4 density; (b) HIV infected cells fuse with CD4-negative human cells transfected with CD4 cDNA, but not with mouse cells transfected with the identical transcript; and (c) capacities of sera from HIV-infected patients to inhibit binding of HIV to CD4-positive cells and to block HIV-induced syncytia formation do not correlate (4-6).

Several recent reports suggest participation of the LFA intercellular adhesion receptor family in HIV-induced syncytia (4,7). The LFA family of adhesion receptors (LFA-1, CR3, and p150,95) are heterodimers of a unique α subunit (CD11a, CD11b, and CD11c) and a common β subunit (CD18). Unlike other integrins, LFA-1 is constitutively and exclusively expressed on all leukocytes. The binding avidity of LFA-1 to its ligand, ICAM-1, is upregulated after any of several reactions including stimulation of resting T lymphocytes with specific antigen (Ag), phorbol myristate acetate (PMA), or mAb against CD2 and CD3 (8,9). Interactions between LFA-1 and ICAM-1 induce cell aggregation integral to Ag-independent lymphocyte-mediated cytotoxicity, and induction of Ag-specific T cell proliferation.

Hildreth and Orentas showed inhibition of syncytia between 8E5 cells, an HIV-infected T cell line, and PHA-stimulated T lymphoblasts by mAb against CD18 and (less effectively) CD11a (4). None of these mAb inhibit the binding of gp120 to CD4-positive CEM cells. Studies by Valentin *et al.* showed inhibition of HIV-induced syncytia by monoclonal anti-CD18 with infectious HIV (HTLV-IIIB) in both T cell and myeloid cell lines (7). In the continuous presence of anti-CD18, the number of syncytia and the frequency of infected cells in the U937 myeloid cell line infected with HIV at 2 to 3 wks were both suppressed: 2 to 5% infected cells in antibody-treated cultures versus 60% infected cells in the controls. The same antibody added to HIV-infected cells 1 wk after infection had little or no effect on either virus replication or cytopathicity. The suppressive effects of monoclonal anti-CD18 were freely reversible after removal of the antibody 1 wk after infection. Both of these studies document participation of intercellular adhesion receptors in cell-to-cell spread of virus. The mechanism for this participation is through facilitation of cell syncytia formation and not by direct interaction with the HIV virion or envelope glycoproteins.

In a series of studies, we have confirmed the initial observations of Hildreth and Orentas and of Valentin *et al.* in T cell and myeloid cell lines in primary cultures of T cells and monocytes derived from peripheral blood mononuclear cells (PBMC). PHA/IL-2 treated T cells and MCSF-treated monocytes were treated with mAb against CD4, CD11a, CD11b, and CD15 for 15 min at 4° C, and then exposed to the HIV isolate, ADA, at a multiplicity of infection of 0.01 infectious virus/cell. After a 2 hr viral adsorption, cultures were washed twice and refed with fresh medium with mAb. Culture fluids was half exchanged every 3 days for 6 wks with medium without mAb. Levels of virus associated reverse transcriptase (RT) activity in culture fluids were assayed at intervals (Table 1). MAb against CD4 inhibited HIV replication in both T cells and monocytes. Cells treated with mAb against CD11a (LFA-1) also failed to support the replication of HIV, but equal concentrations of mAb against CD11b (Mac 1) or CD15 (Leu M1) were ineffective.

Similar experiments with > 20 different mAb against the

Table 1. Effect of mAb against CD4 and CD11a on HIV infection of T cells and monocytes

mAb:	RT activity (cpm/ml x 10^{-4}) in culture fluids of HIV-infected cells at: PHA/IL-2 treated T cells 5 days	10 days	15 days	MCSF treated monocytes 5 days	10 days	15 days
medium	22	94	86	4	90	243
anti-CD4						
10 ug/ml	4	3	2	1	3	15
1 ug/ml	3	3	2	2	3	17
0.1 ug/ml	4	21	90	--	--	--
anti-CD11a						
10 ug/ml	4	3	3	1	3	3
1 ug/ml	4	4	5	1	3	3
0.1 ug/ml	5	80	112	1	4	3
anti-CD11b						
10 ug/ml	60	159	105	4	81	201
anti-CD15						
10 ug/ml	5	28	84	6	95	260

receptors and ligands of distinct groups of leukocyte adhesins appears to document a general phenomenon (Table 2). Inhibition of adhesion-dependent interactions between leukocytes through LFA-1/ICAM-1, CD4/MHC class II, and CD2/LFA-3 each inhibited the replication of HIV in monocytes. Inhibition by any of these mAb may in whole or in part be a direct consequence of blocking cell-to-cell adhesion. For most mAb, inhibition of HIV replication was partial and modest (30 to 90% decrease in RT activity levels at 3 to 4 wks) with no direct correlation to inhibition of PMA-induced homotypic aggregation of PBMC. For example, mAb to CD11a (TS 1/22) and CD18 (TS 1/22) completely inhibited homotypic aggregation of PBMC, yet did not inhibit the replication of HIV in monocytes. Conversely, mAb against CD58 (LFA-3, the ligand for CD2) inhibited HIV replication (80% decrease in RT activity levels at 3 wks with 10 ug/ml mAb), but had little or no effect on PMA-induced homotypic aggregation of PBMC. The interaction between CD4 and MHC class II represents an obvious special case: CD4 is the receptor for HIV on T cells and monocytes; HIV binds to CD4 through the envelope glycoprotein, gp120. The binding sites on CD4 for gp120 and MHC class II partially overlap, so binding of gp120 to CD4 inhibits subsequent binding of MHC class II and completely blocks CD4-dependent lymphokine production (10). Some mAb against MHC class II (HLA-DR, but not HLA-DP or HLA-DQ) directly block HIV infection of T cells (11). HLA-DR and CD4

Table 2. Effect of mAb against leukocyte adhesins on HIV infection of monocytes and homotypic aggregation

Plasma membrane determinant	Clone	Ability of mAb to inhibit: HIV infection of monocytes	Homotypic aggregation
Leukocyte adhesion proteins			
CD11a	TS 1/22	0	++++
(α chain, LFA-1)	25.3.1	+	++++
	SPV-L7	++	+++
	CLB-171	++++	++++
CD11b	D12	0	0
(α chain, Mac-1)	Bear 1	0	0
CD11c	BU15	0	0
(α chain, p150,95)	S.HCL.3	0	0
CD18	TS 1/18	0	++++
(β chain)	BL5	0	0
CD54 (ICAM-1)	RR 1/1	+	+
	84H10	+	+
CD4/MHC class II			
CD4 (Leu 3a)	OKT4a	++++	0
HLA-DR	L243	+	--
CD2/LFA-3			
CD2 (Leu 5b)	S5.2	0	0
CD58 (LFA-3)	TS 2/9	++	0
CD14 (Leu M3)	RM052	0	0
CD15 (Leu M1)	MMA	0	--
CD3 (Leu 4)	SK7	0	--

expression are both transiently decreased during viral attachment and entry. Only CD4 expression and not HLA-DR decreases with gp120 treatment. HLA-DR does not directly interact with viral proteins during viral attachment, but is likely affected by viral entry because of its close proximity to CD4. Finally, results with a mAb against CD11a (clone CLB-171) were conspicuously different from those of 3 other mAb against CD11a. All four mAb against CD11a strongly inhibited the homotypic aggregation of PBMC. One of these mAb (clone TS 1/22) did not inhibit HIV infection of monocytes. Two other mAb (clones 25.3.1 and SPV-L7) were only partially inhibitory. The mAb CLB-171 was as effective for blocking HIV infection of monocytes as an equal concentration (<0.1 ug/ml) of mAb against CD4.

Further analysis of the effects of mAb against CD11a from the CLB-171 clone on HIV infection of monocytes showed complete inhibition of virus infection at <0.1 ug/ml. In T

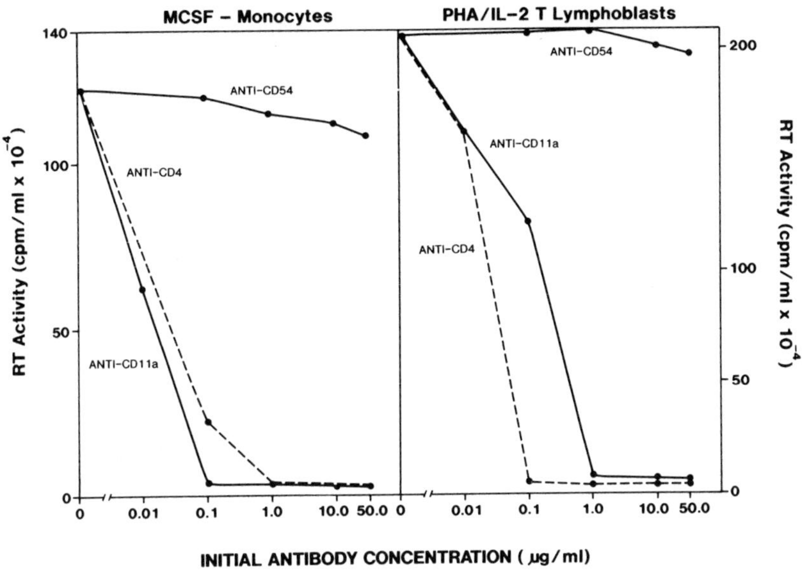

Figure 1.

cells the effective dose was 10 to 50-fold higher (Figure 1). Cells pretreated with mAb and exposed to the HIV inoculum showed no evidence of virus infection: (a) levels of RT activity and p24 Ag were at baseline through 6 wks; (b) HIV-associated cytopathic effects (multinucleated giant cells, cell lysis) were absent in treated cultures; (c) no productively infected cells were detected by *in situ* hybridization for HIV mRNA; and (d) no proviral DNA was detected in cell lysates by polymerase chain reaction amplification with primer pairs for HIV DNA. The absence of HIV proviral DNA in monocytes treated with mAb from the CLB-171 clone strongly suggests that the site of action for this mAb is not through inhibition of cell-to-cell spread of virus, but rather through interference with one or more early events in the viral entry pathway that precedes formation of the provirus. This conclusion is further supported by experiments that dissociate the antiviral effects of this mAb with its interaction in the LFA-1/ICAM-1 complex. The affinity of LFA-1 for ICAM-1 is markedly increased by prior treatment with mAb against CD2 and CD3 in T cells, and by CD14 in monocytes (12). HIV replication is not enhanced in the presence of these mAb, despite the upregulation of cell-to-cell adhesion. Formation of the LFA-1/ICAM-1 complex is dependent upon temperature (37°C) and divalent cations (Mg^{+2}/Ca^{+2}). None of the preceding factors affect the antiviral activity of mAb from clone CLB-171.

The antiviral activity of mAb from the CLB-171 clone might be mediated through direct interaction with binding sites on the HIV virion, or with plasma membrane determinants necessary for virus attachment and entry. Virus interacts with susceptible target cells through both specific and nonspecific attachment sites. Specific viral receptors are characterized for: HIV (CD4), the major human rhinoviruses (ICAM-1), polio virus (an immunoglobulin-like glycoprotein), Epstein-Barr virus (C3d receptor), rabies virus (acetylcholine receptor), reovirus (β-adrenergic receptor), vaccinia virus (epidermal growth factor receptor), and herpes simplex virus type-1 (basic fibroblast growth factor receptor)(1). Only the virus that binds to the specific receptor initiates the sequence of events that result in productive infection. For HIV this sequence includes internalization of the virion by direct membrane fusion or receptor-mediated endocytosis, removal of the outer lipid envelope after fusion with cytoplasmic vacuoles, reverse transcription from the core particle of virion RNA into DNA, translocation into the nucleus and integration of the proviral DNA into the genome of the host cell. Binding sites to the specific receptor on a virus tend to be highly conserved between viral strains or isolates and relatively inaccessible to antibody. In contrast, molecular regions surrounding the receptor binding sites are often hypervariable and frequently the targets for neutralizing antibodies. The nonspecific binding sites on target cells are often more numerous than the specific virus receptors and range from low affinity interactions between viral-associated glycoproteins or lipids and components of the host cell surface to the relatively high affinity interactions of lectin-like receptors for glycosylated proteins, or receptors for complement split products and the Fc portion of immunoglobulins. The role of these nonspecific binding sites as accessory molecules in the anchorage of virus to the host cell membrane varies with viral strain and target cell, but may be considerable:<10% of the binding of HIV to the U937 myeloid cell line is CD4-dependent (13).

Although CD4 is the primary receptor for HIV, other cell surface determinants may be involved in viral entry. It is tempting to speculate that the plasma membrane determinants recognized by mAb from clone CLB-171 participate as viral attachment sites during HIV infection and function either as an alternative receptor for virus or as an accessory molecule that facilitates CD4-mediated infection. In any case, identification of another site at which HIV infection can be inhibited opens new avenues of therapeutic intervention.

REFERENCES

1. Kaner RJ, Baird A, Mansukhani A, Basilico C, Summers BD, Florkiewicz RZ, Hajjar DP (1990). Fibroblast growth factor receptor is a portal of cellular entry for Herpes simplex virus type 1.Science 248: 1410-1413.
2. Lifson JD, Feinberg MB, Reyes GR, Rabin L, Banapour B, Chakrabarti S, Moss B, Wong-Staal F, Steimer KS, Engleman EG (1986).Induction of CD4-dependent cell fusion by the HTLV-III/LAV envelope glycoprotein. Nature 323: 725-728.
3. Dalgleish AG, Beverley PCL, Clapham PR, Crawford DH, Greaves MF, Weiss RA (1984). The CD4 (T4) antigen is an essential component of the receptor for the AIDS retrovirus. Nature 312: 763-767.
4. Hildreth JEK, Orentas RJ (1989). Involvement of a leukocyte adhesion receptor (LFA-1) in HIV-induced syncytium formation. Science 244:1075-1078.
5. Maddon PJ, Dalgleish AG, McDougal JS, Clapham PR, Weiss RA, Axel R (1986). The T4 gene encodes the AIDS virus receptor and is expressed in the immune system and the brain. Cell 47: 333-348.
6. Gomatos PJ, Stamatos NM, Gendelman HE, Fowler A, Hoover DL, Kalter DC, Burke DS, Tramont EC, Meltzer MS (1990).Relative inefficiency of soluble recombinant CD4 for inhibition of infection by monocyte-tropic HIV in monocytes and T cells. J Immunol 144: 4183-4188.
7. Valentin A, Lundin K, Patarroyo M, Asjo B (1990). The leukocyte adhesion glycoprotein CD18 participates in HIV-1-induced syncytia formation in monocytoid and T cells. J Immunol 144:934-937.
8. Dustin ML, Springer TA (1989). T-cell receptor cross-linking transiently stimulates adhesiveness through LFA-1. Nature 341: 619-624.
9. van Kooyk Y, van de Wiel-van Kemenade P, Weder P, Kuijpers TW, Figdor (1989). Enhancement of LFA-1-mediated cell adhesion by triggering through CD2 or CD3 on T lymphocytes. Nature 342: 811-813.
10. Diamond DC, Sleckman BP, Gregory T, Lasky LA, Greenstein JL, Burakoff SJ (1988). Inhibition of CD4+ T cell function by the HIV envelope protein, gp120. J Immunol 141: 3715-3717.
11. Mann DL, Read-Connole E, Arthur LO, Robey WG, Wernet P, Schneider EM, Blattner WA, Popovic M (1988). HLA-DR is involved in the HIV-1 binding site on cells expressing MHC class II antigens. J Immunol 141: 1131-1136.
12. Lauener RP, Geha RS, Vercelli D (1990). Engagement of the monocyte surface antigen CD14 induces LFA-1/ICAM-1 dependent homotypic adhesion. J Immunol 145: 1390-1394.
13. Pauza CD and Price TM (1988). Human immunodeficiency virus infection of T cells and monocytes proceed via receptor-mediated endocytosis. J Cell Biol 107: 959-968.

Cellular and Cytokine Networks in Tissue Immunity, pages 221-227

Nitric Oxide Synthesis from L-arginine: A Cytokine Induced Effector Mechanism that Targets Intracellular Iron

John B. Hibbs, Jr., and Donald L. Granger*

Division of Infectious Diseases, Department of Medicine, Veterans Affairs Medical Center and University of Utah School of Medicine, Salt Lake City, Utah 84148; *Division of Infectious Diseases, Department of Medicine, Duke University, Durham, North Carolina 27710

It was recognized for many years that infection with intracellular pathogens increased the resistance of animals to challenge with an unrelated intracellular pathogen or to transplanted tumor cells (reviewed in Ref 1). In the 1970's activated macrophages from mice with chronic intracellular infections were demonstrated to be nonspecifically cytotoxic for tumor cell *in vitro* (2-6). It was observed in these studies that nonspecific resistance mechanisms for intracellular pathogens and tumor cells appeared to be related and mediated by the same effector cells, e.g., activated macrophages. Macrophages from normal uninfected mice were not activated and were not cytotoxic *in vitro* for intracellular pathogens or tumor cells. Later it was shown the acquisition of cytotoxic activity by activated macrophages required several steps (7-10). The first step produced noncytotoxic activated macrophages or primed macrophages. Primed macrophages were produced *in vivo* by chronic infection with an intracellular pathogen such as the BCG strain of *Mycobacterium bovis* or *in vitro* by exposing peritoneal macrophages from uninfected mice to interferon-γ (IFN-γ). However, expression of cytotoxicity required a second step, e.g., exposure to a microbial product such as lipopolysaccharide (LPS). Later studies showed that tumor necrosis factor (TNF) was a potent second signal (11,12). Microbial products such as muramyl dipeptide or LPS act, at least in part, by inducing TNF synthesis which is a physiologic final inducer of the activated macrophage effector mechanism (11). Therefore, macrophages are activated by classical cell-mediated immune mechanisms to express nonspecific cytotoxicity for microorganisms and tumor cells *in vivo* and *in vitro*.

The first reproducible metabolic effect of activated macrophage induced cytotoxicity recognized was inhibition of DNA replication in tumor target cells (13,14). However, little else was known about the metabolic consequences of this effector mechanism. In the late 1970's studies were initiated with the goal of attaining better understanding of activated macrophage mediated cytotoxic effects at the biochemical level. Results showed that tumor target cells co-cultivated with activated macrophages develop inhibition of mitochondrial respiration and that some tumor cell lines (nonlytic phenotypes) remain viable and continue to synthesize ATP via the glycolytic pathway (15). Granger and Lehninger then demonstrated that this activated macrophage induced effect is due to inhibition of the proximal two oxidoreductases of mitochondrial electron transport system; complex I and complex II (16). Other enzymes of the mitochondrial electron transport system of tumor target cells were not affected. Complex I and complex II are iron-sulfur (Fe-S) flavoprotein dehydrogenases that contain most of the Fe-S complexes of the mitochondrial electron transport chain and which are essential for the catalytic function of these two oxidoreductases. Experiments were then performed to determine if the activated macrophage effector mechanism causes perturbation of intracellular iron metabolism in tumor target cells during cocultivation. Results showed that tumor target cells co-cultivated with activated macrophages released a significant fraction of their intracellular iron content in parallel with development of inhibition of DNA synthesis and inhibition of mitochondrial respiration (17). The target cells remained viable and continued to synthesize ATP via the glycolytic pathway. Kinetic studies showed that specific release of iron-59 from target cells began 4-6 hours after initiating co-cultivation which was the time point that inhibition of DNA synthesis was first detected. Since both DNA replication and mitochondrial respiration are metabolic pathways with enzymatic activity vulnerable to inhibition by depletion of intracellular iron, this observation suggested a link between activated macrophage induced iron mobilization in target cells and activated macrophage induced cytotoxicity. Next aconitase, a citric acid cycle enzyme with a catalytically active (4Fe-4S) cluster, was examined to determine if Fe-S prosthetic groups are targets for activated macrophage induced iron removal (18). Results showed that aconitase activity declined dramatically in target cells after 4 hours of co-cultivation with activated macrophages. Aconitase inhibition occurred simultaneously with arrest of DNA synthesis. Incubation of activated macrophage injured target cells in culture medium supplemented with ferrous ions plus a reducing agent caused near complete reconstitution of aconitase activity. These results showed that removal of a labile iron atom from the (4Fe-4S) cluster, by an activated macrophage-mediated mechanism, is causally related to aconitase inhibition in tumor target cells.

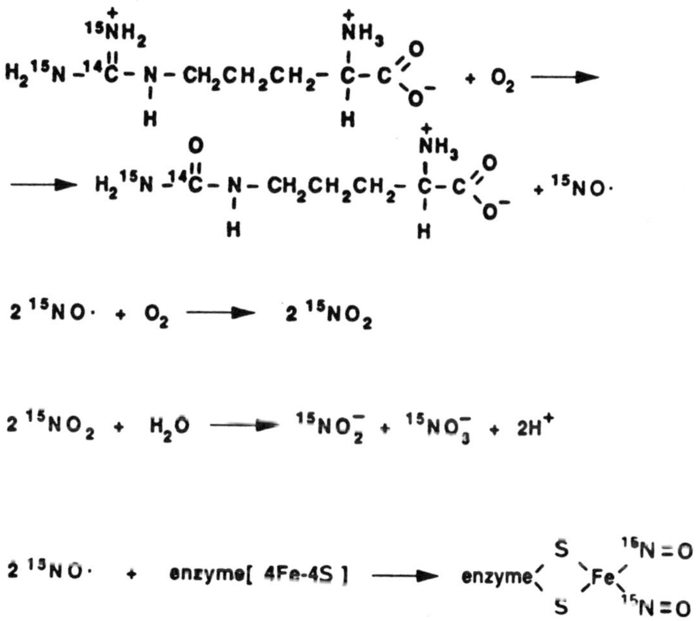

Fig 1. Precursor and products of the biological synthesis of inorganic nitrogen oxides and L-citrulline from L-arginine. Labelled products derived from L-[guanido-$^{15}N_2$ arginine were identified by gas chromatography/mass spectroscopy (21-23) or electroparamagnetic resonance (EPR) spectroscopy (29) except for nitrogen dioxide (NO_2) which was identified by another method (22) involving trapping as NO_2^- in absorbing solution. The direct synthesis of L-citrulline from L-arginine was identified by several techniques (20-23,25). The experiments utilizing L-[guanidino-^{14}C] arginine (22,25) are illustrated in the figure. NO formed by reaction 1 can undergo oxidative degradation in aqueous solution (reactions 2 and 3) or react with non-heme iron associated with sulfur atoms to form nitrosyl-iron-sulfur complexes (reaction 4). Although not shown, certain other forms of intracellular iron also probably form complexes with NO. Adapted from reference 22 with permission of the publisher.

Recently the effector mechanism causing disturbed intracellular iron homeostasis, inhibition of enzymes with iron dependent catalytic activity, and cytostasis was identified. It is a novel mammalian biochemical pathway synthesizing inorganic nitrogen oxides [nitric oxide (NO) nitrite (NO_2^-) and nitrate (NO_3^-)] from a terminal guanidino nitrogen atom of L-arginine (19-27). When L-arginine in the culture medium was replaced with D-arginine activated macrophages did not express cytotoxicity for tumor target cells and inorganic nitrogen oxide synthesis did not occur (19,20). In addition, the L-arginine analogue, NG-monomethyl-L-arginine (N^GMMLA), was found to be a potent competitive inhibitor of activated macrophage induced tumor cell cytostasis and metabolic injury as well as the synthesis of inorganic nitrogen oxides and L-citrulline from L-arginine (19,20). Evidence suggests that NO and L-citrulline are enzymatically synthesized from L-arginine (see Figure 1). Recent experiments demonstrated that authentic NO causes iron loss and the same pattern of biochemical inhibition in tumor cells as that induced by cocultivation with cytotoxic activated macrophages (22,27).

NO, a paramagnetic free radical, degrades to NO_2^- and NO_3^- nonenzymatically in an aerobic aqueous environment. Alternatively, NO can react covalently with intracellular iron. Particularly important, in terms of functional consequences, are nitrosylation reactions with Fe-S prosthetic groups and other forms of catalytically active iron that might occur. Since cytotoxic activated macrophages develop the same pattern of L-arginine dependent metabolic inhibition as is induced in their target cells (28) experiments were performed to identify iron nitrosyl complexes in the cytoplasm of cytotoxic active macrophages. Electron paramagnetic resonances spectroscopy studies demonstrated L-arginine dependent nitrosyl-iron-sulfur complex formation characterized by an axial signal at $g = 2.039$ in macrophages activated by a cell-mediated immune response *in vivo* or by IFN-γ *in vitro* (29,30). This signal was not observed in normal resident macrophages or not in peritoneal macrophages mobilized in response to a sterile inflammatory stimulant such as thioglycollate broth in the absence of an intracellular infection. The formation of nitrosyl-iron-sulfur complexes with Fe-S prosthetic groups of complex I and complex II of the mitochondrial electron transport chain, with the Fe-S prosthetic group of aconitase, and the catalytically active iron of ribonucleotide reductase (rate limiting enzyme of the DNA biosynthetic pathway), provides a molecular explanation for the pattern of enzymatic inhibition caused by nitric oxide synthesis from L-arginine (13-20,22,24,25,28,31,32).

If inducible NO synthesis from L-arginine could inhibit enzymes within macrophage mitochondria (28) it could have a similar cytotoxic effect for facultative and obligate intracellular pathogens that parasitize macrophages. A reasonable hypothesis was that the L-arginine dependent effector pathway which is easily triggered in "primed" or noncytotoxic activated macrophages from mice with chronic intracellular infection must function to inhibit the proliferation or kill the intracellular pathogen in these infected mice. Therefore, experiments were performed to determine if NO synthesis from L-arginine has a role in resistance to microbial pathogens. Results showed that this newly defined effector pathway has potent cytotoxic effects for the fungal pathogen *Cryptococcus neoformans* (33,34), schistosomula of *Schistosoma mansoni* (35,36), intracellular amastigotes of *Leishmania major* (37,38) as well as intracellular trophozoites of *Toxoplasma gondii* (39). It is likely future investigations will expand the number of microbial pathogens sensitive to high output synthesis of NO from L-arginine induced by cytokines.

Although the biochemistry of this pathway (precursor and product molecules) and its relationship to activated macrophage mediated nonspecific cytotoxicity was not identified until 1987, the biological and biochemical consequences of this effector pathway, as well as signals needed for its induction, were studied systematically since the early 1970's and were briefly discussed above. It is now clear that induction of NO synthesis from L-arginine provides a unifying explanation for this earlier work as well as a new understanding of cell-mediated effector function at the biochemical level. The identification of nitrosyl-iron-sulfur complex formation in these studies links iron, which is known to be lost from cells that develop activated macrophage induced cytotoxicity, the inhibition of enzymes with iron dependent catalytic activity, and NO; which is synthesized by activated macrophages capable of expressing cytotoxicity (22,23,26). High output synthesis of NO from L-arginine also has been induced in adenocarcinoma cells (24,25), fibroblasts (25), hepatocytes (40), and endothelial cells (41). These findings suggest that increased levels of cytokines in the tissues can induce the L-arginine dependent effector pathway in somatic cells not specialized for host defense. These results broaden the concept of the cell-mediated immune response against neoplastic cells, intracellular microbes, and certain other pathogens.

Supported by the Department of Veterans Affairs. We are grateful to Colleen Sizemore for manuscript preparation.

References:

1. Hibbs, J.B., Jr., Remington, J.S. and Stewart, C.C. (1980) Pharmoc Ther 8: 37-69.
2. Hibbs, J.B., Jr., Lambert, L.H., Jr. and Remington, J.S. (1971) J Infect Dis 124: 587-592.
3. Hibbs, J.B., Jr., Lambert, L.H., Jr. and Remington, J.S. (1972) Nature New Biology 235: 48-50.
4. Hibbs, J.B., Jr., Lambert, L.H., Jr. and Remington, J.S. (1972) Science 177: 998-1000.
5. Hibbs, J.B., Jr. (1973) Science 180: 868-870.
6. Meltzer, M.S., Tucker, R.W. and Breuer, A.C. (1975) Cell Immunol 17: 30-36.
7. Hibbs, J.B., Jr., Taintor, R.R., Chapman, H.A., Jr. and Weinberg, J.B. (1977) Science 197: 279-282.
8. Russell, S.W., Doe, W.F. and McIntosh, A.T. (1977) J Exp Med 146: 1511-1520.
9. Weinberg, J.B., Chapman, H.A., Jr. and Hibbs, J.B., Jr. (1978) J. Immunol 121: 72-80.
10. Ruco, L.P. and Meltzer, M.S. (1978) J Immunol 121: 2035-2042.
11. Drapier, J-C., Wietzerbin, J., and Hibbs, J.B., Jr., (1988) Eur J Immunol 18: 1587-1592.
12. Ding, A.H., Nathan, C.F., and Stuehr, D.J. (1988) J Immunol 141: 2407-2414.
13. Keller, R. (1973) J Exp Med 138: 625-644
14. Krahenbuhl, J.L. and Remington, J.S. (1974) J Immunol 113: 507-516.
15. Granger, D.L., Taintor, R.R., Cook, J.L. and Hibbs, J.B., Jr. (1980) J Clin Invest 65: 357-370.
16. Granger, D.L. and Lehninger, A.L. (1982) J Cell Biol 95: 527-535.
17. Hibbs, J.B., Jr., Taintor, R.R. and Vavrin, Z. (1984) Biochem Biophys Res Commun 123: 716-723.
18. Drapier, J-C. and Hibbs, J.B., Jr. (1986) J Clin Invest 78: 790-797.
19. Hibbs, J.B., Jr., Vavrin, Z. and Taintor, R.R. (1987) J Immunol 138: 550-565.
20. Hibbs, J.B., Jr., Taintor, R.R. and Vavrin, Z. (1987) Science 235: 473-476.
21. Iyengar, R., Stuehr, D.J. and Marletta, M.A.

(1987) Proc Natl Acad Sci USA 84: 6369-6373.
22. Hibbs, J.B., Jr., Taintor, R.R., Vavrin, Z. and Rachlin, E.M. (1988) Biochem Biophys Res Commun 157: 87-94. (Erratum published Biochem Biophys Res Comm 1989;158:624.)
23. Marletta, M.A., Yoon, P.S., Iyengar, R., Leaf, C.D. and Wishnok, J.S. (1988) Biochemistry 27: 8706-8711.
24. Amber, I.J., Hibbs, J.B., Jr., Taintor, R.R. and Vavrin, Z. (1988) J. Leukoc Biol 43: 187-192.
25. Amber, I.J., Hibbs, J.B., Jr., Taintor, R.R. and Vavrin, Z. (1988) J. Leukoc Biol 44: 58-65.
26. Stuehr, D.J., Gross, S.S., Sakuma, I., Levi, R. and Nathan, C.F. (1989) J Exp Med 169: 1011-1020.
27. Stuehr, D.J. and Nathan, C.F. (1989) J Exp Med 169: 1543-1555.
28. Drapier, J-C. and Hibbs, J.B., Jr. (1988) J Immunol 140: 2829-2838.
29. Lancaster, J.R., Jr. and Hibbs, J.B., Jr. (1990) Proc Natl Acad Sci USA 87: 1223-1227.
30. Pellat, C., Henry, Y. and Drapier, J-C. (1990) Biochem Biophys Res Commun 166: 119-125.
31. Wharton, M, Granger, D.L. and Durack, D.T. (1986) J Immunol 141:1311-1317.
32. Lepoivre, M., Chenais, B., Yapo, A., Lemaire, G., Thelander, L. and Tenu, J-P. (1990) J Biol Chem 265: -14143-14149
33. Granger, D.L., Hibbs, J.B., Jr., Perfect, J.R. and Durack, D.T. (1988) J Clin Invest 81: 1129-1136.
34. Granger, D.L., Hibbs, J.B., Jr., Perfect, J.R. and Durack, D.T. (1990) J Clin Invest 85 264-273.
35. Malkin, R., Flescher, E., Lengy, J. and Keisari, Y. (1987) Immunobiology 176: 63-72.
36. James, S. and Glaven, J. (1989) J Immunol 143: 4208-4212
37. Green, S.J., Meltzer, M.S., Hibbs, J.B., Jr. and Nacy, C.A. (1990) J Immunol 144: 278-283.
38. Liew, F.Y., Millott, S., Parkinson, C., Palmer, R.M.J. and Moncada, S. (1990) J Immunol 144: 4794-4797.
39. Adams, L.B., Hibbs, J.B. Jr., Taintor, R.R. and Krahenbuhl, J.L. (1990) J Immunol 144: 2725-2729.
40. Curran, R.D., Billiar, T.R., Stuehr, D.J., Hoffmann, K. and Simmons, R.L. (1989) J Exp Med 170: 1769-1774.
41. Kilbourn, R.G. and Belloni, P. (1990) J Natl Cancer Inst 82: 772-776.

Cellular and Cytokine Networks in
Tissue Immunity, pages 229-234

DETECTION OF NITROSYL-IRON COMPLEXES IN TUMOR TARGET CELLS AFTER COCULTURE WITH ACTIVATED MACROPHAGES

Catherine Pellat, Yann Henry and Jean-Claude Drapier

Unité 196 INSERM, Institut Curie, Paris (C.P., J.C.D.) and
Unité 219 INSERM, Institut Curie, Orsay (Y.H.), France.

INTRODUCTION

Nitrogen oxides (NO, NO_2^- and NO_3^-) were recently identified as products of L-arginine oxidation in various mammalian cells, including endothelial cells, neutrophils and immunostimulated macrophages (1-3). NO accounts for many biological activities : smooth muscle relaxation, inhibition of platelet aggregation as well as antitumoral and antimicrobial activities (2,3). Murine macrophages activated *in vivo* after BCG infection or *in vitro* by IFN-γ, synthesize NO from the guanido group of L-arginine (1,2). Induction of this metabolic pathway is a prerequisite for selective inhibition of iron-sulfur enzymes, *i.e.*, aconitase of the citric acid cycle and NADH-ubiquinone oxidoreductase (Complex I) and succinate-ubiquinone oxidoreductase (Complex II) of the electron transport chain, both in tumor target cells and in activated macrophages themselves. As gaseous NO is able to induce loss of activity of aconitase , Complex I and Complex II, as well as growth inhibition in L1210 leukemia cells (4,5), we asked whether activated macrophages-derived NO endogenously synthesized from L-arginine could enter tumor cells and directly interact with iron-containing proteins. For this purpose, we used Electron Paramagnetic Resonance (EPR) spectroscopy and we report here evidence for the formation of nitrosyl-iron complexes in L1210 cells after contact with murine activated macrophages.

RESULTS

Unlike macrophages, the murine L1210 leukemia cells are not adherent to plastic culture dishes and were easily removed from macrophage monolayers. Contaminating macrophages removed with L1210 cells (about 5 % of total cells) had a negligible contribution in the further assays.

As expected from earlier experiments (2), L1210 cells cocultivated with BCG-activated macrophages did undergo cytostasis (not shown) and loss of aconitase activity. Nitrogen oxide production was assessed by measurement of nitrite accumulation in the culture medium (Fig. 1). Figure 1 also shows the 77K EPR spectra in the g = 2 region of L1210 cells cultivated in various conditions. No other spectral feature was detected at this temperature. L1210 cells after coculture with BCG-activated peritoneal macrophages (Fig. 1B), exhibited a well resolved spectral absorption centered at g_{av} = 2.03 with g_1 = 2.041, g_2 = 2.015 and all other features earlier ascribed to nitrosyl-iron-thiol complexes (6,7). The presence of these complexes was correlated with nitrite (an end-product of NO) accumulation in the culture medium and with loss of aconitase activity. In contrast, in the presence of mono-methyl-L-arginine (MMA), a competitive inhibitor of NO synthase (2), generation of nitrosyl-iron complexes was prevented (Fig. 1D). Activated macrophage-conditioned medium was without any effect on L1210 cells (Fig.1E).

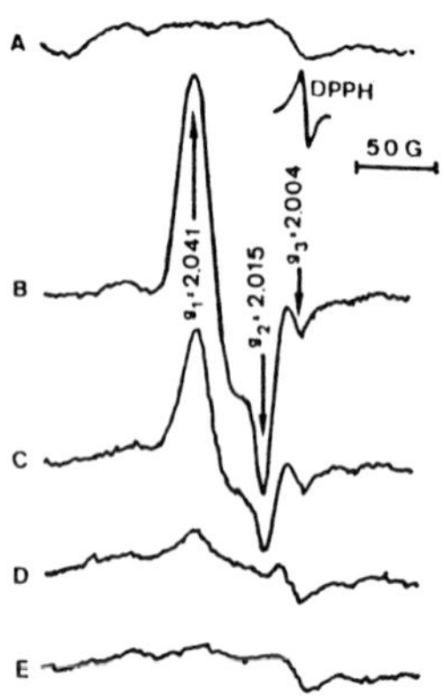

	Aconitase activity (% of control)	NO_2^- (μM)
A	100	und.
B	3	116.1
C	n.a.	n.a.
D	110	10.5
E	115	105.6

Figure 1. EPR spectra (77 K) of L1210 cells under various culture conditions. (A) L1210 cells after culture free of macrophages. (B) L1210 cells removed from BCG-macrophage monolayers. (C) Mitochondria of L1210 cells in B. (D) As B but in the presence of 0.5 mM MMA. (E) L1210 cells cultured in activated macrophage-conditioned medium that, therefore contains NO_2^-. Conditions of EPR spectroscopy : microwave power 10 mW ; modulation amplitude :10 G ; modulation frequency : 9.18 GHz. Field was calibrated with DPPH. Nitrite and aconitase activity were determined as previously described (10). n.a. : non applicable ; und.: undetectable. Representative experiment.

Iron-sulfur enzymes known to be inhibited as a consequence of the L-arginine:NO pathway, are located in mitochondria. Mitochondria, prepared by the digitonin method (8), were assayed for paramagnetic resonance. As shown by Figure 1C, the g_{av} = 2.03 signal was also displayed by mitochondria. The amplitude of the signal, normalized for protein content, was roughly the same as found in the non-permeabilized cells thus showing that the paramagnetic moieties detected are as widespread in mitochondria as in the whole cells.

IFN-γ, a macrophage activator, is the only cytokine so far screened, which alone induces murine macrophages to convert L-arginine into nitrogen oxides (9). Figure 2B shows that NO dependent-paramagnetic complexes were found in L1210 cells removed from IFN-γ-activated macrophages. Again, appearance of this signal was dependent on the opening of the NO:pathway as testified by nitrite release. As expected from previous studies (10,11), activated macrophage monolayers depleted of L1210 cells, displayed identical EPR signal (Fig. 2C).

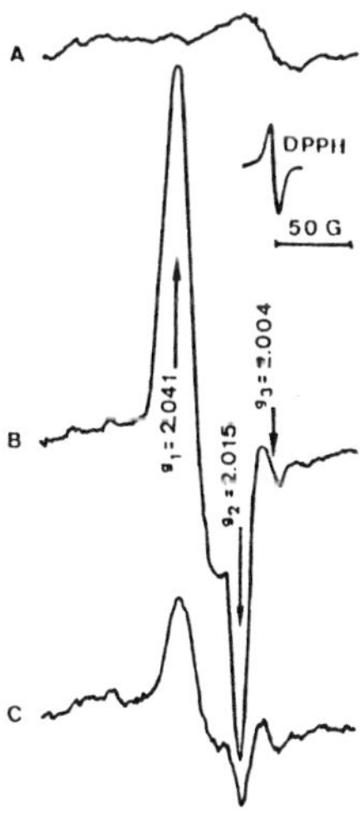

	Aconitase activity (% of control)	NO_2^- (μM)
A	100	und.
B	18	66

Figure 2. EPR spectra of L1210 cells after culture free of macrophages (A) or cultured with macrophages activated with 500 U/ml IFN-γ (B). EPR spectrum of IFN-γ-activated macrophage monolayers (C). Experimental conditions as in Figure 1. und. : undetectable. Representative experiment.

DISCUSSION

In this study, we showed that activated macrophage-injured L1210 cells exhibited the same EPR signal as activated macrophages. This signal was characterized by a g_1= 2.041, a g_2 = 2.015 and a peak to peak width of 42 G. This signal was earlier ascribed to complexes between nitrosyl-iron and thiol proteins (6,7). Detection of this signal correlated with induction of the L-arginine:NO pathway and loss of aconitase activity. Since there was no evidence for intrinsic NO production by L1210 cells, we are left with the only possibility that NO participating in the nitrosyl complex(es) exhibited by L1210 cells was generated by activated macrophages.

NO is a diffusible factor which acts in an isotropic manner and it is quite conceivable that it could have a biological action at sites distal from its origin. However, due to its strong reactivity with oxygen, an action in extracellular spaces is unlikely. Not surprisingly, conditioned medium from activated macrophages was, in our hands, unable to generate paramagnetic nitrosyl complexes in target cells. This is in accordance with the previously reported concept that extracellular targets (cells or large parasites like helminths) require close contact with activated macrophages to be affected by the L-arginine:NO pathway (2,12).

Affinity of NO for iron-proteins is well known. NO binds to heme proteins, e.g. hemoglobin or cytochrome oxidase (13,14) and can disrupt iron-sulfur centers of enzymes like nitrogenase (15,16). Since the nitrosyl-iron complexes were found in L1210 mitochondria, it is likely that iron-sulfur centers in enzymes of the electron transport chain participate in the nitrosyl complexes detected by EPR.

An iron atom can have up to six coordinate ligands. In [4Fe-4S] clusters or in cytochrome a_3 of complex IV, iron is respectively tetra-coordinate and penta-coordinate and may yield one or two additional bonds with a ligand (substrate or cofactor). Regarding aconitase, substrate binding requires coordination of an iron atom of the [4Fe-4S] cluster to one carboxyl group of substrate (17). It is reasonable to expect that binding of NO to this iron atom would prevent enzyme activity. Complex I and complex II, both also depending on at least one [4Fe-4S] center could also be affected in the same way.

In conlusion, the nitrosylation process we described here, might have relevant implications in many aspects of cell behavior including the L-arginine-dependent growth inhibition of various intra- and extra-cellular pathogens, recently reported (12,18,19). Additional experiments aimed at identifying the structure of the nitrosyl-iron complex(es) should help to further delineate the biological consequences of this nitrosylation process.

Acknowledgements. We are grateful to Ms Agnes Géhant for skillfull secretarial assistance. This work was supported from an ARC grant (No 6689). Murine rIFN-γ was a gift from Boehringer-Ingelheim.

REFERENCES

1. Marletta MA (1989) Nitric oxide : biosynthesis and biological significance. TIBS 14: 488-492.
2. Hibbs Jr JB, Taintor RR, Vavrin Z, Granger DL, Drapier JC, Amber I, Lancaster Jr JR (1990) Synthesis of nitric oxide from a terminal guanidino atom of L-arginine : a molecular mechanism regulating cellular proliferation that targets intracellular iron. In "Nitric Oxide from L-arginine : A Bioregulatory System". Moncada S and Higgs EA, eds, Elsevier Science Publishers, pp 189-223.
3. Moncada S, Palmer RMJ, Higgs EA (1989) Biosynthesis of nitric oxide from L-arginine. A pathway for the regulation of cell function and communication. Biochem Pharmacol 38: 1709-1715.
4. Hibbs Jr JB, Taintor RR, Vavrin Z, Rachlin EM (1988) Nitric oxide : a cytotoxic activated macrophage effector molecule. Biochem Biophys Res Commun 157: 87-94.
5. Stuehr DJ, Nathan CF (1989) Nitric oxide. A macrophage product responsible for cytostasis and respiratory inhibition in tumor target cells. J Exp Med 169: 1543-1555.
6. Vanin AF, Kiladze SV, Kubrina LN (1978) Incorporation of non-heme iron into the dinitrosyl complexes in the mouse liver *in vivo*. Biofizika (English translation) 23: 474-478.
7. Woolum JC, Tiezzi E, Commoner B (1968) Electron spin resonance of iron-nitric oxide complexes with amino acids, peptides and proteins. Biochim Biophys Acta 160: 311-320.
8. Granger DL, Lehninger AL (1982) Sites of inhibition of mitochondrial electron transport in macrophage-injured neoplastic cells. J Cell Biol 95: 527-535.

9. Ding A, Nathan CF, Stuehr DJ (1988) Release of reactive nitrogen intermediates and reactive oxygen intermediates from mouse peritoneal macrophages : comparison of activating cytokines and evidence for independent production. J Immunol 141: 2407-2412.
10. Pellat C, Henry Y, Drapier JC (1990) IFN-γ-activated macrophages : detection by electron paramagnetic resonance of complexes between L-arginine-derived nitric oxide and non-heme iron proteins. Biochem Biophys Res Commun 166: 119-125.
11. Lancaster Jr JR, Hibbs Jr JB (1990) EPR demonstration of iron-nitrosyl complex formation by cytotoxic activated macrophages. Proc Natl Acad Sci USA 87: 1223-1227.
12. James S, Glaven J (1989) Macrophage cytotoxicity against schistosomula of *Schistosoma mansoni* larvae involves arginine-dependent production of reactive nitrogen intermediates. J Immunol 143: 4208-4212.
13. Scholler DM, Wang M-YR, Hoffman BM (1979) Resonance Raman and EPR of nitrosyl human hemoglobin and chains, carp hemoglobin and model compounds. J Biol Chem 254: 4072-4078.
14. LoBrutto R, Wei YH, Mascarenhas R, Scholes CP, King TE (1983) Electron nuclear double resonance and EPR study on the structure of the NO-ligated heme a_3 cytochrome C oxidase. J Biol Chem 258: 7437-7448.
15. Meyer J (1981) Comparison of carbon monoxide, nitric oxide, and nitrite as inhibitors of the nitrogenase from *Clostridium pasteurianum*. Arch Biochem Biophys 210: 246-256.
16. Michalski WP, Nicholas DJD (1987) Inhibition of nitrogenase by nitrite and nitric oxide in *Rhodopeudomonas sphaeroides* f sp. *denitrificans*. Arch Microbiol 147: 304-308.
17. Kennedy MC, Werst M, Tesler J, Emptage MH, Beinert H, Hoffman BM (1987) Mode of substrate cartoxyl binding to the $[4Fe-4S]^+$ cluster of reduced aconitase as studied by ^{17}O and ^{13}C ENDOR spectroscopy. Proc Natl Acad Sci USA 84: 8854-8858.
18. Green SJ, Meltzer MS, Hibbs Jr JB, Nacy CA (1990) Activated macrophages destroy intracellular *Leishmania major* amastigotes by an L-arginine-dependent killing mechanism. J Immunol 144: 278-283.
19. Adams LB, Hibbs Jr JB, Taintor RR, Krahenbuhl JL (1990) Microbiostatic effect of murine-activated macrophages from *Toxoplasma Gondii*. Role for synthesis of inorganic nitrogen oxides from L-Arginine. J Immunol 144:2725-2729.

Cellular and Cytokine Networks in Tissue Immunity, pages 235-240

Francisella tularensis IS SUSCEPTIBLE TO NITROGEN OXIDES PRODUCED BY CYTOKINE-ACTIVATED MURINE MACROPHAGES

Shawn J. Green, Anne H. Fortier, Robert M. Crawford, Monte S. Meltzer, and Carol A. Nacy

Dept. of Cell. Immunol., Walter Reed Army Inst. Res., 9620 Medical Center Drive, Rockville MD 20850

Mechanisms of host resistance against bacterial infection vary with the infectious pathogen. Although serum antibodies fully protect against infection with *Salmonella typhimurium* (Hachadel and Keller, 1977), Mackaness (1962) showed that resistance to *Listeria monocytogenes* was independent of such antibodies and instead was mediated by macrophages activated by bacterial antigen-sensitized T cells. Resistance to *Francisella tularensis*, the causative agent of tularemia, is similarly associated with the activation of macrophages by *F. tularensis*-sensitized T cells: passive transfer of spleen cells from *Francisella*-infected mice to recipient control animals protected against a lethal challenge infection with the same microorganism; passive transfer of serum from the identical donor mice was ineffective (Tarnvik, 1989). We use the Live Vaccine Strain (LVS) of *F. tularensis*, a strain lethal for mice, to identify the effector mechanisms by which activated macrophages kill this facultative intracellular bacteria.

Nitric oxide (NO) generated by macrophages exposed to lymphokine activation signals is a potent effector molecule active against a wide spectrum of infectious and neoplastic targets. Such NO sensitive targets include: tumor cells (Hibbs *et al.*, 1987, 1988), fungi (Granger *et al.*, 1990), protozoa (Green *et al.*, 1990; Adams *et al.*, 1990; Liew *et al.*, 1990), helminthic parasites (James and Glaven, 1989), and the macrophage itself (Drapier and Hibbs 1986; Albina *et al.*, 1989). We show in this report that NO is also operative against bacterial pathogens and is the prime effector molecule for the killing of *Franciscella* by lymphokine-activated macrophages.

Stuehr and Marletta (1985,1987) observed that bacillus Calmette-Guerin (BCG) infection of mice results in high levels of nitrite (NO_2^-) and nitrate (NO_3^-) excretion during the course of disease. Urinary NO_3^- levels in BCG infected mice are maximum 8 to 9 days after infection, a time coincident with the appearance of macrophages activated for tumoricidal and microbicidal activity (Nacy *et al.*, 1984). Macrophage activation during BCG infection is mediated by lymphokines released from sensitized T cells. The major activity in lymphokines for the induction of cytotoxic macrophages and NO_2^-/NO_3^- production is interferonγ (IFNγ) (Drapier and Hibbs, 1988; Stuehr and Marletta, 1987). Hibbs and coworkers (1987,1988) found that NO_2^-/NO_3^- production by activated macrophages depends upon extracellular L-arginine and that $NO_2/$ NO_3^- synthesis correlated with the inhibition of iron-dependent enzymes involved in cellular respiration and energy production. NO, an intermediate in the nitrogen oxidation of L-arginine and the oxidative precursor to NO_2^- and NO_3^-, degrades the iron-sulfur prosthetic groups necessary for activity of these vital enzymes (Hibbs *et al.*, 1988). Activated macrophages do not synthesize nitrogen oxides or display tumoricidal or microbial activity when cultured in the presence of N^G-monomethylarginine (MMLA), a specific inhibitor of nitrogen oxidation of L-arginine (Hibbs *et al.*, 1987; Granger *et al.*, 1990).

Earlier work in our laboratory showed that C3H/HeN mice inoculated intraperitoneally (i.p.) with 1 organism of *F. tularensis* died within 7 to 10 days. If BCG was given 8 days prior to such infection, mice were fully protected against a dose of *Francisella* in excess of 10^7 organisms (Fortier *et al.*, 1989). We examined whether the apparent suppression of *Francisella* replication in these mice by BCG-activated macrophages was dependent on L-arginine. Eight days after i.p. inoculation of BCG, peritoneal macrophages were cultured as a cell pellet with an equal number of *Francisella* in the presence or absence of MMLA (Figure 1). Addition of MMLA inhibited both macrophage-mediated antibacterial activity and NO_2^- production in a dose dependent fashion. NO_2^-, an oxidative end product of the short-lived NO effector molecule serves as a marker for macrophage activation and the L-arginine-dependent effector pathway.

Like BCG-activated macrophages, resident peritoneal macrophages from untreated mice exposed to IFNγ also suppressed *Francisella* growth; this suppression required activation of the L-arginine dependent effector pathway. As shown in Table 1, inhibition of *Francisella* growth and NO_2^- production by IFNγ-treated macrophages was blocked by MMLA. While the inhibition of *Franciscella* growth by activated macrophages was unquestionably dependent upon NO, the precise mechanism for this phenomenon is not yet known. NO may have a direct toxic effect on the bacteria itself. Alternatively, macrophages may also by injured by exposure to NO (Drapier and Hibbs, 1988; Albina *et al.*, 1989). We previously showed that growth

Figure 1. Effects of MMLA on BCG-activated macrophage antimicrobial activity against *F. tularensis.*

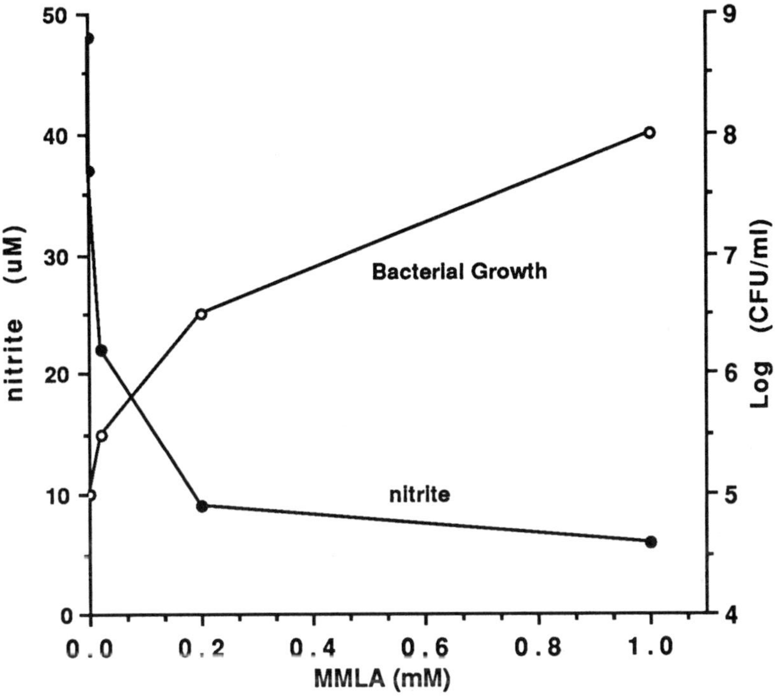

Culture fluids were tested for NO_2^- at 72 hrs using the Griess reagents; cells were lysed in Mueller Hinton broth, serially diluted, and plated on cystine heart agar plates containing 5% rabbit blood.

---

of *Francisella* in tissue culture medium was dependent upon the presence of viable macrophages or medium conditioned by viable and *Franciscella*-infected macrophages for 72 hrs (Fortier *et al.,* 1989). NO may either prevent this conditioning of culture medium for optimal extracellular growth of bacteria or have a direct toxic effect on those *Francisella* residing within the macrophage itself. Regardless of mechanism, these data clearly show that nitrogen oxides derived from L-arginine by lymphokine-activated macrophages suppress the growth of *Francisella*.

Both the virulent and LVS strains of *Franciscella* induce respiratory bursts by neutrophils. These bacteria survive exposure to toxic reactive oxygen products such as H_2O_2,

Table 1. IFNγ induced macrophage anti-*Francisella* activity: Effects of MMLA.

Resident Macrophages treated 72 hrs with:	*Bacterial log growth at 72 hrs:*	*NO_2^- production ($\mu M/10^6/ml$)*
medium +	9.0	0
0.1 mM MMLA	9.0	<1
10 U/ml IFNγ +	6.5	28
0.01 mM MMLA	7.0	15
0.10 mM MMLA	8.5	6

hypochlorous acid, O_2^-, and hydroxyl radicals (Lofgen *et al.*, 1984). Such toxic reactive oxygen products are not only ineffective against *F. tularensis*, but may suppress production of NO by lymphokine-activated macrophages. This double whammy of a survival mechanism may be a major factor in disease pathogenesis. Generation of superoxides decreases toxic effector activities of activated macrophages (Stuehr and Nathan, 1989) and H_2O_2 down-regulates cellular responses to tumor necrosis factorα(TNFα) by reducing TNFα binding capacity (Baud *et al.*, 1990). TNFα is a necessary co-factor for induction of nitrogen oxidation and cytotoxic effector function in IFNγ-treated macrophages (Drapier *et al.*, 1988). TNFα cooperatively interacts with IFNγ in macrophages to inhibit aconitase activity and stimulate NO_2^- production. This interaction is blocked by monoclonal antibody to TNFα (Drapier *et al.*, 1988). Killing of the obligate intracellular protozoan parasite, *Leishmania major*, by macrophages is inhibited by anti-TNFα. Amastigotes of *L. major* directly induce TNFα production in macrophages. TNFα, in turn, acts as an autocrine mediator to initiate the L-arginine effector pathway in IFNγ treated macrophages (Green *et al.*, 1990). Preliminary observations suggest that similar events occur with *Francisella*: monoclonal anti-TNFα suppresses antibacterial activity and NO_2^- production induced by *Franciscella* in IFNγ-treated macrophages. It is likely that *Francisella* LPS provides a required signal to IFNγ-treated macrophages for nitrogen oxidation. As shown in Table 1, *Francisella* infected macrophages (medium) or IFNγ-treated macrophages alone (not shown) were incapable of generating NO_2^- (<1μM $NO_2^-/10^6$ cells). Resident macrophages exposed to both *Francisella* and IFNγ generated 28 μM $NO_2^-/10^5$ cells. Similarly, exogenously added *E. coli* LPS, a potent inducer of TNFα, also enhanced NO production and antibacterial activity by IFNγ-treated macrophages (Crawford *et al.*, 1990).

This report provides further evidence that the L-arginine dependent effector mechanism plays a key role in immunity against infectious pathogens, including bacteria, and that activation of this pathway for toxic effector activity in macrophages is dependent on multiple signals, notably IFNγ and TNFα. *Franciscella* itself participates in this reaction by inducing TNFα and initiating nitrogen oxidation in macrophages exposed to IFNγ.

REFERENCES

Adams LB, Hibbs JB, Jr, Taintor RR, and Krahenbuhl JL (1990). Microbistatic effects of murine-activated macrophages for *Toxoplasma gondii*: Role for synthesis of inorganic nitrogen oxides from L-arginine. J Immunol 144: 2725-2729.

Albina JE, Mills CD, Henry PL, and Caldwell MD (1989). Regulation of macrophage physiology by L-arginine: Role of the oxidative L-arginine deiminase pathway. J Immunol 143: 3641-3645.

Baud L, Affres H, Perez J, Ardaillou R (1990). Reduction in tumor necrosis factor binding and cytotoxicity by hydrogen peroxide. J Immunol 145: 556-560.

Crawford RM, Green SJ, Leiby DA, Nacy CA, and Fortier AH (1990). L-arginine dependent killing mechanism involved in the destruction of Francisella tularensis. J Leukocyte Bio, supplem 1: 48a.

Drapier JC and Hibbs JB, Jr (1988). Differentiation of murine macrophages to express nonspecific cytotoxicity for tumor cells results in L-arginine-dependent inhibition of mitochondrial iron-sulfur enzymes in the macrophage effector cells. J. Immunol 140:2829-2834.

Drapier JC, Wietzerbin J, and Hibbs JB, Jr (1988). Interferon and tumor necrosis factor induced the L-arginine-dependent cytotoxic effector mechanism in murine macrophages. Eur J Immunol 18: 1587-1592.

Fortier AH, Glaser D, Sailor C, Meltzer MS, and Nacy CA (1989). Activated macrophages kill *Francisella tularensis in vitro* and *in vivo*. J Leukocyte Bio 46: 341a.

Granger DL, Hibbs JB, Jr, Perfect, JR, and Durack DT (1990). Metabolic fate of L-arginine in relation to microbistatic capability of murine macrophages. J Clin Invest 85: 264-272.

Green SJ, Meltzer MS, Hibbs JB, Jr, and Nacy CA (1990). Activated macrophages destroy intracellular *Leishmania major* amastigotes by an L-arginine-dependent killing mechanism. J Immunol 144: 278-283.

Green SJ, Crawford RM, Hockmeyer, JT, Meltzer MS, and Nacy CA (1990). *Leishmania major* amastigotes initiate the L-arginine-dependent killing mechanism in IFN-γ-stimulated macrophages by induction of TNFα. J Immunol (in press; Dec 15).

Hachadel JF and Keller KF (1977). Protective effects of passively transferred immune T- or B-lymphocytes in mice infection with *Salmonella typhimurium*. J Infect Dis 135: 813-23.

Hibbs JB, Jr, Taintor R, and Vavrin Z (1987). Macrophage cytotoxicity: Role for L-arginine deiminase and imino nitrogen oxidation of nitrite. Science 235: 473-76.

Hibbs JB, Jr, Taintor R, Vavrin Z, and Rachlin E (1988). Nitric oxide: A cytotoxic activated macrophage effector molecule. Biochem Biophys Res Comm 157: 87-94.

Liew FY, Millott, S, Parkinson, CJ, Palmer, RM, and Moncada S (1990). Macrophages killing of *Leishmania* parasites *in vivo* is mediated by nitric oxide from L-arginine. J Immunol 144: 4794-4797.

Mackaness GB (1962). Cellular resistance to infection. J Exp Med 116: 381-406.

Nacy, CA, Oster CN, James SL, and Meltzer MS (1984). Activation of macrophages to kill *Rickettsia* and *Leishmania*: Dissociation of intracellular microbicidal activities and extracellular destruction of neoplastic and helminth targets. Cont Topics in Immunobiology 13: 147-170.

Lofgren S, Tarnivik A, Thorn M, and Carlsson J (1984). A wild and attenuated strain of *Francisella tularensis* differs in susceptibility to hypochlorous acid: A possible explanation of their different handling by polymorphonuclear leukocytes. Infect Immun 43: 730-734.

Stuehr DJ and Marletta MA (1987). Induction of nitrite/nitrate synthesis in murine macrophages by BCG infection, lymphokines, or interferon-γ. J Immunol 139: 518-525.

Stuehr DJ and Marletta MA (1985). Mammalian nitrate biosynthesis: Mouse macrophages produce nitrite and nitrate in response to *E. coli* LPS. Proc Nat Acad Sci USA 82:7738.

Tarnvik A (1989). Nature of protective immunity to *Francisella tularensis*. Rev Infect Dis 11: 440-451.

Cellular and Cytokine Networks in
Tissue Immunity, pages 241-246

ROLE OF MACROPHAGE NITROGEN OXIDATION METABOLISM AS AN ANTIMICROBIAL HOST DEFENSE MECHANISM

Donald L Granger, J Andrew Alspaugh, Miriam L Cameron and J B Hibbs, Jr.

Department of Medicine, (D.L.G., J.A.A., M.L.C), Duke University School of Medicine, Durham, North Carolina 27710, and Department of Medicine (J.B.H.) University of Utah College of Medicine, Salt Lake City, Utah 84132.

INTRODUCTION

Facultative or obligate intracellular microorganisms may persist in the host for long periods following resolution of a primary infection. Despite persisting organisms the host is asymptomatic and is immune to re-infection. This type of host-parasite relationship suggests the possibility that acquired resistance may have a microbiostatic component, which is distinct from microbicidal mechanisms such as phagocyte based oxidative burst and defensins.

Macrophages may function as repositories of viable, but nonreplicating pathogens. What mechanism(s) are responsible for maintaining intracellular microbes in a dormant state? In this report we summarize findings which indicate that macrophage oxidation of arginine guanidino nitrogen to nitrogen oxides, termed nitrogen oxidation metabolism (NOM), leads to stasis but not killing of the pathogenic fungus, *Cryptococcus neoformans*. NOM in macrophages may be important because failure to maintain microbiostasis could result in reactivation of dormant organisms leading to life-threatening disease.

RESULTS

Murine macrophage fungistasis. Cryptococci replicate freely within, or next to, normal mouse macrophages with a generation time of about three hours. Peritoneal macrophages from mice harboring chronic infection with *Mycobacterium bovis*, strain BCG, (activated macrophages) are fungistatic *in vitro* for *Cryptococcus neoformans* (Granger et al., 1984). Fungistasis occurs in the phagocytic vacuole or extracellularly, but only for yeast in close contact with macrophages. Many inhibited cryptococci form colonies on Sabouraud's agar plates indicating a fungistatic, not cidal action. Replication commenses within 2-3 hours after removing fungi from macrophages. Enumeration and viability assays every two hours after infection of macrophages shows that fungistasis is not the combined results of killing and replication of two populations of cryptococci.

Dependence on nitrogen oxidation metabolism. Wild type strains of *C. neoformans* are not auxotrophic for L-arginine. Glutamine, asparagine and glycine serve as nitrogen sources for fungal proliferation in cell culture medium. Activated macrophage-mediated fungistasis fails when L-arginine is deleted from the medium (Granger et al., 1987). The degree of fungistasis achieved by macrophages depends on L-arginine concentration with complete inhibition of replication requiring about 100 micromolar L-arginine per 24 hours. This correlates with the amount of L-arginine metabolized by macrophages to nitrite, an end-product of NOM (Granger et al., 1990). The arginine analogue., N(guanidino)monomethyl-L-arginine (NMMA), competatively inhibits both fungistasis and nitrite production. There is a close temporal correlation between the onset of fungistasis and nitrite appearance. All strains of *C. neoformans* tested are susceptible to fungistasis by macrophages carrying out NOM.

Macrophages from other species. Activated peritoneal and alveolar macrophages from rats exhibit high level NOM and this activity correlates with fungistatic capability. Activated macrophages from rabbit lung are highly fungistatic *in vitro* but in this case NOM is not usually detectable as assayed by nitrite/nitrate production and/or L-arginine consumption. Resident human alveolar macrophages, peritoneal macrophages and blood monocytes possess partial fungistatic capability yet NOM is not present in these phagocytes (Cameron et al., 1990). As yet we are not able to induce NOM in human mononuclear phagocytes by treatment with activating cytokines. Rabbit and human macrophages apparently have NOM-independent microbiostatic mechanisms.

Fungistasis by gaseous nitrogen oxides. Evidence suggests that an intermediate nitrogen oxide gas mediates mouse macrophage NOM cytotoxicity (Hibbs et al., 1989); the end-products, nitrite, nitrate and citrulline are not toxic at neutral pH. A dual chamber apparatus is used to investigate potential fungistatic intermediates of NOM (Alspaugh and Granger, 1990). The lower chamber contains a nitrogen oxides generating solution (nitrous acid) separated by a gas permeable, but ion impermeable membrane, from an upper chamber which is filled with cell culture medium, pH 7.4.

Cryptococci resting upon this membrane in the upper chamber stop dividing when nitrogen oxides are produced below the membrane. Nitrite and nitrate anions appear in the upper chamber, but the pH gradient is not perturbed. This indicates that proliferation of cryptococci can be blocked by a substance capable of traversing a gas permeable membrane and that this substance ultimately yields nitrite and nitrate.

NOM *in vivo.* Mice with chronic BCG infection, ingesting a nitrite/nitrate-free diet, excrete large amounts of nitrate in their urine (Stuehr and Marletta, 1985). We find a similar phenomenon which continues for at least 45 days after intraperitoneal infection (Granger et al., 1990). It is likely that nitrate excretion under these conditions reflects NOM occurring *in vivo.* When L-arginine is deleted from the rodent chemically-defined diet, urinary nitrate excretion is not altered and nitrogen balance is maintained. This suggests that arginine is synthesized from other nutrients in the mouse. Mice ingesting approximately 100 micromoles NMMA per day per mouse show a markedly reduced nitrate excretion in response to BCG infection. Thus oral NMMA may inhibit macrophage NOM *in vivo.*

Mice given an LD_{50} dose of *Listeria monocytogenes* excrete nitrate in their urine with a time course which correlates with resolution of the infection in surviving animals. Current studies are examining whether oral NMMA blocks this response and whether this inhibition leads to immunosuppression.

CONCLUSIONS AND FUTURE WORK

There is good evidence in rodent species that NOM is an effective macrophage mechanism for blocking proliferation of, and possibly killing, intracellular microorganisms. This evidence is based largely on *in vitro* cell culture assays. Further studies strongly suggest that NOM occurs in the intact rodent in response to intracellular infection. *In vivo* NOM is likely to include macrophage based metabolism in part. Work is needed to assess the importance of NOM *in vivo* in acquired cellular immunity. An animal model in mice or rats should be developed to determine whether NOM is essential for preventing re-activation of a latent infection. Insight is needed toward understanding the mechanisms of microbiostasis by activated macrophages from other mammalian species, including humans.

REFERENCES

Alspaugh JA, Granger DL (1990). Inhibition of *Cryptococcus neoformans* replication by nitric oxide supports this molecule's role as an effector of macrophage-mediated cytostasis. Submitted for publication.

Cameron ML, Granger DL, Weinberg JB, Kozumbo WJ, Koren HS (1990). Human alveolar and peritoneal macrophages mediate fungistasis independently of L-arginine oxidation to nitrite or nitrate. Amer Rev Resp Dis. In press.

Granger DL, Perfect JR, Durack DT (1986). Macrophage-mediated fungistasis *in vitro* : requirements for intracellular and extracellular cytotoxicity. J Immunol 136:672-680.

Granger DL, Hibbs JB, Perfect JR, Durack DT (1987). Specific amino acid (L-arginine) requirement for the microbiostatic activity of murine macrophages. J Clin Invest 81:1129-1187.

Granger DL Hibbs JB Perfect JR Durack DT (1990). Metabolic fate of L-arginine in relation to microbiostatic capability of murine macrophages. J Clin Invest 85:264-273.

Granger DL Hibbs JB Broadnax LM (1990). Urinary nitrate excretion in relation to macrophage activation: influence of dietary L-arginine and oral N(guanidino)monomethyl-L-arginine. Submitted for publication.

Hibbs JB Taintor RR Vavrin Z Rachlin EM (1988). Nitric oxide: a cytotoxic activated macrophage effector molecule. Biochem Biophys Res Comm 157:87-94.

Stuehr DJ Marletta MA (1985). Mammalian nitrate biosynthesis: mouse macrophages produce nitrite and nitrate in response to *Escherichia coli* lipopolysaccharide. Proc Natl Acad Sci USA 82:7738-7742.

Cellular and Cytokine Networks in
Tissue Immunity, pages 247-252

REGULATORY EVENTS IN ACTIVATION OF NADPH OXIDASE

Daniel Rotrosen, Michael E. Kleinberg, Thomas L. Leto, and Harry L. Malech

Laboratory of Clinical Investigation, National Institute of Allergy and Infectious Diseases, Bethesda, MD 20892

INTRODUCTION

Polymorphonuclear neutrophils and other professional phagocytes reduce molecular oxygen to superoxide on exposure to particulate and soluble stimuli (1). Superoxide is the obligate precursor for generation of hydrogen peroxide and other microbicidal oxidants. The NADPH oxidase responsible for production of superoxide is dormant in the resting cell. Its activation during phagocytosis requires interaction of components in the cytosol and membranes of resting cells resulting in assembly of a multicomponent electron transport chain on the membrane of the nascent phagolysosome. Recently developed cell-free systems for activation of the oxidase have aided identification of several of its individual components (2-5). These studies have led to the recognition of cytosolic proteins of 47 kDa (p47phox) and 67 kDa (p67phox) which complex with a membrane-associated cytochrome b558 (6). An additional, as yet uncharacterized cytosolic protein is also required for oxidase activity (2,4,7). Cytochrome b558 is a heterodimer composed of a 22 kDa α-subunit and a glycosylated ≈91 kDa ß-subunit. Cytochrome b558 is thought to be the terminal electron carrying component of the oxidase and the immediate donor of electrons to molecular oxygen (1). We analyzed activation pathways in intact neutrophils and in a cell-free system to provide evidence that the cytochrome also plays a regulatory role in events leading to oxidase assembly.

MATERIALS AND METHODS

Human neutrophils were isolated from peripheral blood, and cytosol and membrane fractions were prepared as described (8). NADPH oxidase activity was determined by superoxide dismutase inhibitable reduction of acetylated ferricytochrome c in a cell-free system using 10^6 cell equivalents of neutrophil cytosol and 2.5-5 x 10^5 cell equivalents of neutrophil membrane in 100 ul of buffer containing 75 mM potassium phosphate (pH 7), 40 uM arachidonic acid, 150 uM acetylated ferricytochrome c, 10 uM GTPτS, 4 mM $MgCl_2$, 1 mM EGTA, 10 uM FAD, 200 uM NADPH ± 25 ug/ml superoxide dismutase (9). In certain experiments membranes were preincubated in rabbit antisera raised against synthetic peptides corresponding to a sequence in the cytochrome ß-subunit carboxylterminus. In other experiments the cell-free system was perturbed by addition of inhibitory synthetic peptides (100 uM) corresponding to the same region of the cytochrome ß-subunit (9).

Neutrophils were loaded with ^{32}P orthophosphate, treated with phorbol myristate acetate (PMA, 0.5 ug/ml) and p47phox phosphoproteins in cytosol and membrane fractions were analyzed by immunoprecipitation and nonequilibrium pH gradient electrophoresis followed by SDS-PAGE and autoradiography (10).

RESULTS AND DISCUSSION

Identification of cytochrome ß-subunit functional domain

A polyclonal antiserum raised against a 19-residue synthetic peptide containing residues 552-570 in the carboxylterminus of the cytochrome b558 ß-subunit recognizes the denatured cytochrome ß-subunit as assessed by immunoblotting (9). The ß-subunit behaves as an integral membrane protein (1) and has several potential membrane-spanning regions based on hydrophobicity analysis. The carboxylterminus antiserum also recognizes native epitopes present only on the cytoplasmic face of plasma membrane sheets, as determined by indirect immunofluorescence (9). These results established the transmembrane topography of the ß-subunit carboxylterminus and indicated that this region of the ß-subunit could potentially interact with cytosolic proteins during assembly of the oxidase.

Membranes were incubated with anticarboxylterminus serum, washed, and added to reaction mixtures containing cytosol and the remaining components required for cell-free activation of the oxidase. These membranes showed a specific loss of cytosol- and arachidonate-dependent oxidase activity (Fig 1a), a result we attributed to steric hindrance of a ß-subunit domain essential for oxidase activity. In the next series of experiments we asked whether the free synthetic peptide, corresponding to the same region of the ß-subunit could compete in the interaction of oxidase components required for activity. The ß-subunit synthetic peptides inhibited oxidase activity in a concentration dependent fashion with near complete inhibition seen at 100-200 uM peptide and half-maximal inhibitory activity at ≈30 uM peptide (Fig.1b).

The inhibitory activity was specific for the ß-subunit carboxylterminus peptide compared to control peptides matched for size, net charge, and hydrophobicity (Table 1). We assayed a family of truncated ß-subunit carboxylterminus

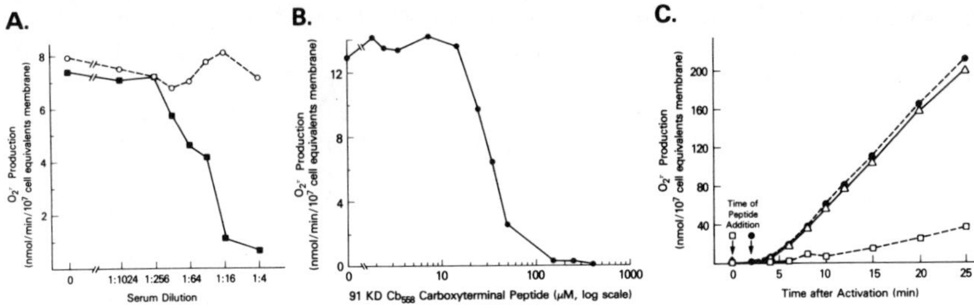

Fig. 1: Inhibition of NADPH oxidase by cytochrome ß-subunit antiserum (A) or synthetic peptides added to the cell-free assay before activation by arachidonate (B) and (C, open squares) or 2 min after activation (C, closed circles). Reprinted from ref. 9, with permission.

---

peptides to identify the minimum amino acid sequence responsible for inhibitory activity. Peptides containing the seven amino acid sequence RGVHFIF (residues 559-565 of the ß-subunit) were as inhibitory as the parent 19-residue peptide (Table 1), but further truncations were accompanied by substantial or total loss of inhibitory activity (data not shown). Inhibition by peptide was noted only when the peptides were introduced early after activation by arachidonate (Fig.1c), indicating that the peptides interfere with a step in oxidase assembly rather than blocking enzymatic turnover of the fully assembled oxidase or simply scavenging superoxide.

To delineate the peptide-sensitive stage of oxidase assembly we reconstituted the otherwise complete reaction mixture by sequential addition of chronic granulomatous

---

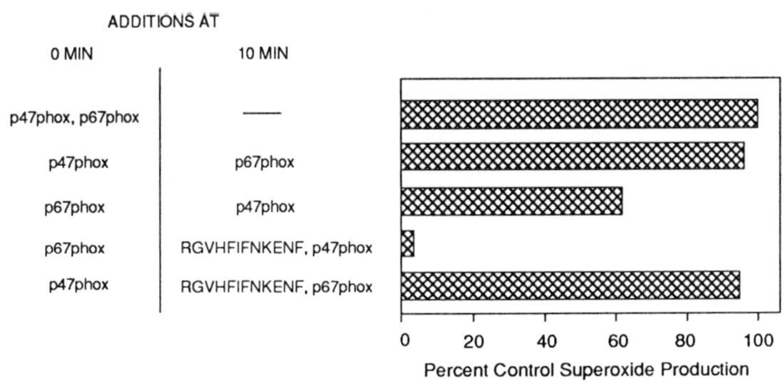

Fig. 2: Inhibition of NADPH oxidase by synthetic peptide during sequential activation with cytosol factor-deficient CGD cytosols. 5 x 10^5 cell equivalents of each cytosol ± synthetic peptide were added at the indicated time to reaction mixtures containing membrane and arachidonate (see text).

disease (CGD) cytosols deficient in either p47phox or p67phox. Under these conditions superoxide generation begins only after the system is fully reconstituted upon inclusion of both cytosols. In these experiments RGVHFIFNKENF was added with the second CGD cytosol, following a 10 min preincubation of membranes, arachidonate, and the complementary CGD cytosol. RGVHFIFNKENF was not inhibitory if the prior incubation included p47phox (Fig. 2). In contrast, when only p67phox was present during the initial incubation and RGVHFIFNKENF was added at 10 min with p47phox-containing cytosol, the peptide blocked oxidase activation. These results indicate that the cytochrome ß-subunit carboxylterminus participates at a stage of oxidase activation during which p47phox interacts with membrane. The data also suggest that the arachidonate stimulated interaction of p47phox and membrane leads to formation of an intermediate complex which on addition of p67phox goes on to form a functional oxidase.

Regulation of p47phox phosphorylation by cytochrome b558

With most stimuli the kinetics of oxidase activation correspond to the kinetics of phosphorylation of p47phox (11), suggesting that p47phox phosphorylation may be important in regulating assembly of the oxidase. In cytochrome b-deficient forms of CGD, p47phox phosphorylation is incomplete (12) and p47phox fails to translocate to membrane (13). With evidence in the cell-free system that the cytochrome modulates an early, p47phox dependent step in oxidase assembly we turned to the intact cell to more specifically address the role of

TABLE I: Inhibition of NADPH oxidase by cytochrome ß-subunit peptides

peptide source		peptide sequence	*percent inhibition
cytochrome ß-subunit			
residues	552-570	SNSESGPRGVHFIFNKENF	96
	559-570	RGVHFIFNKENF	93
	559-565	RGVHFIF	97
	552-558	SNSESGP	-8
	2-9	GNWAVNEGC	-17
	119-126	HLFNVEWC	-17
non-cytochrome peptides			
		RPPGFSPFR	-8
		RKRAHAGFQATI	-5
		VFSMFQGEES	10
		CQTNEENWRVLP	-3
		CDDSDDDLLHI	7

*Percent inhibition derived from Vmax (expressed as nmol superoxide production/min) in the presence of peptides vs. buffer control. Data in part from ref. 9, with permission.

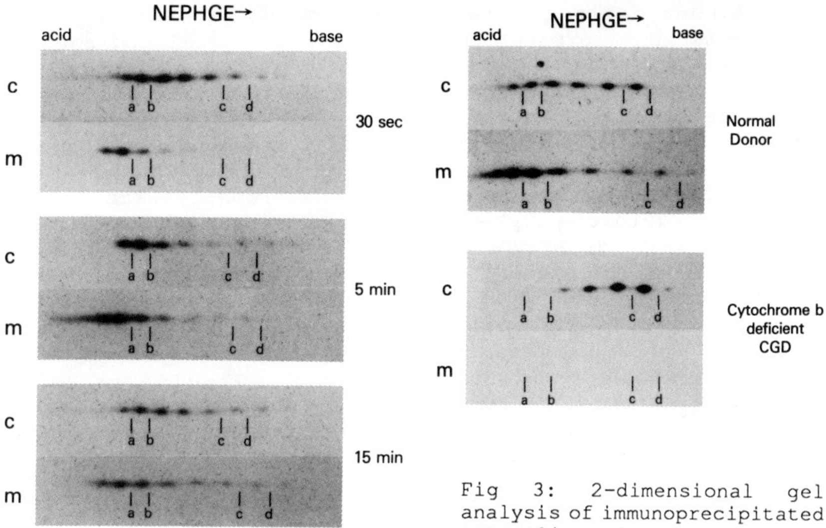

Fig 3: 2-dimensional gel analysis of immunoprecipitated cytosolic and membrane associated p47phox phosphoproteins. Subcellular fractions were prepared from normal neutrophils at the indicated times after stimulation with PMA (left panel) or after stimulation of normal and cytochrome b-deficient CGD neutrophils for 3 min (right panel), and analyzed by 2-dimensional gel electrophoresis and autoradiography. Letters a-d indicate mobilities of pI marker proteins included in electrofocussing gels to facilitate alignment of autoradiographs. reprinted in part from ref. 10, with permission.

---

the cytochrome in modulating p47phox phosphorylation and translocation to membrane. Native p47phox is a basic protein that undergoes stepwise charge shifts with successive phosphorylation events. p47phox was not phosphorylated in resting cells and migrated as a single isoform on immunoblots (data not shown). Fig. 3 (left panel) shows the immunoprecipitated p47phox phosphoproteins in cytosol and membrane fractions of PMA stimulated neutrophils after resolution in electrofocussing gradients. The more acidic cytosolic p47phox phosphoproteins were present in increasing relative amounts over the first 5 minutes, but by 15 min the more basic forms of p47phox were again apparent. Only the more acidic forms of membrane p47phox were seen at 30 sec after exposure to PMA, and only at later times were the basic p47phox phosphoproteins present in the membrane fraction, suggesting that these arise by dephosphorylation of the p47phox species in membrane immediately after translocation. A striking finding is the presence of a single more acidic p47phox phosphoprotein in membrane, compared with cytosol. This indicates that a distinct phosphorylation event occurs only on membrane-associated forms of p47phox, or if it occurs in cytosol, addition of this phosphate confers rapid and stable binding of p47phox to membrane.

p47phox fails to translocate to membrane in cytochrome b558-deficient forms of CGD (Fig 3, right panel and ref. 13). We took advantage of this observation to identify those p47phox phosphorylation events that are indicative of p47phox interaction with membrane. The four most acidic p47phox species seen in normal neutrophils were either absent or greatly diminished in the CGD neutrophils. Thus, at early times after stimulation of normal neutrophils with PMA only the more acidic p47phox phosphoproteins, whose formation requires or is greatly enhanced by interactions involving the cytochrome, were present in the membrane fraction.

The temporal correlation between specific p47phox phosphorylation events and p47phox translocation to membrane is consistent with a model of oxidase activation in which p47phox phosphorylation events, which occur in cytosol, may be critical determinants of the initial interaction of p47phox and membrane. Once membrane association occurs, p47phox becomes phosphorylated at additional sites. Further studies will be required to determine whether the ß-subunit carboxyl-terminus functional domain, identified via the cell-free approach, is also involved in the translocation of p47phox to membrane and in control of the p47phox phosphorylation events in the intact cell.

REFERENCES

1. Segal, A.W. (1989) J. Clin. Invest. 83, 1785-1793
2. Pick, E., Kroizman, T., and Abo, A. (1989) J. Immunol. 143, 4180-4187
3. Babior, B.M., Kuver, R., and Curnutte, J.T. (1988) J. Biol. Chem. 263, 1713-1718
4. Nunoi, H., Rotrosen, D., Gallin, J.I., and Malech, H.L. (1988) Science 242, 1298-1301
5. Volpp, B.D., Nauseef, W.M., and Clark, R.A. (1988) Science 242, 1295-1297
6. Clark, R.A., Volpp, B.D., Leidal, K.G., and Nauseef, W.M. (1990) J. Clin. Invest. 85, 714-721
7. Bolscher, B.G.J.M., Denis, S.W., Verhoeven, A.J., and Roos, D. (1990) J. Biol. Chem. 265, 15782-15787
8. Kleinberg, M.E., Malech, H.L., and Rotrosen, D. (1990) J. Biol. Chem. 265, 15577-15583
9. Rotrosen, D., Kleinberg, M.E., Nunoi, H., Leto, T.L., Gallin, J.I., and Malech, H.L. (1990) J. Biol. Chem. 265, 8745-8750
10. Rotrosen, D., and Leto, T.L. (1990) J. Biol. Chem. 265, in press
11. Heyworth, P.G., and Badwey, J.A. (1990) J. Bioenerg. Biomembr. 22, 1-26
12. Okamura, N., Curnutte, J.T., Roberts, R.L., and Babior, B.M. (1988) J. Biol. Chem. 263, 6777-6782
13. Heyworth, P.G., Shrimpton, C.F., and Segal, A.W. (1989) Biochem. J. 260, 243-248

Cellular and Cytokine Networks in Tissue Immunity, pages 253-257

Mg^{2+} Binding Epitope on Leukocyte Integrin α Subunits

Nancy Hogg and Ian Dransfield

Macrophage Laboratory, Imperial Cancer Research Fund, Lincoln's Inn Fields, London, WC2A 3PX

INTRODUCTION

LFA-1 is a receptor mediating adhesive interactions between monocytes and T cells during the early stages of an immune response. There is a requirement for a reciprocal interaction for LFA-1 on both cell types which results in T cell proliferation (Dougherty & Hogg, 1987; Dransfield *et al*, 1990) (see Fig 1). LFA-1 is a heterodimer with noncovalently associated α and β subunits and together with CR3 and p150,95, these molecules comprise the β_2 family (CD11/CD18; leukocyte integrins) of adhesion molecules which form a subset of the family known as integrins (for review, see Springer, 1990). These receptors require divalent cations such as Mg^{2+} to function and each leukocyte integrin has three putative "EF hand"-like cation binding domains. The two identified ligands or counter-receptors for LFA-1 are termed intercellular adhesion molecule-1 (ICAM-1, CD54) and ICAM-2. Both molecules are members of another family, the immunoglobulin superfamily, and for ICAM-1 which has five Ig-like domains, the two membrane distal domains contain the sequences that interact with LFA-1. ICAM-2 has only two Ig-like domains which share sequence homology with the two LFA-1 interactive domains of ICAM-1, suggesting that LFA-1 may bind both molecules in a similar manner. Expression of LFA-1 is confined to leukocytes, whereas ICAM-1 is relatively widespread and can be further induced by cytokines. How the interaction between these two molecules is controlled, is of interest. If LFA-1 were readily able to interact with ICAM-1 expressing cells, random cellular clustering or aggregation ought to be a feature of systems involving leukocytes. However, this is not observed and there has been much recent interest in how the affinity/avidity of leukocyte integrin binding is increased in order to permit an adhesive event to occur. Earlier work suggested that the avidity of the leukocyte integrin CR3 for ligand could be increased by cellular activation and was a transient phenomenon (Wright and Meyer, 1986; Buyon *et al*, 1988; Lo *et al*, 1989). More recently, increased avidity of LFA-1 for ICAM-1 has been demonstrated to be inducible in a transient manner after cross-linking of CD3 molecules (Dustin and Springer, 1989). Interestingly, avid LFA-1/ICAM-1 binding is also responsible for the increased clustering observed when leukocytes are treated with mAbs to CD2 (van Kooyk *et al*, 1989), CD14 (Lauener *et al*, 1990), CD43 (Axelsson *et al*, 1988) and CD44 (S.Pals; D.Katz - personal communication) suggesting a common mechanism of activation involving intracellular signal transmission.

RESULTS

We have recently described mAb 24 which blocks antigen presentation by monocytes to T cells (Dougherty *et al*, 1988). This mAb reacts with a novel epitope present on leukocyte integrin α subunits (Dransfield and Hogg, 1989; Dransfield *et al*, 1990). Our evidence so far suggests that this epitope is expressed on activated β_2-type leukocyte integrins. In addition recognition of the epitope by mAb 24 is Mg^{2+}-dependent which is of interest because of the evidence that Mg^{2+} is required

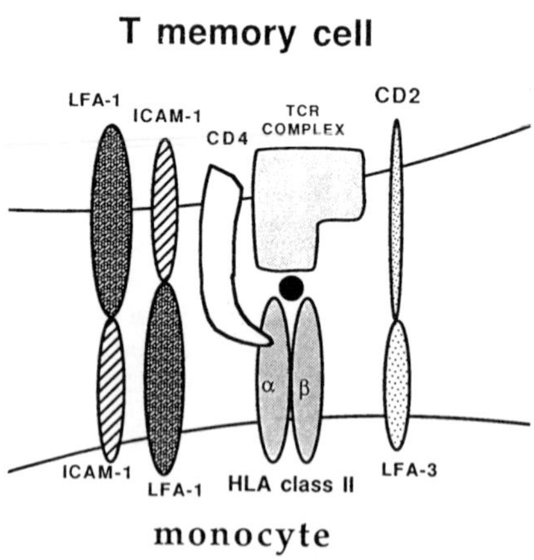

Figure 1. Schematic representation of the interactions that occur between monocytes and memory T cells at the early stages of immune responsiveness. Monoclonal antibody specific for LFA-1α (CD11a) or ICAM-1 inhibits T cell proliferation if added within 8-12 hours of addition of antigen.

for leukocyte integrin function (Martz, 1980). Thus expression of the 24 epitope by LFA-1 (or other leukocyte integrins) can act as a marker for cation binding. We do not yet know the location of the 24 epitope but speculate that it may be within or closely associated with the cation binding sites of leukocyte integrins. For intact cells, expression of the 24 epitope requires active cellular metabolism which confirms the suggestion that activation of LFA-1 is generated from within the cell (Dransfield & Hogg, 1989). A second implication of these findings is that regulation of the receptor function may be achieved simply by controlling cation binding. This suggests that some intracellular event causes an alteration in LFA-1 which has the effect of causing the exposure of a Mg^{2+} binding site in the extracellular domain allowing Mg^{2+}, found in medium or cellular fluids, to bind to integrin. Possible intracellular events that might cause alterations in LFA-1 are phosphorylation of the β_2 or α subunit cytoplasmic "tails" (although the α subunit is constitutively phosphorylated) and/or altered association of LFA-1 with the cytoskeleton.

We are now analysing how mAb 24 effects LFA-1 function with the knowledge that LFA-1-dependent antigen presentation to PPD and to influenza virus is inhibited by this antibody (Dougherty *et al*, 1989). Studies with the β_3-type integrins such as IIbIIIa and the vitronectin receptor (VNR) have suggested that ligand binding is associated with the cation binding sites (D'Souza *et al*, 1990; Smith and Cheresh, 1990). Thus cross-linking studies have shown that the RGD sequence recognised in matrix proteins by the β_3 receptors, binds within the cation binding domains. In spite of the fact that neither ICAM-1 nor -2 possess such an RGD sequence, we wondered whether mAb 24 would directly block LFA-1 binding to ICAM-1 or ICAM-2. However, the result has been that binding of LFA-1 to ICAM-1 or ICAM-2 is unaffected by the presence of mAb 24 (Dransfield *et al*, submitted). This suggests that the mode of binding of ligand by integrins may differ depending on the type of (integrin and/or) target protein. Thus matrix molecules such as fibronectin and Ig-superfamily members such as ICAM may be bound in different ways. In fact it has already been shown that the β_1-type integrin, VLA-4, which has specificity for the CS-1 site of fibronectin as well as the Ig superfamily member, VCAM-1, binds these two ligands at distinct sites (Elices *et al*, 1990). However, another explanation for the inability of mAb 24 to block LFA-1/ICAM bindng could be that the 24 epitope, although behaving as an indicator of Mg^{2+} binding, is not actually physically located within the cation binding domains and may not be affected by ligand binding.

We have now asked whether mAb 24 might block some type of post-receptor occupancy change in the LFA-1 molecule that is necessary for T cell proliferation to occur. To test this possibility we have made use of the CD3 crosslinking model of transient LFA-1/ICAM-1 adhesion (Dustin and Springer, 1990). These experiments have indicated that mAb 24 may be "locking" LFA-1 in the high affinity or adhesive mode if ICAM-1 binding and preventing receptor/ligand "deadhesion" (Dransfield *et al*, submitted). Why "transient" adhesion between LFA-1 and ICAM-1 is important for progress in an immune response is not yet certain. It may be simply a logistical problem, allowing access of large numbers of T cells to antigen presenting cells for a brief period of time. Alternatively, there is present interest in the possibility that LFA-1 mediates crucial intracellular signalling required for the T cell programming leading to proliferation.

REFERENCES

Axelsson B, Youseffi-Etemad R, Hammarström S, Perlman P (1988). Induction of aggregation and enhancement of proliferation and IL-2 secretion in human T cells by antibodies to CD43. J Immunol 141: 2912-2197.

Buyon JP, Abramson SB, Philips MR, Slade SG, Ross GD, Weissman G, Winchester, RJ (1988). Dissociation between increased surface expression of Gp165/95 and homotypic neutrophil aggregation. J Immunol 140: 3156-3160.

Dougherty GJ, Hogg N (1987). The role of monocyte lymphocyte function-associated antigen 1 (LFA-1) in accessory cell function. Eur J Immunol 17: 943-947.

Dougherty GJ, Dransfield I, Hogg N (1988). Identification of a novel monocyte cell surface molecule involved in the generation of antigen-induced proliferative responses. Eur J Immunol 18: 2067-2071.

Dransfield I, Hogg N (1989). Regulated expression of Mg^{2+} binding epitope on leukocyte integrin α subunits. EMBO J 8: 3659-3765.

Dransfield I, Buckle A-M, Hogg N (1990). Early events of the immune response mediated by leukocyte integrins. Immunol Rev 114: 29-44.

D'Souza SE, Ginsberg MH, Burke, TA, Plow EF (1990). The ligand binding site of the platelet integrin receptor GPIIb-IIIa is proximal to the second bindign domain of its α subunit. J Biol Chem 265: 3440-3446.

Dustin ML, Springer TA (1989). T-cell receptor cross-linking transiently stimulates adhesiveness through LFA-1. Nature 341: 619-624.

Elices MJ, Osborn L, Takada Y, Crouse C, Luhowskyi S, Hemler ME, Lobb RR (1990). VCAM-1 on activated endothelium interacts with the leukocyte integrin VLA-4 at a site distince from the VLA-4/fibronectin binding site. Cell 60:577-584.

van Kooyk Y, van de Wiel-van Kemanade P, Weder P, Kuijpers TW, Figdor CG (1989). Enhancement of LFA-1-mediated cell adhesion by triggering through CD2 or CD3 on T lymphocytes. Nature 342: 811-813.

Martz E (1980). Immune T lymphocyte to tumor cell adhesion. Magnesium sufficient, calcium insufficient. J Cell Biol 84: 584-598.

Lauener RP, Geha RS, Vercelli, D. (1990). Engagement of the monocyte surface antigen CD14 induces lymphocyte function-associated antigen-1/intercellular adhesion molecule-1-dependent homotypic adhesion. J Immunol 145: 1390-1394.

Lo SK, Detmers PA, Levin SM, Wright SD (1989). Transient adhesion of neutrophils to endothelium. J Exp Med 169: 1779-1793.

Smith JW, Cheresh DA (1990). Integrin ($\alpha_v\beta_3$)-ligand interaction. Identification of a heterodimeric RGD binding site on the vitronectin receptor. J. Biol. Chem. 265: 2169-2172.

Springer TS (1990). Adhesion receptors of the immune system. Nature 346: 425-434.

Wright, SD, Meyer BC (1986). Phorbol esters cause sequential activation and deactivation of complement receptors on polymorphonuclear leukocytes. J Immunol 136: 1758-1764.

Cellular and Cytokine Networks in Tissue Immunity, pages 259-264

β_1 AND β_2 INTEGRIN SUBUNIT REGULATION OF THE MONOCYTE INFLAMMATORY RESPONSE

David F. Eierman and Stephen Haskill

Departments of Obstetrics and Gynecology, Microbiology and Immunology, and Lineberger Comprehensive Cancer Center. University of North Carolina at Chapel Hill, Chapel Hill, NC 27599.

INTRODUCTION

Understanding of the mechanisms controlling the expression of the monocyte adherence response is important in view of the pivotal role which these cells play in mediating inflammation. As monocytes *in vivo* interact adherently with both cellular and matrix-derived adherence substrates, it is these interactions which determine the expression of the monocyte phenotype and the subsequent response of the monocyte to inflammatory agents and aberrant cells. These cell-cell and cell-matrix interactions are likely to provide specific and discrete signals to the monocyte dependent upon the specific receptor/ligand interactions at the specific sites of adherence.

Cell adherence to extracellular matrix components is via the cytoadhesion integrin subfamily. This subfamily consists of receptors comprised of specific α subunits and a common β_1 subunit which bind fibronectin ($\alpha_4\beta_1$ and $\alpha_5\beta_1$), collagen ($\alpha_2\beta_1$)and laminin ($\alpha_6\beta_1$) (Hynes, 1987).

Cell adhesion to endothelial cell substrates is via the leukocyte adhesion integrin sub-family consisting of CD11a/CD18 (LFA-1), CD11b/CD18 (Mac-1) and CD11c/CD18 (p150,95). All three members of this sub-family share a common β_2 chain (CD18) necessary for the functional integrity of the α_x/β_2 complex (Hynes, 1987).

As we have previously reported, monocyte adherence to plastic (Haskill *et al.*, 1988), extracellular matrix components (Eierman *et al.*, 1989) and endothelial and connective tissue cells (Johnson, 1989) results in distinct patterns of expression of a number of important monocyte inflammatory mediator genes. These findings have led us to investigate the specific role of β_1 and β_2 integrins in the regulation of the monocyte adherence response.

RESULTS AND DISCUSSION

We first examined the influence of antibodies directed against these subunits on steady-state mRNA levels. Treatment of non-adherent monocytes with the monoclonal antibody AIIB2, specific for β_1 rapidly induced IL-1β, c-fos and TNFα mRNA expression (Figure 1). In contrast, treatment of non-adherent monocytes with the β_2 specific monoclonal antibody 60.3 had no effect on steady-state mRNA levels. PMA stimulated controls expressed all of the examined mRNA species.

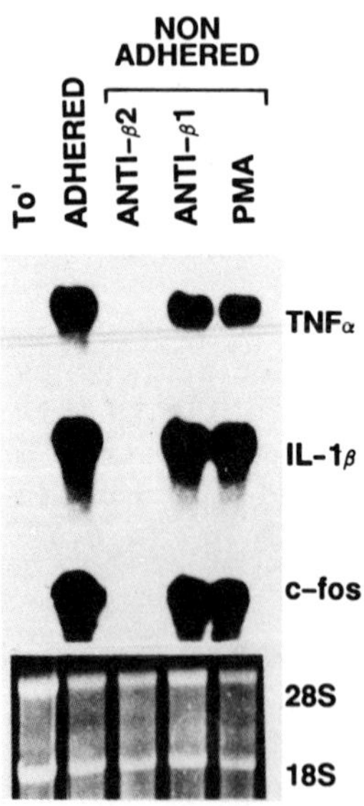

As adherence to endothelial cell substrates is inhibited by pretreatment with anti-β_2 (Wallis *et al.* 1986), we examined the influence of anti-β_2 upon the adherence induced expression of monocyte inflammatory mediator mRNAs. Adherent monocyte culture in the presence of anti-β_2 resulted in decreased steady state levels of mRNAs coding for TNFα, IL-1β, CSF-1 and c-fos (Figure 2).

Figure 1. Density isolated monocytes were either adhered to plastic or cultured non-adherently for 1 h in the presence of anti-β_1 or -β_2 at 1 μg/ml/10^6 cells or 10 ng/ml PMA. mRNA expression was determined by Northern analysis.

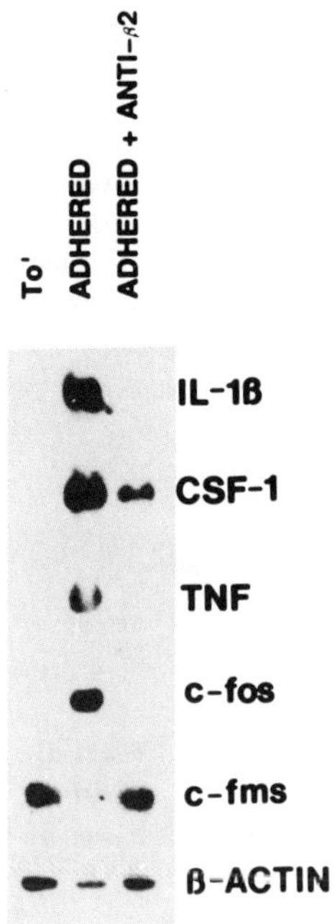

Figure 2. Density isolated monocytes were adhered to plastic for 1 h following 30′ pretreatment with anti-β_2 at 1 μg/ml/10^6 cells at 4°. mRNA expression was determined by Northern analysis.

As low levels of LPS (1 ng/ml) are sufficient to effect cytokine secretion following an initial adherence stimulus (Haskill *et al.*, 1988), we examined the influence of low levels of LPS on secretion of TNFα following stimulation with β_1 and β_2 antibodies. As shown in Figure 3, non-adhered control monocytes were unable to secrete TNFα either in the presence or absence of LPS while adhered monocytes secreted large quantities of this monokine only when adhered in LPS supplemented medium. When monocytes were exposed to either anti-β_1 or anti-β_2 in the presence of LPS under non-adhered culture conditions we observed secreted TNFα levels higher than adhered + LPS controls. Surprisingly, adhering monocytes in the presence of LPS following anti-β_2 exposure resulted in the almost total loss of TNFα secretion while no inhibition of TNFα secretion was observed in adherent

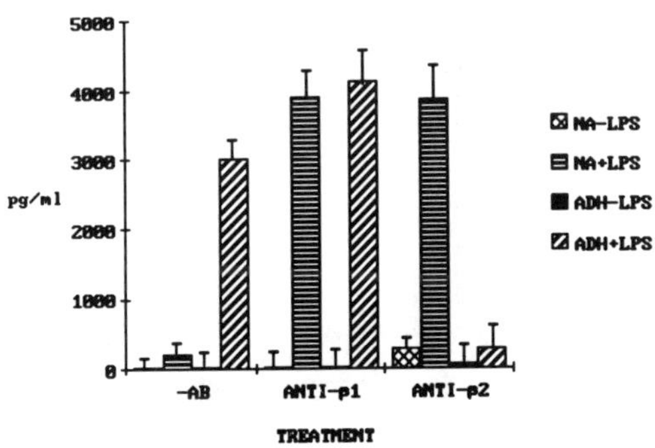

Fig. 3. Density isolated monocytes were adhered to plastic or cultured non-adherently for 4 h in the presence of anti-β_1 or -β_2 at 1 μg/ml/10^6 cells either with or without LPS at .01 μg/ml. TNF activity in culture supernatants was determined by IRMA.

monocytes following anti-β_1 exposure and secreted TNFα levels were highest under this condition.

Monocyte adherence induces high levels of TNFα and IL-1β mRNA which is readily inhibited by specific PKC inhibitors (Eierman, D. and Haskill, S. 1990. Manuscript submitted). Since anti-β_1 stimulates expression of these mRNAs, we examined the the influence of anti-β_1 and anti-β_2 upon PKC activation. As shown in Figure 4, both anti-β_1 and anti-β_2 binding to non-adherent monocytes triggered PKC activation with slightly higher levels of PKC activity observed following monocyte treatment with the β_1 specific antibody.

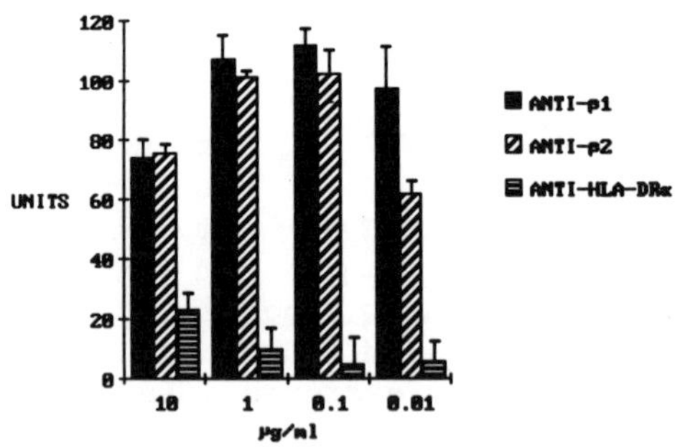

Fig. 4. Density isolated monocytes were pretreated for 30′ in the presence of anti-β_1 or -β_2 or anti-HLA-DR at the indicated concentrations and then adhered to plastic for 30′. Cell membranes were isolated and solubilized and PKC activity was determined by histone phosphorylation.

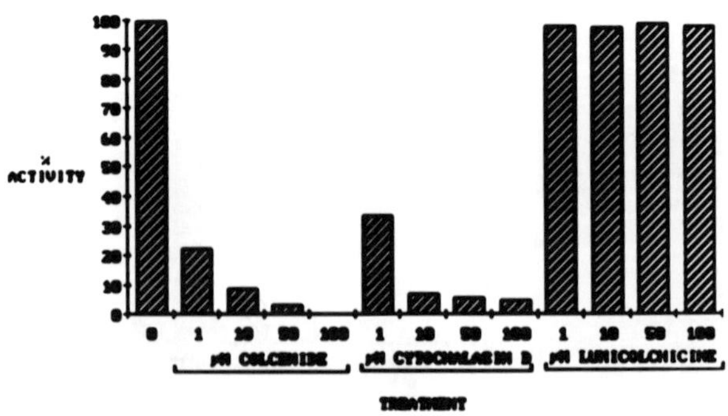

Fig. 5. Density isolated monocytes were pretreated with the cytoskeletal inhibitors colchecine or cytochalasin D, or as a control lumicolchicine, for 30′ at the indicated concentrations and then adhered to plastic culture dishes for 1 h. PKC activity was determined as described above.

As we have previously shown, cytoskeletal inhibitors also mediate the expression of monocyte inflammatory mediator mRNAs (Eierman, et al., 1990). Both colcemide and cytochalasin D inhibit the adherence induction of IL-1β and TNFα while lumicolchicine controls have no effect. Neither inhibitor has an inhibitory effect on mRNA levels in monocytes cultured non-adherently in the presence of PMA (Data not shown). To further understand the mechanisms by which adherence mediates monocytes and because of the close association of integrins with the cytoskeleton, we assessed the influence of cytoskeletal inhibitors upon the adherence activation of PKC. As shown in Figure 5, both colcemide and cytochalasin D inhibited PKC activation activation following adherence. Lumicolchicine, which exhibits similar toxicity to colcemide but does not interact with cytoskeletal components had no influence upon PKC activity.

In summary: Antibody binding to β_1 integrin but not to β_2 is a sufficient signal for the induction of monocyte c-fos, TNFα and IL-1β steady-state mRNA levels under non-adherent culture conditions while anti-β_2 inhibits the adherence mediated expression of monocyte mRNAs. Engagement of β_1 in non-adherent monocytes both activates PKC and effects TNFα secretion in the presence of LPS. Unlike β_1, antibody binding to β_2 integrins, although inducing PKC, does not induce changes in mRNA levels in non-adherently cultured monocytes but does synergize with nanogram levels of LPS to induce secretion of TNFα. β_2 integrins are therefore capable of exerting both stimulatory and inhibitory effects on monocytes. β_1 and β_2 receptor/ligand interactions play an important role in the expression of the monocyte/macrophage phenotype and the resultant inflammatory response. It will be important to see if this pattern of β_1 and β_2 mediated gene expression is similar in other cell types.

REFERENCES

Eierman, D.F., Johnson, C.E., and Haskill, J.S. (1989). Human monocyte inflammatory mediator gene expression is selectively regulated by adherence substrates. J. Immunol. 142:1970-1976.

Eierman, D., C. Johnson, S. Sporn, C. Rinehart, Jr. and S. Haskill. (1990). Monocyte gene expression of cellular adherence substrates. in Molecular and Cellular Biology of Cytokines. J.J. Oppenheim, et.al. eds. Wiley-Liss, New York. pp. 415-420.

Haskill, S., Johnson, C., Eierman, D., Becker, S., and Warren, K. (1988). Adherence induces selective mRNA expression of monocyte mediators and proto-oncogenes. J. Immunol. 140:1690-1694.

Hynes, R.O. (1987). Integrins: a family of cell surface receptors. Cell 48:549-554.

Johnson, C.E. (1989). Characterization of inflammatory gene expression in monocytes and in vascular and connective tissue cells. Doctoral dissertation. The University of North Carolina at Chapel Hill.

Wallis, W.J., Hickstein, D.D., Schwartz, B.R., June, C.H., Ochs, H.D., Beatty, P.G., Klebanoff, S.J. and Harlan, J.M. (1986). Monoclonal antibody-defined functional epitopes on the adhesion-promoting glycoprotein complex (CDw18) in human neutrophils. Blood 67:1007-1013.

Cellular and Cytokine Networks in
Tissue Immunity, pages 265-270

TUMOR NECROSIS FACTOR-INDUCED DEGRANULATION IN ADHERENT HUMAN NEUTROPHILS IS DEPENDENT ON CD11b/CD18-INTEGRIN TRIGGERED OSCILLATIONS OF CYTOSOLIC FREE CALCIUM

Johan Richter*, Janet Ng-Sikorski**, Inge Olsson* and Tommy Andersson**.
Department of Medicine, University Hospital, Lund*, and Department of Cell Biology, University of Linköping, Linköping, Sweden**

Cytokines are potent activators of neutrophil granulocytes. Recent work has showed that while cells in suspension respond poorly to cytokines, adherent neutrophils are capable of mounting a massive respiratory burst in response to tumor necrosis factor (TNF) and other cytokines (1,2). TNF-induced degranulation was also much more pronounced in adherent neutrophils compared to neutrophils in suspension (3). Thus it is clear that adherent neutrophils exhibit quite different functional characteristics in comparison with cells in suspension. We have demonstrated a crucial role of cytosolic free calcium changes in TNF-induced secretion from adherent neutrophils (4). It is intriguing that 50% of neutrophils adhering to albumin or fibronectin coated surfaces exhibit "spontaneous" oscillations of the cytosolic free calcium (5), a phenomenen never seen in non-adherent cells. Recently we were able to show that the dependency on calcium is not due to a TNF-induced calcium signal but rather to a requirement of adherence-induced changes in cytosolic calcium for the subsequent TNF-stimulated secretion in adherent neutrophils (6). The mechanism(s) reponsible for triggering the oscillatory activity of calcium in adherent neutrophils is not known.

At least part of the molecular basis for the different responses of adherent and non-adherent neutrophils to TNF has been shown to involve ligation of CD11/CD18 integrins (7). Integrins are a superfamily of heterodimeric glycoproteins which act as receptors on the cell surface (8). One group of integrins found on leukocytes is the LFA-family (Leukocyte Function Associated) which includes LFA-1 (CD11a/CD18),

Mac-1 or (CD11b/CD18) and p150,95 (CD11c/CD18) (9). These integrins share a common beta chain, CD18, but have different alpha chains (CD11a,b and c). Using monoclonal antibodies to these adherence proteins, their role for various neutrophil functions has been investigated (10). Superoxide generation and granule protein secretion in response to soluble stimuli have until recently been considered to be adherence-independent granulocyte functions (10). Nathan et al, however, showed that TNF-induced respiratory burst of adherent human neutrophils could be inhibited if the cells were incubated with an anti-CD18 antibody (IB4) (7).

The present study was undertaken to determine whether also TNF induced secretion from adherent neutrophils is dependent on the CD11/CD18 integrins, and if so, if this dependency is related to the oscillatory activity of cytosolic free calcium found in adherent neutrophils. A previously described hemolytic plaque assay (4) that measures granule protein secretion from single adherent neutrophils was used to in-

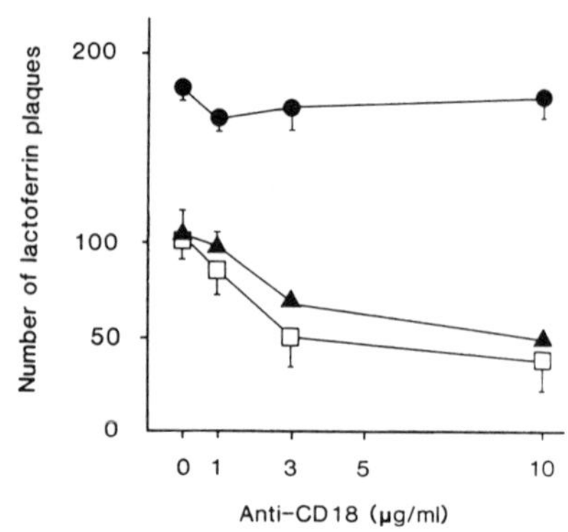

Figure 1. Effect of different concentrations of anti-CD18 on TNF-, FMLP- and PMA-induced lactoferrin secretion. Neutrophils were preincubated with the indicated concentrations of anti-CD18 for 60 min. The cells were then added to the plaque assay with the same concentrations of the MoAb and exposed to 1,000 U/ml of TNF (□), 100 nM fMet-Leu-Phe (▲) or 10 ng/ml PMA (●). The results are expressed as number of plaques (lactoferrin secernating cells) per dish. The values given are mean±SEM from three different determinations.

vestigate the effect of monoclonal antibodies to the leukocyte integrins on degranulation. To determine the effects of the same antibodies on the adherence-induced calcium oscillations we used a sensitive microflurometer technique (6) which allows the continous registration of changes in the cytosolic free calcium concentration in single cells.

The effects of an antibody to CD18, the common beta-chain of leukocyte integrins, on lactoferrin secretion induced by TNF, the chemotactic peptide FMLP, and the phorbolester PMA can be seen in fig 1. Neutrophils were preincubated with the respective concentrations of the antibody at 37°C for 1 hour prior to the degranulation assay. Both TNF and FMLP induced secretion was inhibited in a dose-dependent manner, while PMA-induced degranulation was unaffected, arguing against a deteriorating effect of the antibodies on cellular functions. Similar results were obtained when an antibody to

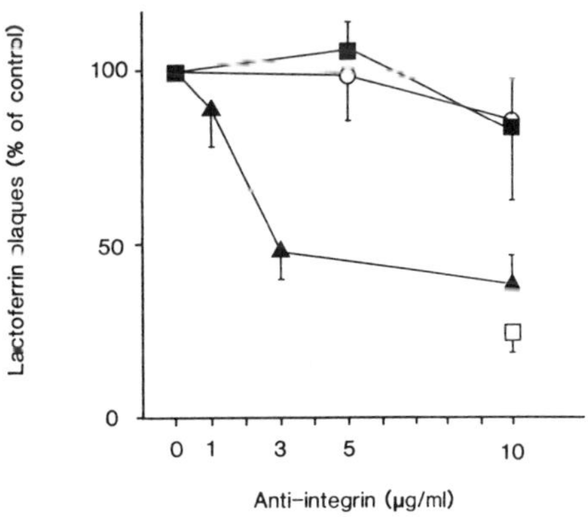

Figure 2. Effect of different integrin antibodies on TNF induced lactoferrin secretion. Neutrophils were preincubated with anti-CD18 (▲), anti-CD11a (■) or anti-CD11c (○) with the concentrations indicated in the figure or with anti-CD18 together with anti-CD11b in a 1:10 dilution (□). The cells were then added to the plaque assay with the same concentration of the MoAbs and stimulated with 1,000 U/ml of TNF. Lactoferrin plaques are expressed as percentage of plaques formed by cells not preincubated with any MoAb but otherwise treated in the same way. The values given are mean±SEM from 3-5 separate experiments.

CD11b, anti-Mac-1 was used, (data not shown). The effects of antibodies to CD11a, alpha-chain of LFA1 and CD11c, which is the alpha-chain of p150.95 are shown in fig 2. These two antibodies did not significantly inhibit degranulation induced by TNF. The combination of anti-CD18 and anti-CD11b was even more effective in inhibiting secretion than anti-CD18 alone.

Antibody	Percentage of cells exhibiting calcium oscillations	Representative calcium trace from single neutrophil exhibiting calcium oscillations
None	65 %	A
anti-CD18	29 %	B
anti-CD11b	28 %	C
anti-CD11c	44 %	D

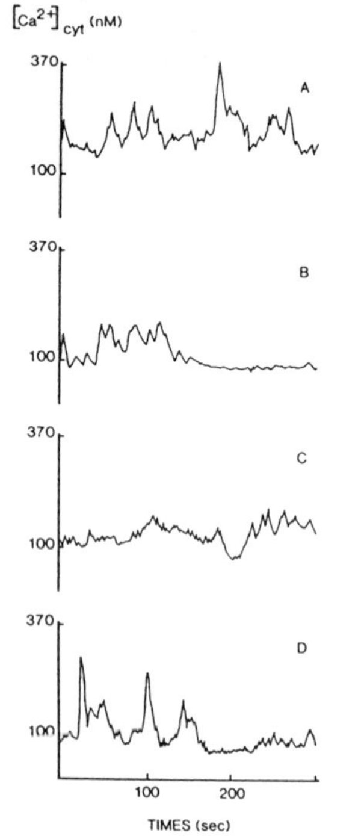

Figure 3. Modulation of oscillatory activity of cytosolic free calcium in single adherent neutrophils by different MoAb. Neutrophils were preincubated for 1 hour without MoAbs (A) or with either of the following MoAbs: CD18 (10 ug/ml; B), CD11b (dilution 1:10; C) or CD11c (10 ug/ml; D). The cells were then loaded with fura2 and allowed to adhere to cover slips coated with human serum albumin. All traces shown are representative single cell registrations from numerous similar experiments.

Having established that TNF-induced secretion from adherent neutrophils is dependent both on an intact integrin function and the calcium oscillations, a natural question to pose was of course whether the spontaneous oscillations of cytosolic free calcium are mediated via CD11/CD18 integrins. Fig 3. summarizes our findings on that particular point. Neutrophils were incubated with three different anti-integrin antibodies, namely anti-CD18, anti-CD11b and anti-CD11c at a concentration of 10ug/ml and then the cytosolic free calcium concentration in single adherent cells was monitored. Controll cells without antibody were treated the same way. CD18 and CD11b antibodies reduced the number of cells responding with calcium oscillations to less then half. However, not only was the number of responding cells reduced, but the oscillatory activity in the responding cells was also reduced as can be seen from representative calcium traces in fig 3. This activity was quantified by measuring the level of highest peak and the area under the calcium curve, and a decrease of 40-50% in the calcium activity of the cells incubated with anti-CD18 and anti-CD11b was found.

In accordance with the degranulation experiments anti-CD11c was found to reduce the number of reponding cells only slightly but no definite reduction of the calcium activity in the responding cells was seen. It should be noted that the inhibitory effect of the antibodies was reversible as the calcium oscillations returned to the normal level if the cells were washed free of antibodies (data not shown). Further support for the calcium signalling capacity of the in-

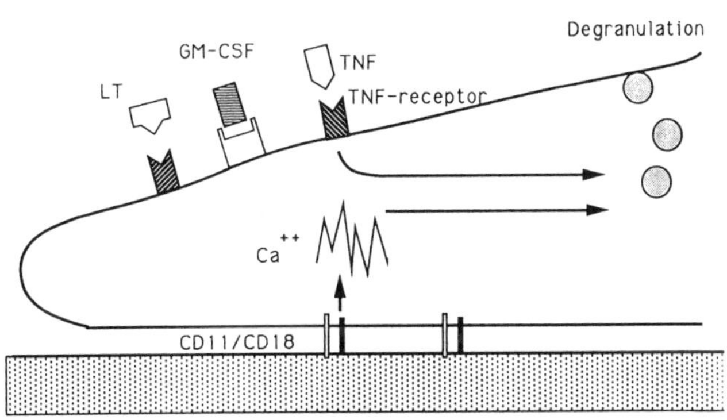

Figure 4. Cytokine-induced exocytosis requires CD11/CD18-integrin-triggered calcium oscillations.

tegrins in neutrophils has recently been obtained as cross-linking of anti-CD11b or anti-CD18 antibodies with a secondary antibody on the neutrophil surface was shown to induce a rapid calcium transient in the cytosol (11).

Our current view of cytokine-induced exocytosis in adherent neutrophil granulocytes is summarized in fig 4. Binding of TNF to its receptor alone does not trigger degranulation. Another signal is also needed. This signal involves the CD11/CD18 integrins which trigger the calciums oscillations in adherent neutrophils. Together these two signals are capable of inducing degranulation in adherent neutrophils. We have found that also secretion induced by lymphotoxin and granulocyte/macrophage colony-stimulating factor is inhibited by calcium chelators, and that these two cytokines do not induce any changes in cytosolic free calcium (4,12). This suggests that the mechanism described here does not apply only to TNF but is of a more general nature, and applicable to activation of neutrophils by several cytokines.

REFERENCES

1. Nathan, C. 1987. J. Clin. Invest. 80,1550-1560.
2. Nathan, C. 1989. Blood. 73,301-306.
3. Luedke, E. S., and Humes, J. L. 1989. Agents and actions 27,451-454.
4. Richter, J., Andersson, T., and Olsson, I. 1989. J. Immunol. 142,3199-3205
5. Jaconi, M. E. E., Rivest, R. W., Schlegel, W., Wollheim, C. B., Pittet, D., and Lew, P. D. 1988. J. Biol. Chem. 263,10557-10560.
6. Richter, J., Olsson, I. and Andersson, T. 1990. J. Biol. Chem. 265,14358-14363
7. Nathan, C., Srimal, S., Farber, C., Sanchez, E., Kabbash, L., Asch, A., Gailit, J., and Wright, S. D. 1989. J. Cell Biol. 109,1341-1349.
8. Hynes, R.O. 1987. Cell 48,549-554.
9. Sanchez-Madrid, F., Nagy, J., Robbins, E., Simon, P. and Springer, T. A. 1983. J. Exp. Med. 158,1785-1803.
10. Springer, T. A. and Andersson, D. C. (1986) In: Biochemistry of macrophages. (Ciba Foundation Symposium 118) Pitman, London 102-126.
11. Ng-Sikorski, J., Andersson, R., Patarroyo, M. and Andersson, T. 1990. Submitted
12. Richter, J. 1989. J. Leuk. Biol. 47,506-513.

Footnote: The complete version of this work was published in Proc. Natl. Acad. Sci. USA, December 1990.

Cellular and Cytokine Networks in Tissue Immunity, pages 271-276

CYTOKINE NETWORKS AND REGULATION OF MACROPHAGE ANTIMICROBIAL ACTIVITIES

Carol A. Nacy, Barbara J. Nelson, and Shawn J. Green and Anda I. Meierovics

Department of Cellular Immunology, Walter Reed Army Institute of Research, 9620 Medical Center Drive, Rockville, MD 20850

INTRODUCTION

Macrophages infected with amastigotes of *Leishmania major* and treated with lymphokines *in vitro* develop an impressive capacity to destroy these intracellular parasites. During the first 48 h, replication of the microorganism is suppressed; between 48 and 72 h, the macrophage actually kills and digests the parasites (Nacy, *et al.*, 1981). When we survey a number of cloned or purified cytokines for induction of macrophage killing of *L. major*, we find that only lymphokines depleted of IFNγ by immunoaffinity chromatography, and IFNγ itself, are able to induce this effector reaction (Nacy, *et al.*, 1985). Nono of the other purified cytokines are effective. In murine studies, as little as 5 U/ml of recombinant IFNγ is sufficient by itself to induce the intracellular destruction of *L. major*, and plateau levels of intracellular killing activity are obtained with >10 U/ml *in vitro* (Nacy, *et al.*, 1985).

Macrophages are activated for most cytotoxic effector activities by a two-stage reaction process known as priming and triggering (Ruco and Meltzer, 1978b). While IFNγ is the best characterized priming signal, the nature of the trigger signal remains controversial, and very system dependent. Several endogenous cytokines perform this function for induction of different effector reactions. TNFα is involved in the activation cascade as a trigger signal for intracellular killing by macrophages. The combination of IFNγ and TNFα is essential for the induction of a novel effector molecule, nitric oxide (NO), that is involved in the destruction of *Leishmania* (Green, *et al.*, 1990b). The basic biochemical pathway for nitrogen oxidation is as follows: the terminal guanido nitrogen of L-arginine is oxidized and released as an unstable, highly reactive intermediate, NO. Citrulline is formed as a byproduct, and NO, with a half-life of milli-seconds, is further oxidized to NO_2^- and NO_3^-. The labile NO intermediate is incredibly toxic to both eukaryotic and prokaryotic cells. NO toxicity is mediated through inactivation of iron-dependent enzyme systems, such as the oxidoreductases of the mitochondrial electron transport chain, the Krebs' citric acid cycle enzyme aconitase, and still other enzymes necessary for DNA replication. Each of these enzymes contains a catalytically active iron molecule linked to a sulfur group that is degraded by NO and released as an iron-nitrosyl complex.

To demonstrate that IFNγ activated macrophages use NO as an effector molecule in the destruction of intracellular amastigotes, we used a specific inhibitor of the nitrogen oxidation of L-arginine, N^G-monomethyl-L-arginine (N^GMMLA). Microbicidal activity by macrophages in cultures treated with IFNγ in the presence of N^GMMLA is completely blocked (Green, *et al.*, 1990a). Macrophage cytotoxicity against *Leishmania* amastigotes directly correlates with the metabolic breakdown of L-arginine to NO_2^-, the oxidative and stable end product of the short-lived NO intermediate. Levels of NO_2^- in culture media, then, are quantitative indices of macrophage activation and cytotoxic effector function.

Macrophages treated with IFNγ, endotoxin, or amastigotes alone produce minimal quantities (<5 μM/72h) of NO_2^- and fail to develop the capacity to kill extracellular tumor targets (Green, et al, 1990b). In contrast, the combination of IFNγ and endotoxin, or IFNγ and amastigotes, induces high levels (>40 μM/72h) of NO_2^- production and macrophage cytotoxicity against both intracellular and extracellular targets. For macrophages treated with IFNγ and infected with *L. major in vitro*, the parasite itself provides the second signal for nitrogen oxidation by activated macrophages. This amastigote-associated activation signal is not LPS or a component of the parasite membrane. In a survey of several different cytokines that the parasite might induce in the macrophage it infects, only TNFα participated in regulation of NO production in IFNγ treated macrophages (Green, *et al.*, 1990b; Drapier, Wietzerbin, and Hibbs, 1988). To test whether TNFα is the amastigote-induced second signal, we infected macrophages in the presence of anti-TNFα antibodies, and then treated these infected cells with IFNγ (Table 1). Anti-TNFα Ab, but not control Ab, totally abrogated NO_2^- production and microbicidal activity. Further, the anti-TNFα inhibition of both activities was reversed by the addition of excess TNFα. Thus, amastigotes trigger the synthesis and release of TNFα, which then acts as an auto-

TABLE 1. Induction of nitrogen oxidation and intracellular killing in macrophages cultured in the presence of ant-TNFα antibodies.

Culture Conditions:	Microbicidal Activity (%):	NO_2^- (μM/ml;72h):	TNFα (U/(ml/1.5 h)
Macrophages:		0	0
+ Amastigotes		0	4
+ Amastigotes + IFNγ	97	40	20
+ anti-TNFα Ab	3	7	< 1
+ anti-TNFα + TNFα	87	41	--
+ control MAb	91	42	25

crine signal to induce NO-dependent microbicidal activity in the IFNγ-activated macrophages (Green, *et al.*, 1990b).

Every cytotoxic reaction generated by an immune response is carefully regulated at the cellular level to prevent leakage of the toxic effector molecules (i.e., reactive oxygen and nitrogen intermediates) into normal tissues. Control of these reactions include limiting the expression of cytotoxic reactions to certain maturational stages of the macrophage (Ruco and Meltzer, 1978a; Hoover and Nacy, 1984), limiting the time that these cells remain responsive to activation signals (Ruco and Meltzer, 1978b; Nacy, *et al.*, 1981), and limiting the expression of cytotoxic activity to cells that actually encounter a pathogen (Green, *et al.*, 1990b). There must also be active pathways for regulation of the expression of these cytotoxic activities at the molecular level: cellular signals that shut down cytotoxic effector function and redirect the energy of the effector cell into the next, repair phase of restoring homeostasis. A while ago, we reported that factors in culture fluids from PMA-stimulated EL-4 thymoma cells, a continuous T cell line, suppress lymphokine-induced activation of macrophages for intracellular killing (Nacy, 1984). Attempts to purify this suppressor factor have been uniformly unsuccessful. In an effort to identify the factor in EL-4 fluids that specifically blocks intracellular killing, we examined the activity of other cytokines that demonstrate inhibitory activity on immune responses.

TGFβ, a 25 kD homodimeric protein secreted by both transformed and nontransformed cells, was originally defined by its ability to induce phenotypic transformation on non-neoplastic cells. It is now known to be a powerful immunomodulatory agent, as well. TGFβ has profound suppressive effects on intracellular destruction of *L. major* amastigotes by activated macrophages (Nelson, *et al.*, 1991). These effects are exerted at the level of NO production: cells treated with TGFβ fail to produce NO, and the only cytotoxic effector reactions sensitive to TGFβ are those that rely on the synthesis of NO (intracellular killing, cytotoxicity against certain tumor targets). Whether TGFβ blocks nitrogen oxidation somewhere in the biochemical pathway for release of the terminal guanido nitrogen of L-arginine, or blocks TNFα-mediated initiation of this pathway, remains to be resolved.

When we examine the production of TGFβ by macrophages, we find that peritoneal cells in culture produce TGFβ constitutively at low (1-30 pg/ml/10^6 cells) levels. Infection of these cells with amastigotes increases the production of TGFβ by 100-fold, to ng quantities in 24-48 h. Macrophage production of a cytokine that inhibits the intracellular destruction of the parasite may represent an evolutionary defense mechanism of *L. major* for intracellular survival: autocrine action of this amastigote-induced suppressor factor could dramatically increase parasite survival within the cells, and may also be the underlying cause of the broad immunosuppression observed in leishmanial disease.

When macrophages are treated with different cytokines, most of the cytokines increase TGFβ production 2-3 fold. One cytokine, however, is phenomenally active: IL-2. The increase in TGFβ production following 24-48 h treatment with 100 U/ml of IL-2 is well over 500-fold. The EL-4 clone ($EL\text{-}4_{Farrar}$) that produces the elusive suppressor factor (Nacy, 1984) was selected originally for its capacity to secrete enormous quantities of IL-2 for purification. Using antibodies to TGFβ, we can show that TGFβ is *not* the suppressor factor in EL-4 fluids. Since IL-2 is such a potent stimulant of TGFβ production, however, the suppressive effects of the EL-4 fluids may be due to an indirect effect of the IL-2 produced by these cells (Table 2). Microbicidal activity of IL-2-pretreated cells is less than half that of the cells pretreated with medium and then infected and activated (82%). IL-2, then, can act as a suppressor factor indirectly through its actions on macrophages to produce TGFβ. Since TGFβ is produced by activated macrophages, the signal for downregulation of cytotoxic effector functions in the natural evolution of an immune reaction may be under autocrine control.

A summary of the events and sequence of cytokines that regulate macrophage intracellular killing activities is presented in Figure 1. Macrophages infected with amastigotes of *L. major* are induced by the parasite to secrete two competing cytokines: TNFα and TGFβ. If the macrophage remains

TABLE 2. Induction of intracellular killing in macrophage cultures treated with IL-2.

Macrophages Treated with:	Infected Macrophages (%):	Intracellular Killing (%):	Suppression of Intracellular Killing (%):
Media	56		
Lymphokines	10	82	0
IL-2 (100 U/ml)	51	9	0
Lymphokines After IL-2 Pretreatment For			
4 hours	32	43	**50**
1 hour	32	43	**50**
0 hours	38	32	**60**

unexposed to IFNγ, TGFβ shuts down the capacity of the infected macrophage to become activated. If IFNγ is present, it both initiates the activation cascade by priming the cell, and enhances the production of TNFα triggered by infection with the parasite. As TNFα reaches the threshhold for acting as a second signal, it turns on the pathway for nitrogen oxidation of L-arginine, and toxic levels of NO accumulate inside the cell. When the NO levels are sufficiently high, the parasite succumbs, and the macrophage is victorious.

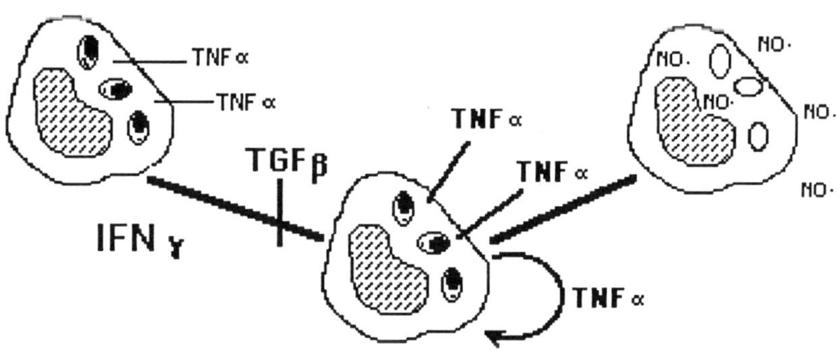

Figure 1.Cytokines that regulate microbicidal activities.

REFERENCES

Green SJ, Meltzer MS, Hibbs JB Jr, Nacy CA (1990a). Activated macrophages destroy intracellular *Leishmania major* amastigotes by an L-arginine-dependent killing mechanism. J. Immunol. 144:278-285.

Green SJ, Crawford RM, Hockmeyer JT, Meltzer MS, Nacy CA (1990b). *Leishmania major* amastigotes initiate the L-arginine-dependent killing mechanism in IFNγ-stimulated macrophages by induction of TNFα. J. Immunol. 145 (in press).

Hoover DL, Nacy CA. (1984) Macrophage activation to kill *Leishmania tropica*: defective intracellular killing of amastigotes by macrophages elicited with sterile inflammatory agents. J. Immunol. 132:1487-1492.

Nacy CA (1984) Macrophage activation to kill *Leishmania tropica*: identification of a soluble T cell factor that suppresses lymphokine-induced intracellular killing of amastigotes. J. Immunol. 133:448-453.

Nacy CA, Meltzer MS, Leonard EJ, Wyler DJ, (1981) Intracellular replication and lymphokine-induced destruction of *Leishmania tropica* in C3H/HeN mouse macrophages. J. Immunol 127:2381-2385.

Nacy CA, Fortier AH, Meltzer MS, Buchmeier NA, Schreiber RD, (1985) Macrophage activation to kill *Leishmania major*: Activation of macrophages for intracellular destruction of amastigotes can be induced by both interferonγ and non-interferon lymphokines. J. Immunol. 135:3505-3512.

Nelson BA, Ralph P, Nacy CA (1991) Differential susceptibility of activated macrophage cytotoxic effector reactions to the suppressive effects of Transforming Growth Factor β, J. Immunol. (in press)

Ruco L, Meltzer MS (1978a) Macrophage activation for tumor cytotoxicity: increased lymphokine responsiveness of peritoneal macrophages during acute inflammation. J. Immunol. 120:1054-1060.

Ruco L, Meltzer MS (1978b) Macrophage activation for tumor cytotoxicity: development of macrophage cytotoxic activity requires the completion of a series of short-lived intermediary interactions, J. Immunol. 121:2035-2040.

Cellular and Cytokine Networks in Tissue Immunity, pages 277-282

REGULATION OF MURINE INFECTIONS WITH *Francisella tularensis* (LVS) BY ALTERING THE ACTIVITY OF T_H1 AND T_H2 CELL POPULATIONS WITH ANTI-CYTOKINE ANTIBODIES

David A. Leiby, Anne H. Fortier, Robert D. Schreiber and Carol A. Nacy

Dept of Cellular Immunology, Walter Reed Army Inst of Res, Rockville, MD 20850, (D.A.L., A.H.F., C.A.N.), and Pathology Dept., Washington Univ., St. Louis, MO 63110 (R.D.S.)

INTRODUCTION

Francisella tularensis, a gram-negative bacterium, is described as a facultative intracellular parasite (1). Recent studies in our laboratory demonstrated that the live vaccine strain (LVS) of *F. tularensis* preferentially infects macrophages of mice. Once sequestered within the macrophage, bacteria can be eliminated only by cytokine induced macrophage activation resulting from antigenic stimulation of T-helper (T_H) cells. Recently, it has been proposed that two subpopulations of T_H cells exist which are differentiated solely on cytokine production (2): T_H1 cells secrete interferon-γ (IFN-γ), lymphotoxin/TNFβ, and interleukin-2 (IL-2), while T_H2 cells secrete IL-4, IL-5, and IL-6. Both subsets secrete IL-3, tumor necrosis factor-α (TNF-α) and granulocyte macrophage colony stimulating factor, but the latter two are produced primarily by T_H1 cells. For several pathogens, in particular *Leishmania major*, murine resistance or susceptibility to infection is correlated with the predominate T_H cell population found in the host: T_H1 cells confer resistance, while T_H2 cells confer susceptibility (3,4). In this study, we present preliminary observations on the role cytokines, and thus T_H cell subpopulations, play in the establishment of protective immunity to *F. tularensis*.

RESULTS AND DISCUSSION

The LD_{50} for C3H/HeN mice infected intraperitoneally (IP) with *F. tularensis* (LVS) is approximately 1 bacterium. When bacteria are introduced intradermally (ID), however, the LD_{50} is considerably higher, approximately 1 x 10^5 bacteria (5). Mice which survive an ID infection develop solid immunity: they are unaffected by an IP challenge with 10^4 bacteria, a dose lethal for non-immune mice. To evaluate the roles several cytokines play in establishment of protective immunity, mice infected ID with *F. tularensis* were treated IP with one of the following anti-cytokine mAb: α-IL-4, α-IFN-γ, or α-TNF-α (6,7,8) Table 1 demonstrates that anti-cytokine treatment has a profound effect on the LD_{50} of mice infected with *F. tularensis*: mice treated with α-IFN-γ or α-TNF-α had dramatically lower LD_{50}'s compared to untreated mice or to those receiving an irrelevant control mAb. In contrast, the LD_{50} for mice treated with α-IL-4 was dramatically higher than mice left untreated or treated with the irrelevant mAb.

TABLE 1. Survival of C3H/HeN mice infected intradermally with *F. tularensis* (LVS).

Treatment[a]	LD_{50} (x 10^2)
none	330.00
control mAb	270.00
α-IL-4 (11B11)	14000.00
none	1900.00
control mAb	> 100.00
α-IFN-γ (H22)	0.04
none	360.00
control mAb	> 100.00
α-TNF-α (TN3-19.12)	0.01

[a] Mice were treated with a single IP infection (500 μg) of an anti-cytokine mAb at the time of bacterial infection.

To investigate if the dramatic decrease in the LD_{50} observed following α-IFN-γ or α-TNF-α treatment was dependent upon Ab dose, we infected mice with *F. tularensis* and treated them with different concentrations of these anti-cytokines. As demonstrated in Figure 1, α-IFN-γ and α-TNF-α do indeed lower the LD_{50}'s in a dose dependent manner. Even when only 12.5 μg of α-TNF-α and α-IFN-γ were used, the corresponding LD_{50}'s were approximately 1 and 2 logs lower, respectively, compared to untreated mice.

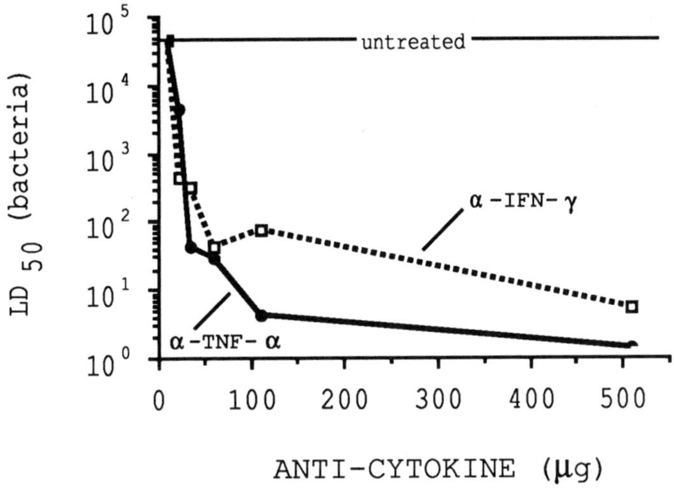

Figure 1. Effects of single IP treatment with α-IFN-γ or α-TNF-α on the LD_{50} of C3H/HeN mice infected ID with *F. tularensis* (LVS).

IFN-γ and TNF-α play essential roles in the establishment of protective immunity during a primary infection with *F. tularensis*. Similar observations have been reported for several other pathogens, including *L. major* and *Listeria monocytogenes* (9,10,11,12). In these infections, IFN-γ is assumed to play a central role in the activation of macrophage intracellular destruction of the parasite. The mechanisms by which TNF-α influences protective immunity are less clear. Like IFN-γ, TNF-α activates macrophages for certain effector activities (12). TNF-α can also recruit monocytes to the site of inflammation (10). In both instances, TNF-α appears to interact with macrophages for pathogen destruction. IL-4, on the other hand, may negatively influence establishment of protective immunity to *F. tularensis* by down-regulating the T_H1 cell population, and thereby limit production of IFN-γ. This explanation, however, may not suffice for all model systems. BALB/c mice are normally susceptible to infection with *L. major*, but weekly treatment with α-IL-4 results in parasite clearance and a concomitant fourfold increase in IFN-γ mRNA (13). However, when α-IL-4 is coadministered with a neutralizing dose of α-IFN-γ no effect on resistance to disease is observed. This suggests that increased production of IFN-γ by T_H1 cells is of little consequence in this system (13). The mechanism by which IL-4 contributes to the suppression of protective immunity warrants further investigation.

Our results suggest that resistance or susceptibility to *F. tularensis* is influenced by subpopulations of T_H cells. In this bacterial system, resistance is conferred by T_H1 cells which produce IFN-γ and TNF-α, while susceptibility correlates with the presence of IL-4, which is produced by T_H2 cells. What is not clear, however, is whether treatment with an anti-cytokine specific for a cytokine of one subpopulation leads to increased production of cytokines by the opposing subpopulation.

While IFN-γ and TNF-α play an important role in the development of a primary immune response to *F. tularensis*, their roles, if any, during a secondary immune response to *F. tularensis* are unclear. Immune mice (ID infected animals, 28 days postinfection) were treated with either α-TNF-α or α-IFN-γ (500 μg, IP) and challenged with an IP inoculum lethal for non-immune mice. This treatment had no effect: all mice survived despite the anti-cytokine treatment. The lack of effect in the immune *Francisella* model system was surprising, since secondary immunity to both *L. monocytogenes* (10) and *L. major* (12) can be totally blocked by treatment with α-TNF-α. Abrogation of secondary immunity to *L. major* was accomplished using 2 mg of α-TNF-α (12), a dose fourfold higher than we used. However, immunity to *Leishmania*, unlike *F. tularensis*, is not sterile, and anti-cytokine treatment may merely allow quiescent parasites to begin replication. Alternatively, pretreatment of immune mice with anti-cytokines may be necessary, as demonstrated for *L. monocytogenes*.(10). Lastly, cytokines and the cellular immune response may indeed play a role in secondary immune reactions to *F. tularensis*, but elucidation of their precise roles and importance may be masked by the simultaneous presence of specific immune products such as Ab.

To determine if macrophages from immune mice are exposed to cytokines during the secondary challenge, we measured the ability of peritoneal cells (PC) from ID inoculated *Francisella*-immune mice to produce nitrite and inhibit bacterial growth *in vitro*. Recent evidence suggests that nitrogen oxides synthesized from L-arginine are important effector molecules for the killing of several pathogens (14). As demonstrated in Table 2, PC from immune mice generate significant nitrite when cultured with *Francisella* compared to cells from control mice. This generation of nitrite was concomitant with significant inhibition of bacterial growth. Addition of IFN-γ to cultures had little additional effect on immune cells, suggesting that the macrophages were primed for nitrite production *in vivo*. Control cells from naive mice demonstrated significant increases in nitrite production and inhibition of bacterial growth with the addition of IFN-γ. N^G-monomethyl-L-arginine, an L-arginine analogue that competitively inhibits nitric oxide synthesis, inhibited nitrite production and led to increased bacterial growth in both control macrophage populations and cells from immune mice. Furthermore, the addition of 100 µg of α-IFN-γ to cultures completely abrogated the nitrite response and inhibition of bacterial growth (data not shown). Taken together, these results suggest that nitrogen oxides are important effector molecules for the elimination of *F. tularensis*, and that IFN-γ produced *in vivo* during secondary challenge constitutes an important part of the protective immune response.

TABLE 2. Production of nitrite (NO_2^-) and related inhibition of bacterial growth by peritoneal cells from control and immune mice cultured with *F. tularensis*, with or without IFN-γ or N^G-monomethyl-L-arginine (N^GMMLA).

	Mice	NO_2^- Production (µM/5x10^5cells/72h)	Bacteria (10^6/ml)
peritoneal cells + Francisella	control	0	66
	immune	78	<1
peritoneal cells + Francisella + IFN	control	26	5
	immune	83	<1
peritoneal cells + Francisella + N^GMMLA	control	0	22
	immune	1	20

In conclusion, protective immunity to *F. tularensis* is clearly influenced by opposing subpopulations of of T_H cells. IFN-γ and TNF-α, produced by T_H1 cells, contribute to the establishment and maintenance of immunity to *F. tularensis*. In contrast, IL-4 produced by T_H2 cells has a deleterious effect on development of protective immunity, since its removal enhances the ability of mice to withstand infectious challenge. Thus, this *F. tularensis*-model represents an ideal system for examining the influence of T_H cell subpopulations on the establishment of protective immunity to an acute bacterial infection.

REFERENCES

1. Tarnvik, A (1989). Nature of protective immunity to *Francisella tularensis*. Rev Infect Dis 11: 440-451.
2. Mosmann TR, Coffman RL (1989). TH1 and TH2 cells: different patterns of lymphokine secretion lead to different functional properties. Ann Rev Immunol 7: 145-173.
3. Scott P, Pearce E, Cheever AW, Coffman RL, Sher A (1989). Role of cytokines and CD4+ T-cell subsets in the regulation of parasite immunity and disease. Immunol Rev 112: 161-182.
4. Kierszenbaum F., Sztein MB (1990). Mechanisms underlying immunosuppression induced by *Trypanosoma cruzi*. Parasitology Today 8: 261-264.
5. Fortier A, Slayter MV, Ziemba R, Meltzer M, Nacy CA. Live vaccine strain of Francisella tularensis infection and immunity in mice (submitted).
6. Ohara J, Paul WE (1985). Production of a monoclonal antibody to and molecular characterization of B-cell stimulatory factor-1. Nature (London) 315: 333-336.
7. Schreiber RD, Hicks LJ, Celada A, Buchmeier NA, Gray PW (1985). Monoclonal antibodies to murine γ-interferon which differentially modulate macrophage activation and antiviral activity. J Immunol 134: 1609-1618.
8. Sheehan KCF, Ruddle NH, Schreiber RD (1989). Generation and characterization of hamster monoclonal antibodies that neutralize murine tumor necrosis factors. J Immunol 142: 3884-3893.
9. Buchmeier NA, Schreiber RD (1985). Requirement of endogenous interferon-γ production for resolution of *Listeria monocytogenes* infection. Proc Natl Acad Sci 82: 7404-7408.
10. Havell EA (1989). Evidence that tumor necrosis factor has an important role in antibacterial resistance. J Immunol 143: 2894-2899.
11. Belosevic M, Finbloom DS, Van der Meide PH, Slayter MV, Nacy CA (1989). Administration of monoclonal anti-IFN-g antibodies in vivo abrogates natural resistance of C3H/HeN mice to infection with Leishmania major. J Immunol 143: 266-274.
12. Liew FY, Parkinson C, Millott S, Severn A, Carrier M (1990). Tumor necrosis factor (TNFα) in leishmaniasis. I. TNFα mediates host protection against cutaneous leishmaniasis. Immunology 69: 570-573.
13. Sadick MD, Heinzel FP, Holaday BJ, Pu RT, Dawkins RS, Locksley RM (1990). Cure of murine leishmaniasis with anti-interleukin 4 monoclonal antibody. Evidence for a T cell-dependent, interferon γ-independent mechanism. J Exp Med 171: 115-127.
14. James SL, Hibbs Jr JB (1990). The role of nitrogen oxides as effector molecules of parasite killing. Parasitology Today 9: 303-305.

Cellular and Cytokine Networks in Tissue Immunity, pages 283-288

INTERLEUKIN 1β: STRUCTURE-FUNCTION RELATIONSHIP

Diana Boraschi, Paolo Ghiara and Aldo Tagliabue

Sclavo Research Centre, Siena, Italy (D.B., P.G.), and Dompe' S.p.A., Milano, Italy (A.T.)

INTRODUCTION

Interleukin 1 (IL-1) is a family of related cytokines which have an important role in the onset and development of the host immune and inflammatory reaction to invading events (Dinarello, 1989). At least two members of the IL-1 family have been identified, IL-1α and IL-1β, which share low amino acid homology (about 26%), but possess an overlapping spectrum of biological activities and bind to the same two types of IL-1 receptors (IL-1R_I, on T cells and fibroblasts; IL-1R_{II} on B cells, PMN and macrophages) (Lomedico et al., 1987; Dower & Urdal, 1987; Dinarello et al., 1989). The pleiotropic activities of IL-1 have fostered a series of studies on the structure-function relationship in the IL-1 proteins (reviewed by Boraschi & Tagliabue, 1989). Based on the hypothesis that the common biological activities of IL-1α and IL-1β might be brought about by conserved domains, the amino acid sequences of the two IL-1 polypeptides have been compared, to reveal some regions of high homology (A, B, C-D, E; Auron et al., 1985). Indeed, a synthetic peptide corresponding to the sequence 163-171 of human IL-1β within the C-D region can mimic some of the immunostimulatory activities of IL-1β, but does not possess IL-1-like inflammatory capacities (Boraschi et al., 1988; Rao & Nayak, 1990).

In the present study, we will summarize recent data on the analysis of the structure-function relationship of human IL-1β by the use of synthetic peptides and of mAbs with defined specificity, in the attempt to identify regions of the molecule involved in different functions.

RESULTS AND DISCUSSION

A series of mAbs raised against hu rIL-1β or to synthetic IL-1β peptides has been mapped for their specificity by recognition in immunoblot or in solid-phase RIA of truncated recombinant IL-1β fragments and synthetic peptides (Massone et al., 1988; Bigio et al., 1989; Boraschi et al., 1989; Herzbeck et al., 1989). Affinities of mAbs for the entire mature IL-1β were similar (data not shown), thus mAbs have been used to inhibit different IL-1β functions and binding of IL-1β to the two IL-1R types. As shown in Table 1, antibodies directed to epitope(s) within the IL-1β region 133-147 were effective in neutralizing several IL-1β activities _in vitro_ and _in vivo_ and were also able to inhibit binding of IL-1β to both IL-1R_{I} and IL-1R_{II}. IL-1β domains within the stretch 161-186 have no relevance for IL-1β binding to IL-1R_{I}, but are partially involved in binding to IL-1R_{II}, with epitopes in the region 174-186 also important T cell activation _in vitro_. Epitopes within the sequence 218-243 are apparently relevant for several IL-1β bioactivities and for binding to both IL-1R types. Eventually, the region 251-269 is involved in IL-1β effects and, possibly, in binding to IL-1R_{I}. It can be thus concluded that some IL-1β regions are important for binding to both IL-1R_{I} and IL-1R_{II} (e.g., 133-147 and 218-243), while others are involved in binding to a single IL-1R type (e.g., 166-186 for IL-1R_{II} and 251-269 for IL-1R_{I}). In any case, no clear correlation could be found between IL-1R binding and biological activities, suggesting that IL-1β sites involved in bioactivities may be distinct from IL-1R-binding site.

Along this line, the synthetic peptide corresponding to the sequence in position 163-171 of human IL-1β (VQGEESNDK) was found able to mimic a restricted range of immune system-directed IL-1β activites, while devoid of most inflammatory effects of the entire molecule (Table 2). That this fragment is in fact selectively important for the immunostimulatory activities of IL-1β was

TABLE 1

Specificity and IL-1β inhibitory capacity of anti-IL-1β mAbs

mAb[a]	IL-1β fragment recognized[b]	Neutralization of IL-1β-induced: T cell proliferation[c]	fibroblast PGE_2[d]	Adjuvanticity[e]	Fever	Inhibition of IL-1β binding to $IL\text{-}1R_I$[f]	$IL\text{-}1R_{II}$[f]
MhC1	133-147	++	++	+	n.t.	+	n.t.
BRhC3	133-147	++	n.t.	++	n.t.	++	++
MhD1	161-164	-	-	+++	n.t.	-	-
Vhp20	166-169	-	-	+	-	-	+/-
FIB1	174-186	+	n.t.	++	n.t.	-	-
BRhD2	177-186	++	n.t.	++	n.t.	-	+/-
MhG1	218-243	+	+	n.t.	n.t.	+/-	n.t.
MhG2	218-243	+	+	n.t.	n.t.	+/-	n.t.
BRhG5	218-243	+	n.t.	++	n.t.	+	+
MhI	251-269	++	++	+	n.t.	+/-	-

[a] MhC1, MhD1, MhG1, MhG2, MhI were provided by Dr. A. Massone (Massone et al., 1988); BRhC3, BRhD2 and BRhG5 by Drs. R. Rossi and M. Bigio (Bigio et al., 1989); FIB1 by Dr. H-D. Flad (Herzbeck et al., 1989).

[b] Determined with recombinant IL-1β fragments and synthetic peptides.

[c] Proliferation of murine thymocytes to 1-5 ng/ml of IL-1β; ++, IC_{50} 30-50 μg/ml; +, 100-300 μg/ml.

[d] PGE_2 production from human fibroblasts to 1-5 ng/ml of IL-1β; ++, IC_{50} 100-200 μg/ml; +, 300-600 μg/ml.

[e] Enhancement of immune response to SRBC by 100 pg/Kg of IL-1β; +++, ID_{80} 5 ng/Kg; ++, 50-200 ng/Kg; +, around 1 μg/Kg.

[f] Binding of ^{125}I IL-1β (0.1-0.3 nM) to $IL\text{-}1R_I^+$ EL4-6.1 cells and to $IL\text{-}1R_{II}^+$ RAJI or 1H7 cells ; ++, IC_{50} 2-4 μg/ml; +, 30-90 μg/ml; +/-, >200 μg/ml or only partial inhibition.

TABLE 2

Biological relevance of the IL-1β fragment 163-171

Function	IL-1β	163-171 peptide
Immunostimulation[a]	+	+
Inhibited by Vhp20	yes	yes
Inflammation[b]	+	-
Inhibited by Vhp20	no	n.d.
Binding to IL-1R_I[c]	+	-
Binding to IL-1R_{II}[c]	+	-
IL-1R-independent uptake[c]	+	+
Intracellular localization[d]		
cytoplasm	++	++
membranes	+/-	+/-
nucleus	+	+

[a] Enhancement of immune responses in vivo (Boraschi et al., 1988; Rao & Nayak, 1990; Gahring & Weigle, 1990).

[b] Induction of fever and acute phase-related responses in vivo (Boraschi et al., 1988).

[c] Binding of ^{125}I labeled IL-1β and 163-171 peptide to IL-1R_I^+ cells (EL4-6.1, D10.G4.1), IL-1R_{II}^+ cells (RAJI, 1H7, STS25) or to IL-1R^- cells (DAUDI, CTLL-2, THP-1, HL60, etc.), in the absence or in the presence of excess amounts of unlabeled IL-1β.

[d] After 6 h of radioactive 163-171 peptide uptake, cells were homogenated and fractionated by isopycnic gradient centrifugation.

confirmed by the finding that Vhp20 (a mAb raised against the 163-171 peptide and recognizing the stretch 166-169) could inhibit the adjuvant effect of IL-1β but not its pyrogenicity, besides inhibiting immunostimulation by the 163-171 peptide itself (Table 2). This fragment was unable to displace IL-1β from either IL-1R$_I$ or IL-1R$_{II}$, thus is not an IL-1R-binding domain. However, the 163-171 peptide could bind to cells and, possibly by passive diffusion, be internalized in significant amounts. Inside the cell, the 163-171 fragment localizes mainly to the soluble cytoplasmic fractions, with a small but significant amount of peptide associated to the nucleus, in agreement with the intracellular distribution of internalized IL-1β (Qwarnstrom et al., 1989). Thus, despite its inability to trigger the IL-1R, and therefore to stimulate the IL-1R-dependent IL-1β functions, the 163-171 fragment maintains the ability to stimulate some IL-1β effects which possibly do not depend on IL-1R but which are activated by interaction of the IL-1β active domains with distinct cytoplasmic and/or nuclear receptor-like structures.

In conclusion, analysis of the structure-function relationship of the human IL-1β protein indicates that active domains can be distinct from receptor-binding domains and that activation of cellular functions by IL-1β can take place through different mechanisms, some dependent on IL-1R triggering and others dependent on distinct intracellular pathways.

REFERENCES

Auron PE, Rosenwasser LJ, Matsushima K, Copeland T, Dinarello CA, Oppenheim JJ, Webb AC (1985). Human and murine interleukin 1 possess sequence and structural similarities. J Mol Cell Immunol 2:169-177.

Bigio M, Rossi R, Borri MG, Casagli MC, Nucci D, Baldari C, Volpini G, Boraschi D (1989). One-step immunoaffinity purification of bioactive human recombinant IL-1β with a monoclonal antibody directed to a well-exposed domain of the protein. J Immunol Meth 123:1-8.

Boraschi D, Nencioni L, Villa L, Censini S, Bossu' P, Ghiara P, Presentini R, Perin F, Frasca D, Doria G,

Forni G, Musso T, Giovarelli M, Ghezzi P, Bertini R, Besedovsky HO, del Rey A, Sipe JD, Antoni G, Silvestri S, Tagliabue A (1988). In vivo stimulation and restoration of the immune response by the noninflammatory fragment 163-171 of human interleukin 1β. J Exp Med 168:675-686.

Boraschi D, Tagliabue A (1989). Structure-function relationship of interleukin-1 giving new insights for its therapeutic potential. Biotherapy 1:377-389.

Boraschi D, Volpini G, Villa L, Nencioni L, Scapigliati G, Nucci D, Antoni G, Matteucci G, Cioli F, Tagliabue A (1989). A monoclonal antibody to the IL-1β peptide 163-171 blocks adjuvanticity but not pyrogenicity of IL-1β in vivo. J Immunol 143:131-134.

Dinarello CA (1989). Interleukin-1 and its biologically related cytokines. Adv Immunol 44: 153-205.

Dinarello CA, Clark BD, Puren AJ, Savage N, Rosoff PM (1989). The interleukin 1 receptor. Immunol Today 10:49-51.

Dower SK, Urdal DL (1987). The interleukin-1 receptor. Immunol Today 8:46-51.

Herzbeck H, Blum B, Ronspeck W, Frenzel B, Brandt E, Ulmer AJ, Flad H-D (1989). Functional and molecular characterization of a monoclonal antibody against the 165-186 peptide of human IL-1β. Scand J Immunol 30:549-562.

Gahring LC, Weigle WO (1990). The regulatory effects of cytokines on the induction of a peripheral immunologic tolerance in mice. J Immunol 145:1318-1323.

Lomedico PT, Gubler U, Mizel SB (1987). Cloning and expression of murine, human, and rabbit interleukin 1 genes. Lymphokines 13:139-150.

Massone A, Baldari C, Censini S, Bartalini M, Nucci D, Boraschi D, Telford JL (1988). Mapping of biologically relevant sites on human IL-1β using monoclonal antibodies. J Immunol 140:3812-3816.

Qwarnstrom EE, Page RC, Gillis S, Dower SK (1988). Binding, internalization, and intracellular localization of interleukin-1β in human diploid fibroblasts. J Biol Chem 263:8261-8269.

Rao KVS, Nayak AR (1990). Enhanced immunogenicity of a sequence derived from hepatitis B virus surface antigen in a composite peptide that includes the immunostimulatory region from human interleukin 1. Proc Natl Acad Sci USA 87:5519-5522.

Cellular and Cytokine Networks in
Tissue Immunity, pages 289-294

IL-1/TNF alpha PRODUCTION CORRELATES WITH ELAM-1 EXPRESSION BY ENDOTHELIAL CELLS IN HUMAN TISSUES

Luigi P. Ruco, Antonella Stoppacciaro, Donatella Pomponi, Alberto Pisacane, Andrea Baiocchini and Carlo D. Baroni

II Pathological Anatomy, Department of Human Biopathology University "La Sapienza", Rome, Italy 00161.

INTRODUCTION

Interleukin 1 (IL-1) and Tumor Necrosis Factor (TNF) alpha are pleiotropic molecules which play a pivotal role in inflammatory and immune reactions (Dinarello 1984; Oppenheim et al. 1986; Beutler and Cerami 1988). Cells containing IL-1 or TNF alpha can be demonstrated on sections of human tissues by immunocytochemical methods (Ruco et al. 1989). IL-1 and/or TNF alpha has been demonstrated in lymph nodes with paracortical activation, in immune granulomas, and in neoplastic cells of Hodgkin's disease (Hsu and Zhao 1986; Chilosi et al. 1988; Ruco et al. 1990).

Endothelial leukocyte adhesion molecule 1 (ELAM-1) is an inducible protein expressed by activated endothelial cells which is mainly involved in granulocyte adhesion and extravasation (Cotran et al. 1986; Bevilacqua et al. 1987). Normal endothelial cells do not express ELAM-1. In vitro exposure of umbelical vein endothelial cells to IL-1/TNF results in de novo synthesis and expression of ELAM-1 (Bevilacqua et al. 1985). Similarly, intradermal injection of IL-1/TNF in Papio anubis is followed by ELAM-1 expression in dermal blood vessels, and by perivascular accumulation of granulocytes (Munro et al. 1989).

We have recently investigated the relationship between

production of IL-1/TNF and vascular activation in vivo (Ruco et al. 1990). For this purpose, cryostat sections of normal and pathological human tissues were immunostained to correlate the presence of cells containing IL-1/TNF alpha with the expression of the activation antigen ELAM-1 by vascular endothelial cells.

RESULTS

Cryostat sections of 89 samples of lymphoid tissues, and of 56 non-lymphoid organs were immunostained using avidin-biotin-peroxidase complexes and mAbs directed to IL-1 alpha (Vmp 18), IL-1 beta (Vhp20, BRhC3), TNF alpha (B 154.7), or ELAM-1 (29F2, 5D11).

In normal non-lymphoid tissues, cells containing IL-1 and/or TNF alpha were extremely rare. In sections of skin, kidney, heart, skeletal muscle, liver, ovaries, lung, esophagus, stomach, small and large intestine, thyroid, breast, testis, hypophisis, adrenals, and brain, IL-1+ve cells were absent, and immunoreactivity for TNF alpha was confined to a few interstitial macrophages and to mast cells. In non-lymphoid tissues, absence of cytokine containing cells was well correlated with negative staining of blood vessels for ELAM-1 (Table 1).

In normal spleen and lymph nodes IL-1/TNF+ve cells were not detected and blood vessels were ELAM-1-ve. In fetal thymus, a weak reactivity for ELAM-1 was observed in rare high endothelium venules (HEVs) located at the cortico-medullary junction. ELAM-1 expression in junctional HEVs was associated with marked presence of IL-1 alpha in the medullary interdigitating reticulum cells (IDRCs).

Reactive hyperplastic lymph nodes are characterized by different histological pictures depending on the functional compartment undergoing major activation (Butler 1969; Dorfman and Warnke 1974). Immunoreactivity for ELAM-1 was

Table 1.: Expression of ELAM-1 and production of IL-1 alpha, IL-1 beta, and TNF alpha in human tissues

TISSUE	n	ELAM-1	CYTOKINES
Non-lymphoid	23	Absent	TNF+ mast cells and rare macrophages
Fetal thymus	10	Few junctional HEVs	IL-1 in IDRCs
Spleen	4	Absent	Absent
Lymph node Normal	5	Absent	Absent
Lymph node Foll. hyperpl.	12	Few HEVs in 6 cases	Rare IL-1+ cells
Lymph node Parac. hyperpl.	5	Some to many HEVs in 5/5 cases	IL-1+ mac./IDRCs Some TNF+ cells
Granuloma	6	Small blood vessels around granulomas	Epithelioid mac. are IL-1+/TNF+
Hodgkin's dis.	20	Some to many vessels in 17 cases	IL-1 and/or TNF in mac., IDRCs, H/R-S
NHLs B-cell	16	Few vessels in a single case	Rare IL-1+ cells
NHLs T-cell	7	Some to many vessels in 7 cases	IL-1 and/or TNF in and IDRCs

Acetone-fixed cryostat sections were immunostained for ELAM-1 (29F2), IL-1 alpha (Vmp18), IL-1 beta (Vhp20), and TNF alpha (B154.7) using avidin-biotin-peroxidase complexes. The immunoreaction product was developed with H_2O_2 and diaminobenzidine.

mainly observed in cases of diffuse lymphadenitis with activation of the T-dependent area. Moreover, ELAM-1+ve HEVs were often located near macrophages/IDRCs+ve for IL-1/TNF. These findings provide circumstantial evidence of the existence of a paracrine mechanism of endothelial activation in the lymph node paracortex. In 12 cases of lymph node follicular hyperplasia, characterized by prominent activation of the B-cell compartment, cells containing IL-1/TNF were extremely rare, and HEVs were ELAM-1-ve.

A strict correlation between vascular expression of ELAM-1, and presence of IL-1/TNF+ve cells was observed in granulomatous lymphadenitis (sarcoidosis and tuberculosis), and in Hodgkin's disease, a neoplastic condition mimicking a granulomatous reaction. Sarcoid and tuberculous granulomas were formed from epithelioid macrophages often immunoreactive for IL-1/TNF; small blood vessels located near granulomas were frequently ELAM-1+ve. A high frequency of IL-1/TNF+ cells associated with ELAM-1+ blood vessels was also observed in Hodgkin's disease. A puzzling tumour in which few neoplastic cells, Hodgkin's and Reed-Sternberg cells (H/RS cells), lie in an inflammatory background. Immunoreactivity for IL-1 alpha and TNF alpha was detected in neoplastic H/RS cells and in reactive macrophages as well. ELAM-1+ve blood vessels were often present in areas in which perivascular macrophages and neoplastic H/RS cells were markedly immunoreactive for IL-1/TNF.

Non-Hodgkin's lymphomas (NHLs) derive from clonal neoplastic proliferations of B lymphocytes, T lymphocytes, or much less frequently, histiocytes. In 16 cases of B-cell NHLs, representative of all the major histological variants, cells producing IL-1/TNF were extremely rare and blood vessels were generally negative for ELAM-1. In 7 cases of T-cell NHLs, immunoreactivity for IL-1 and/or TNF was observed in reactive macrophage/IDRCs; in T-NHLs, some tumor blood vessels were ELAM-1+ve.

In conclusion, tissue immunocytochemistry may provide important information concerning the role that cytokines play in the pathogenesis of neoplastic and inflammatory diseases. Our survey of a variety of normal, flogistic and neoplastic tissues strongly suggest that ELAM-1 expression is well correlated with presence of perivascular cells containing IL-1/TNF. Moreover, cytokine-induced ELAM-1 expression was observed in tissue lesions characterized by scanty neutrophils, and by massive involvement of macrophages and T lymphocytes. In these latter conditions it seems likely that ELAM-1 molecule is involved in functions other than promoting neutrophil adhesion to endothelial cells.

REFERENCES

Butler, J.J. (1969). Non neoplastic lesions of lymph nodes of man to be differentiated from lymphomas. Natl. Cancer Inst. Monogr. 32: 233-255.

Bevilacqua, M.P., Pober, J.S., Wheeler, M.E., Contra, R.S., and Gimbrone, M.A. Jr. (1985). Interleukin 1 acts on cultured human vascular endothelium to increase the adhesion of polymorphonuclear leukocytes, monocytes and related cell lines. J. Clin. Invest. 76: 2003-2011.

Bevilacqua, M.P., Pober, J.S., Mendrick, D.L., Cotran, R.S., and Gimbrone, M.A. Jr. (1987). Identification of ani inducible endothelial leukocyte adhesion molecule. Proc. Natl. Acad. Sci. USA 84: 9238-9242.

Chilosi, M., Menestrina, F., Capelli, P., Montagna, L., Lestani, M., Pizzolo, G., Cipriani, A., Agostini, C., Trentin, L., Zambello, R., and Semenzato, G. (1988). Immunohistochemical analysis of sarcoid granulomas. Evaluation of Ki67+ cells and interleukin 1+ cells. Am. J. Pathol. 131: 191-198.

Cotran, R.S., Gimbrone, M.A. Jr., Bevilacqua, M.P., Mendrick, D.L., and Pober, J.S. (1986). Induction and detection of a human endothelial activation antigen in vivo. J. Exp. Med. 164: 661-666.

Dorfman, R.F., and Warnke, R. (1974). Lymphadenopathy simulating the malignant lymphomas. Hum. Pathol. 5:

519-550.

Hsu, S.M., and Zhao, X. (1986). Expression of Interleukin 1 in Reed Sternberg cells and neoplastic cells from true histiocytic malignancies. Am. J. Pathol. 125: 221-225.

Munro, S.M., Pober, J.S., and Cotran, R.S. (1989). Tumor necrosis factor and interferon gamma induce distinct patterns of endothelial activation and associated leukocyte accumulation in skin of Papio anubis. Am. J. Pathol. 135: 121-133.

Ruco, L.P., Stoppacciaro, A., Pomponi, D., Boraschi, D., Santoni, A., Tagliabue, A., Uccini, S., and Baroni, C.D. (1989). Immunoreactivity for IL-1 beta and TNF alpha in human lymphoid and non-lymphoid tissues. Am. J. Pathol. 135: 889-897.

Ruco, L.P., Pisacane, A., Pomponi, D., Stoppacciaro, A., Pescarmona, E., Rendina, E.A., Santoni, A., Boraschi, D., Tagliabue, A., Uccini, S., Baroni, C.D. (1990). Macrophages and interdigitating reticulum cells in normal thymus and thymomas: immunoreactivity for interleukin 1 alpha, interleukin 1 beta, and tumor necrosis factor alpha. Histopathology, in press.

Ruco, L.P., Pomponi, D., Pigott, R., Stoppacciaro, A., Monardo, F., Uccini, S., Boraschi, D., Tagliabue, A., Santoni, A., Dejana, E., Mantovani, A., and Baroni, C.D. (1990). Cytokine production (IL-1 alpha, IL-1 beta, and TNF alpha) and endothelial cell activation (ELAM-1 and HLA-DR) in reactive lymphadenitis, Hodgkin's disease, and in non-Hodgkin's lymphomas: an immunocytochemical study. Am. J. Pathol., (in press).

Cellular and Cytokine Networks in Tissue Immunity, pages 295-300

ENHANCED EXPRESSION OF INTERFERON-BETA DURING THE TRIGGERING PHASE OF MACROPHAGE CYTOCIDAL ACTIVATION.

David W.H. Riches.

Division of Basic Sciences, Department of Pediatrics, National Jewish Center for Immunology and Respiratory Medicine, Denver, CO 80206.

INTRODUCTION

Macrophage cytocidal activation is a pathway of development that enables macrophages to recognize and destroy neoplastically-transformed target cells. Observed in the early 1970s as a single response of macrophages to μg quantities of naturally occurring and synthetic double stranded RNAs such as poly [I:C] or to bacterial LPS (1), work conducted in the late 1970s (2) revealed this pathway to comprise two distinct stages (Fig. 1). In the first stage, macrophages become primed in response to a suitable stimulus, the most thoroughly characterized being the IFNs, which serve to increase the sensitivity of the cells to a second triggering stimulus. Full cytocidal activity is induced when IFN-primed macrophages are exposed to pg ng quantities of a triggering stimulus which can also take the form of double-stranded RNAs, LPS and heat-killed *Listeria monocytogenes*.

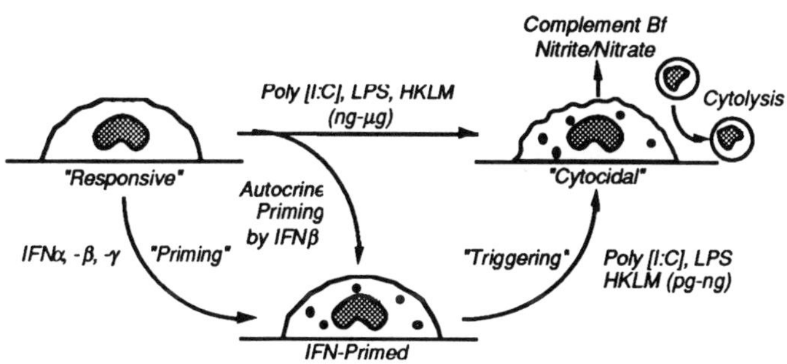

Figure 1. Pathways of macrophage development of cytocidal activity and the autocrine/paracrine role of endogenously-derived IFN.

The relationship between the single step pathway and the two step pathway has been revealed in studies collectively conducted in several laboratories. These studies have shown that one of the early responses of macrophages to moderate (μg) quantities of activating stimuli is the expression of IFNα/β, which serves to prime the cells in an autocrine or paracrine fashion thereby rendering the macrophages sensitive to triggering stimuli (Fig. 1). Nevertheless, even when macrophages have been primed with IFNs, there still exists a striking parallelism between the triggering activity and the IFN-inducing activity of many stimuli including double-stranded RNAs, LPS and heat-killed *Listeria monocytogenes*. This led us to question if, in addition to initially priming macrophages for cytocidal activation, IFN may be expressed during the triggering phase where it may contribute to the expression of full cytocidal activity. By quantifying the level of synthesis by mouse bone marrow macrophages of the complement component Bf, and the reactive nitrogen intermediates, NO_2/NO_3, that previous studies have demonstrated to be associated with the development of cytocidal activity (3,4), we show that IFNβ is expressed during the triggering phase of cytocidal activation and provide evidence to support a role in the regulation of full cytocidal activity.

RESULTS

IFNβ Expression During The Triggering Phase.

We initially determined if IFNβ was being expressed during the triggering phase of cytocidal activation. Macrophage monolayers were primed with IFNβ or incubated in medium alone for 3 hr, washed in HBSS, and then exposed to a triggering concentration of poly [I:C] (2 ng/ml) for various time intervals up to 18 hr before isolating total cellular RNA and quantifying the level of expression of IFNβ mRNA by Northern blotting and hybridization with a $[^{32}P]$-labeled IFNβ cDNA probe. Exposure of unprimed macrophages to poly [I:C] for 4 hr led to a minimal expression of IFNβ mRNA. (Fig. 2). However, a dramatic increase in the level of expression of the IFNβ mRNA was detected when IFN-primed macrophages were exposed to a triggering concentration of poly [I:C] (Fig. 2). Optimal expression of IFNβ mRNA during the triggering phase of cytocidal activation was transient being maximal at 3-4 hr after the addition of the triggering stimulus. Priming activity was also seen when macrophages were primed with IFNγ (1-10 U/ml) and triggered with poly [I:C]. Hybridization of Northern blot with an $IFN\alpha_2$ cDNA probe failed to detect expression of this IFN subtype.

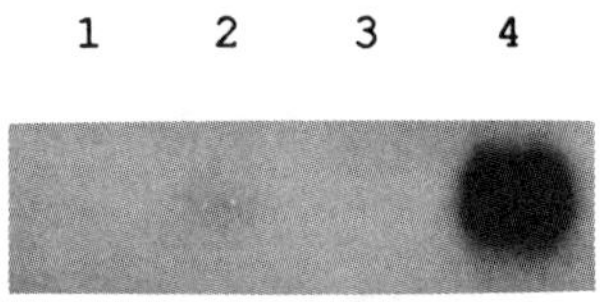

Figure 2. Expression of IFNβ during the triggering phase of macrophage cytocidal activation. Macrophages were primed with IFNβ (100 U/ml, 3 hr) and triggered with poly [I:C] (2 ng/ml) for 4 hr. Lane 1=medium alone; lane 2=IFN-primed alone; lane 3=poly [I:C] triggered alone; lane 4=IFN-primed and poly [I:C] triggered.

Involvement of Macrophage-Derived IFNβ in the Triggering Stage of Cytocidal Activation.

The ability of IFNs to prime their own production has been previously reported in other cell types (5) and hence it was important to determine if the triggering-associated transient expression of IFNβ played a role in the expression of cytocidal activity by macrophages. We addressed this question in two ways. Firstly, we have applied genetic differences in the ability of different strains of mice to produce IFN in response to poly [I:C] to question the potential role of IFN during the triggering phase. The mice selected for study consisted of four strains, C3H/HeJ, BALB/c, C57BL/6 and A/J, which, while differing at the *If-1* locus (6) which controls IFN induction by Newcastle Disease virus (NDV) bore a standard phenotype with respect to IFN induction by poly [I:C] (7). The fifth strain, B10.A(2R) was deficient in its capacity to produce IFN in response to poly [I:C]. All strain bore a standard Bf phenotype (8). As expected, when monolayers of unprimed macrophages were exposed to poly [I:C], macrophages derived from B10.A(2R) mice showed a diminished capacity to synthesize Bf compared to the other strains of mice studied (Fig. 3).

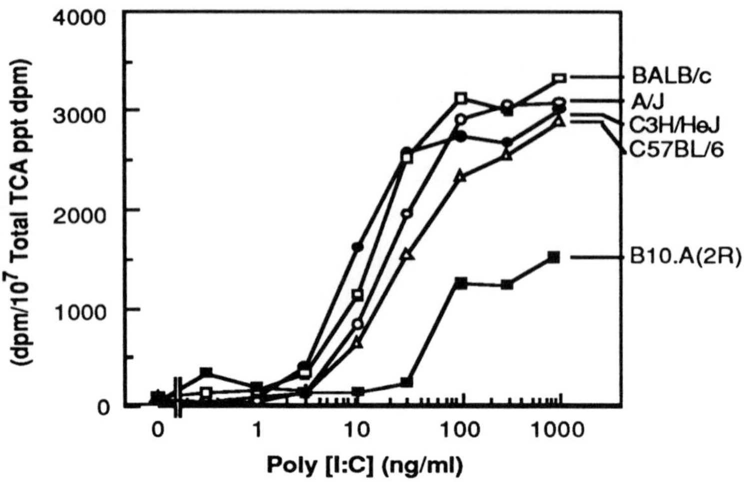

Figure 3. Synthesis of Bf by macrophages derived from different stains of mice differing in IFN responsiveness to poly [I:C].Bf synthesis is shown as the dpm incorporated into Bf protein/10^7 total TCA precipitable protein.

The diminished expression of Bf in macrophages from B10.A(2R) mice persisted when the cells were first primed with IFNβ (100 U/ml, 4 hr), washed in HBSS, and triggered with poly [I:C] in the absence of added IFN (data not shown). These data thus suggest that the triggering associated expression of IFNβ contribute to the full expression of the triggering stage.

Secondly, we determined if anti-IFNα/β antibodies, present during the triggering stage, modulated the triggering response of macrophages to poly [I:C]. Macrophage monolayers were primed with either IFNβ (100 U/ml) or IFNγ (10 U/ml) for 2 hr, washed to remove the priming stimulus, and then triggered with a suboptimal concentration of poly [I:C] (10 ng/ml) for 48 hr in the presence of absence of 5000 neutralizing Units of anti-IFNα/β antibody before quantifying NO_2/NO_3 accumulation in the culture supernatants. As will be seen in Table I, in the absence of priming, a low level of accumulation of NO_2/NO_3 was detected, which, in confirmation of previous studies using Bf as a marker of cytocidal activity (3), was completely inhibited by anti-

IFNα/β antibody. When IFNγ-primed macrophages were washed and triggered with poly [I:C], there was a marked increase in the accumulation of NO_2/NO_3 in the culture supernatants. However, this was substantially inhibited, when macrophages were triggered with poly [I:C] in the presence of anti-IFNα/β antibody. Similar data were obtained when macrophages were primed with IFNβ. These data provide a second compelling line of evidence supporting an active role of IFNβ in the triggering stage of macrophage cytocidal activation.

Table I. Inhibition of triggering of NO_2/NO_3 synthesis by anti-IFNα/β anti body. * NO_2/NO_3 levels are reported as nmol NO_2/NO_3 per 10^6 cells/48 hr.

	Unprimed	IFNγ-Primed
No Ab	7.4±1.6	22.3±1.2
Anti-IFNα/β Ab	0.0±1.4	1.3±2.0

DISCUSSION

The hypothesis of this study was that IFN expression is be induced during the triggering stage of cytocidal activation where it could potentially contribute to the expression of this activity. The results of this study provide two lines of evidence to indicate this hypothesis to be correct. Firstly, we have shown that IFNβ is expressed when IFN-primed macrophages are exposed to a concentration of poly [I:C] sufficient to induce macrophages to develop cytocidal activity. IFNβ mRNA was not expressed in response to either the priming stimulus alone or the triggering stimulus alone. Secondly, using two independent experimental approaches, we have shown that the IFNβ produced during the triggering phase is actively involved in the full expression of the cytocidal state.

The precise role that IFNβ plays during the triggering phase remains to be fully elucidated. However, hints have emerged from other studies in which our laboratory has been investigating the mechanism of transmembrane signaling leading to cytocidal activation.We have observed that when IFN-primed macrophages are exposed to the calcium ionophores A23187 or ionomycin, there is a marked induction of both Bf and NO_2/NO_3 synthesis. However, unlike the situation with poly [I:C], the response is much briefer in its duration (9). Importantly, unlike ligand triggering stimuli such as poly [I:C], calcium ionophores fail to induce IFNβ expression during the triggering stage. Based on the findings, we speculate that a potential role for the IFNβ produced during the triggering phase may be to maintain macrophages in the primed state.

ACKNOWEDGEMENTS

This work was supported by PHS grant CA 50107.

REFERENCES

(1) Alexander, P and Evans, R. (1971). Endotoxin and double-stranded RNA render macrophages cytotoxic. Nature New Biol. 232: 76-78.

(2) Russell, S.W., Doe, W.F. and McIntosh, A.T. (1977) Functional characterization of a stable, noncytolytic stage of macrophage activation in tumors. J. Exp. Med. 146:1511

(3) Riches, D.W.H., Henson, P.M., Remigio, L.K., Catterall, J.F and Strunk, R.C. (1988) Differential regulation of gene expression during macrophage activation with a polyribonucleotide. The role of endogenously-derived IFN. J. Immunol. 141:180

(4) Hibbs Jnr, J.B., Taintor, R.R. and Vavrin, Z.(1987) Macrophage cytotoxicity: role for L-arginine deiminase and imino nitrogen oxidation to nitrite. Science 235:473

(5) Stewart, W.E., Gosser, L.B. and Lockart, R.Z. (1971) Priming: a nonantiviral function of interferon. J. Virol. 7:792

(6) De Maeyer, E., De Maeyer-Guignard, J. and Bailey, D.W. (1975) Effect of mouse genotype on interferon production. Lines congenic at the *If-1* locus. Immunogenetics. 8:257

(7) Pugliese, A., Cortese, D. and Forni, G. 1980. Polygenic control of interferon production induced by poly [I:C] in vivo. Arch. Virol. 65:83

(8) Paolucci, E.S. and Shreffler, D.C. (1983) H-2-linked murine factor B phenotypes. Immunogenetics. 17:67

(9) Underwood, G.A. and Riches, D.W.H. Transmembrane-mediated changes in $[Ca^{2+}]_i$ are involved in the signalling pathway leading to macrophage cytocidal differentiation. Implications of localized changes in $[Ca^{2+}]_i$ and of IFN-primed on Ca^{2+} utilization. Submitted for publication.

Cellular and Cytokine Networks in Tissue Immunity, pages 301-306

Expression and Function of Interleukin-2 Receptors on Human Monocytes and Murine Macrophages

George W. Cox, Igor Espinoza-Delgado, Dan L. Longo and Luigi Varesio

Biological Response Modifiers Program, National Cancer Institute, Frederick, Maryland 21702-1201

INTRODUCTION

The expression of the interleukin-2 (IL-2) receptor (IL-2R) is not restricted to lymphoid cells. Several reports have indicated that normal human monocytes or monocytic cell lines express IL-2R mRNA and IL-2R protein following treatment with interferon gamma (IFN-γ) [1,2]. Although investigators generally examined the expression of only the p55 subunit of the IL-2R, they demonstrated that the IL-2R on human monocytes is functional. Accordingly, treatment of human monocytes with IL-2 induces hydrogen peroxide and superoxide anion production, interleukin-1 beta and tumor necrosis factor alpha mRNA expression, and microbicidal and tumoricidal activity [2-6].

Because p55 alone does not mediate the biologic activity of IL-2 in T lymphocytes, we questioned whether human monocytes, like T lymphocytes, also express the p70-75 subunit of the IL-2R complex [7]. Our studies were also designed to determine the ability of IL-2 to specifically induce monocyte-mediated tumoricidal activity and c-*fms* proto-oncogene expression [7,8]. Inasmuch as circulating monocytes typically migrate to tissues where they terminally differentiate into macrophages (Mϕ), we investigated the expression and role of IL-2R on murine Mϕ [9]. In this brief review, we compare and contrast the results of our studies of IL-2R expression and function on human monocytes and murine Mϕ.

MATERIALS AND METHODS

Human monocytes were purified (93 ± 3%) from leukophoresed PBMC by centrifugal elutriation. The murine Mϕ cell lines ANA-1 (C57BL/6) and GG2EE (C3H/HeJ) were established previously in our laboratory and retain functions of normal Mϕ as well as genetically determined responses to external stimuli [10,11]. Thioglycollate-elicited peritoneal Mϕ were obtained from either C57BL/6 or C3H/HeJ mice. All materials and methods have been reported previously [7-9].

RESULTS

Initial experiments were designed to analyze the expression of the p55 subunit of the IL-2R on human monocytes and murine Mϕ. Neither human monocytes [12], nor the murine Mϕ cell line ANA-1 expressed detectable levels of p55 mRNA as determined by Northern blot analysis (Table 1).

<u>TABLE 1</u>. Constitutive or stimulated expression of IL-2R subunits on human monocytes or the murine Mϕ cell line ANA-1

	p55[a]		p55[b]			p75[c]		
Cells	M	γ	M	I	γ	M	I	γ
Monocytes	n	n	-	-	+	+	+	+
Mϕ (ANA-1)	-	+	+	n	++	+	n	+

[a]=mRNA, [b]=protein, [c]=protein, M=medium, I=IL-2, γ=IFN-γ, n=not tested

However, like human monocytes, the murine Mϕ cell line ANA-1 expressed p55 mRNA after a brief (5 hour) incubation in medium supplemented with 100 U/ml of IFN-γ. As indicated in Table 1, human monocytes did not express constitutive levels of p55 protein, as determined using anti-Tac monoclonal antibody (mAb) and flow cytometry analysis (FCA). In contrast, the murine Mϕ cell line ANA-1 expressed very low constitutive levels of p55 protein, as determined using 7D4 or 3C7 mAb and

FCA. Overnight incubation of human monocytes in medium supplemented with IFN-γ (500 U/ml) but not IL-2 (1,000 U/ml) induced the expression of p55 protein. Similarly, overnight incubation of the murine Mϕ cell line ANA-1 in medium supplemented with IFN-γ (100 U/ml) augmented the cell surface expression of p55 protein.

We examined the expression of the p75 subunit of the IL-2R on monocytes and Mϕ. As assessed using TU27 mAb and FCA, human monocytes expressed p75 constitutively (Table 1). Affinity binding and chemical crosslinking experiments with $[^{125}I]$IL-2 confirmed that the murine Mϕ cell line ANA-1 expressed constitutive levels of p55 protein. Furthermore, the appearance of proteins with M_r of 82-93 kD upon SDS-PAGE analysis of the affinity binding and crosslinking experiments indicated that the murine Mϕ cell line ANA-1 also constitutively expressed p70-75. Treatment of either normal human monocytes or the murine Mϕ cell line ANA-1 with IFN-γ did not augment significantly their expression of p70-75.

The functional significance of the IL-2R subunits expressed on human monocytes and murine Mϕ was investigated. As reported previously [6], human monocytes responded to IL-2 alone (1,000 U/ml) with the induction of tumoricidal activity (Table 2).

TABLE 2. Induction of c-*fms* mRNA expression or tumoricidal activity by IL-2 and/or IFN-γ

	c-*fms*[a]			Tumoricidal Activity[b]			
Cells	M	I	γ	M	I	γ	I+γ
Monocytes	+	++	+	-	+	+	n
ANA-1 Mϕ	n	n	n	-	-	-	+
GG2EE Mϕ	n	n	n	-	-	-	+
Peritoneal Mϕ[c]	n	n	n	-	-	-	+

[a]=mRNA, [b]=tumor targets were: HT29 with monocytes or P815 with Mϕ, [c]=from either C57BL/6 or C3H/HeJ mice, n=not tested

We utilized mAbs to either p55 or p75 to determine which subunit was responsible for mediating the effect of IL-2 on monocyte tumoricidal activity. Our results revealed that p75 but not p55 mediated this effect of IL-2 (data not shown). In contrast to human monocytes, the murine Mϕ cell lines ANA-1 and GG2EE or normal murine peritoneal Mϕ did not become tumoricidal in response to IL-2 alone (up to 10,000 U/ml). However, murine Mϕ did become tumoricidal when they were incubated with IL-2 (1,000 U/ml) and a suboptimal concentration of IFN-γ (100 U/ml). Therefore, IL-2 was a costimulator of murine Mϕ tumoricidal activity. Experiments with the murine Mϕ cell line GG2EE or murine peritoneal Mϕ that are not stimulated to tumoricidal activity by IFN-γ and lipopolysaccharide (i.e. derived from genetically defective C3H/HeJ mice) also indicated that IL-2 in combination with IFN-γ but neither agent alone induced tumoricidal activity. These data indicate that IL-2 circumvented the genetic defect in C3H/HeJ mice and suggest that IL-2 may be an important physiologic counterpart of lipopolysaccharide or endotoxin.

Studies of IL-2R expression and function in human monocytes have extended previous observations of the effects of IL-2 on gene expression. We found that IL-2 (1,000 U/ml) but not IFN-γ (500 U/ml) enhanced the expression of c-*fms* mRNA and the expression of colony stimulating factor-1 receptor protein in human monocytes (Table 2). Perhaps as a consequence, CSF-1 treatment of monocytes sustained the tumoricidal activity induced by IL-2 but not IFN-γ (data not shown).

DISCUSSION

We demonstrated that human monocytes expressed p75 constitutively and p55 following treatment with IFN-γ. The murine Mϕ cell line ANA-1 also expressed p75 constitutively and, in contrast to human monocytes, also expressed p55 constitutively. The results of our functional studies suggest that the differentiation of monocytes into Mϕ may be associated with an altered expression of IL-2R subunits and a decreased responsiveness of the cells to IL-2. Although IL-2 alone was sufficient to induce human monocyte tumoricidal activity, IL-2 alone was unable to induce murine Mϕ tumoricidal activity. We are intrigued by this observation because both cell types expressed p75 constitutively. Therefore, the expression of only the p75 subunit of the IL-2R may have been sufficient for mediating the IL-2-induced tumoricidal activity of monocytes. However, neither p75 alone nor p75 in combination with low levels of p55 was sufficient to mediate the same IL-2-induced activity in murine Mϕ. Our data suggest that increased levels of p55 may have been required for the response of murine Mϕ to IL-2. In fact, IFN-γ augmented p55 expression and the ability of IL-2 to induce murine Mϕ tumoricidal activity was dependent upon a second stimulus provided by IFN-γ. An additional possibility is that IFN-γ may have been required for the physical association of p55 and p75 into a functional IL-2R complex in Mϕ. IFN-γ may also have been necessary for the expression of another IL-2R subunit that may have been required for mediating the effects of IL-2 in Mϕ. Alternatively, the intracellular events that occurred subsequent to the binding of IL-2 alone in human monocytes may have been necessary but not sufficient to mediate the effect of IL-2 alone in murine Mϕ. It will be interesting to determine the individual contributions of IFN-γ and IL-2 to the development of murine Mϕ tumoricidal activity.

REFERENCES

1. **Herrmann, F., S. A. Cannistra, H. Levine, and J. D. Griffin.** 1985. Expression of interleukin 2 receptors and binding of interleukin 2 by gamma interferon-induced human leukemic and normal monocytic cells. *J.Exp.Med. 162*:1111.

2. **Holter, W., C. K. Goldman, L. Casabo, D. L. Nelson, W. C. Greene, and T. A. Waldmann.** 1987. Expression of functional IL 2 receptors by lipopolysaccharide and interferon-γ stimulated human monocytes. *J.Immunol. 138*:2917.

3. **Wahl, S. M., N. McCartney-Francis, D. A. Hunt, P.D. Smith, L. M. Wahl, and I. M. Katona.** 1987. Monocyte interleukin 2 receptor gene expression and interleukin 2 augmentation of microbicidal activity. *J.Immunol. 139*:1342.

4. **Strieter, R. M., D. G. Remick, J. P. III Lynch, R. N. Spengler, and S. L. Kunkel.** 1989. Interleukin-2-induced tumor necrosis factor-alpha (TNFα) gene expression in human alveolar macrophages and blood monocytes. *Amer.Rev.Respir.Dis. 139*:335.

5. **Herrmann, F., S. A. Cannistra, A. Lindemann, D. Blohm, A. Rambaldi, R. H. Mertelsmann, and J. D. Griffin.** 1989. Functional consequences of monocyte IL-2 receptor expression. Induction of IL-1ß secretion by IFN and IL-2. *J.Immunol. 142*:139.

6. **Malkovsky, M., B. Loveland, M. North, G. L. Asherson, L. Gao, P. Ward, and W. Fiers.** 1987. Recombinant interleukin-2 directly augments the cytotoxicity of human monocytes. *Nature 325*:262.

7. **Espinoza-Delgado, I., J. R. Ortaldo, R. Winkler-Pickett, K. Sugamura, L. Varesio, and D. L. Longo.** 1990. Expression and role of p75 interleukin 2 receptor on human monocytes. *J.Exp.Med. 171*:1821.

8. **Espinoza-Delgado, I., D. L. Longo, G. L. Gusella, and L. Varesio.** 1990. IL-2 enhances c-fms expression in human monocytes. *J.Immunol. 145*:1137.

9. **Cox, G. W., B. J. Mathieson, S. L. Giardina, and L. Varesio.** 1990. Characterization of IL-2 receptor expression and function on murine macrophages. *J.Immunol. 145*:1719.

10. **Cox, G. W., B. J. Mathieson, L. Gandino, E. Blasi, D. Radzioch, and L. Varesio.** 1989. Heterogeneity of hematopoietic cells immortalized by v-myc/v-raf recombinant retrovirus infection of bone marrow or fetal liver. *JNCI 81*:1492.

11. **Blasi, E., D. Radzioch, S. K. Durum, and L. Varesio.** 1987. A murine macrophage cell line, immortalized by v-raf and v-myc oncogenes, exhibits normal macrophage functions. *Eur.J. Immunol. 17*:1491.

12. **Rambaldi, A., D. C. Young, F. Herrmann, S. A. Cannistra, and J. D. Griffin.** 1987. Interferon-γ induces expression of the interleukin 2 receptor gene in human monocytes. *Eur.J. Immunol. 17*:153.

Cellular and Cytokine Networks in
Tissue Immunity, pages 307-312

SELECTIVE INDUCTION OF PDGF A CHAIN AND B CHAIN GENE EXPRESSION IN RAT PERITONEAL MACROPHAGES BY INTERLEUKIN-2

Elizabeth J. Kovacs and Judith E. Neuman
Department of Cell Biology, Neurobiology and Anatomy and Molecular Biology Program, Loyola University Stritch School of Medicine, Maywood, IL 60153

INTRODUCTION

We have previously shown that cytokines produced by IL-2 activated peripheral blood leukocytes (PBL) stimulate fibroblast proliferation and collagen gene expression in vitro (1). Several cytokines, including interleukin-1 (IL-1) (2), tumor necrosis factor α (TNFα) (3), platelet derived growth factor (PDGF) (4), fibroblast growth factor (FGF) (5), and transforming growth factor β (TGFß) (6), which are elaborated by activated leukocytes have been reported to influence fibroblast growth and metabolism. However, evidence suggests that, TGFß and PDGF are the most highly fibrogenic (7), i.e. can stimulate either the proliferation of fibroblasts and the production of collagen.

Patients who undergo the intraperitoneal (i.p.) administration of lymphokine-activated killer (LAK) cells and IL-2 to combat ovarian tumors develop peritoneal adhesions (8). Preliminary observations reveal that immuno-reactive TGFß and PDGF A chain and B chain are present in the peritoneal fluid of these cancer patients who develop abdominal adhesions (EJ Kovacs, unpublished). Since the genes which code for TGFß and PDGF B chain are expressed in IL-2-treated PBL (9), the production and release of these mediators in the abdominal cavity may play a role in the development of peritoneal adhesions. To determine the role of IL-2 in the formation of the connective tissue in the abdominal cavity, we chose to ascertain whether the expression of genes which code for fibrogenic cytokines could be induced in peritoneal macrophages following treatment with IL-2. Herein, we report that IL-2 induces the expression of PDGF A chain and B chain mRNAs in rat peritoneal macrophages, but not TGFβ.

MATERIALS AND METHODS

Resident peritoneal macrophages were obtained from adult male (Harlan Sprague Dawley) rats. Adherence purified macrophages were plated at 1 x 10^6 cells/ml of AIM V medium containing 50 u/ml penicillin sulfate, 50 ug/ml streptomycin, 50 ug/ml gentamicin sulfate, 2 mM glutamine (GIBCO, Grand Island, NY) and "rested" overnight in the absence of exogenous stimulants to diminish the plastic adherence-induced cytokine gene expression (10). The following morning, IL-2 (100 units/ml) or LPS (1 ug/ml) were added for various periods of time.

Northern blot analysis was performed (11) and blots were hybridized with cDNA probes for TGF-ß (R Derynk, Genentech, S San Francisco, CA), PDGF A chain (C Betsholtz, Univ of Uppsala, Uppsula, Sweden) and v-sis (PDGF B chain, ATCC, Rockville, MD).

RESULTS

PDGF A chain and B chain mRNAs are minimally expressed in peritoneal macrophages in the absence of stimulation, but were induced as soon as 2 hours after treatment with IL-2. The level of PDGF A chain mRNA expression in macrophages after 5 hours of culture with IL-2 ranged from 3- to 6-fold that of untreated cells (Table 1). PDGF B chain mRNA expression stimulated by IL-2 was elevated to 2- to 6-fold that of untreated cells. The induction of expression of the PDGF A chain and B chain mRNAs by IL-2 represents 25% -

100% of the levels of the PDGF genes induced by LPS. In contrast to the expression of the PDGF genes, TGFß mRNA is constitutively expressed at a high level by peritoneal macrophages and can not be upregulated by treatment with either IL-2 or LPS.

TABLE 1. DENSITOMETRIC ANALYSIS OF CYTOKINE mRNA EXPRESSION BY RESIDENT PERITONEAL MACROPHAGES

TREATMENT[a]	PDGF A chain[b]	PDGF B Chain	TGFβ
none	1.0	1.0	10.3
IL-2	3.6	5.2	11.2
LPS	4.8	6.6	10.6

[a]Peritoneal macrophages were cultured with or without LPS or IL-2 for 5 hours. Blots were initially hybridized with a probe for PDGF B chain (v-sis), then stripped and sequentially hybridized with probes for PDGF A chain and TGFβ.

[b]mRNA levels are expressed as arbitrary optical density units obtained from scanning densitometric analysis of xray filters.

DISCUSSION

Herein, we report that the exposure of peritoneal macrophages to IL-2 selectively induces the expression of both PDGF A chain and B chain mRNAs, and not TGFß. These data taken with our earlier work on the production of fibrogenic cytokines by IL-2 treated PBL (1), suggest that the excessive amount of connective tissue production in cancer patients given i.p. IL-2/LAK cell therapy could be a result of these mediators.

Although other cytokines including IL-1α, IL-1ß, and TNFα are expressed by IL-2 treated leukocytes (12), they do not directly stimulate the production of connective tissue in vitro (1), and therefore may not be important mediators triggering the development of peritoneal adhesions. Alternatively TNFα and IL-1 may induce fibrosis indirectly by stimulating the production of secondary cytokines such as PDGF.

The role of fibrogenic cytokines, such as PDGF, in the production of connective tissue is not unique to this system. Several laboratories have reported on the role of PDGF and TGFß in wound healing (13-15) and pulmonary fibrosis (16).

The observations reported herein for peritoneal macrophages differ from those of our earlier work performed in PBL and purified blood monocytes (9). In contrast to peritoneal macrophages in which TGFβ mRNA is constitutively expressed and cannot be upregulated, in PBL it is not spontaneously expressed by PBL and can be induced within 2 hours of IL-2 treatment. Both non-adherent and adherent populations of PBL can be induced by IL-2 to express TGFß mRNA. Like PBL, blood monocytes express TGFß mRNA following IL-2 treatment, however the peak levels of expression are not achieved until 18 hours.

In contrast to TGFß mRNA which can be induced in both adherent and non-adherent PBL, only the adherent population of PBL expressed the PDGF mRNAs. Neither adherent PBL nor blood monocytes spontaneously expressed PDGF mRNAs but can be following treatment with IL-2.

These data suggest that peritoneal macrophage-derived PDGF induced by IL-2 may play a critical role in the development of peritoneal adhesions in patients receiving intra-abdominal adoptive immunotherapy. Since TGFß mRNA expression is not enhanced by treatment with IL-2, it suggests that, if TGFβ is involved in the production of adhesions, the peritoneal macrophages is not the source of the mediator in the abdominal cavity.

An understanding of the signals responsible for the production of fibrogenic cytokines by leukocytes may aid in the development of therapeutic regimens by which the aberrant production of connective tissue which is the hallmark of a variety of diseases including atherosclerosis and pulmonary fibrosis can be controlled.

ACKNOWLEDGEMENTS

This work was supported by ONR #N00014-89-J-1130.

REFERENCES

1. Kovacs, EJ, B Brock, I Silber, and JE Neuman. Fibroblast proliferation and connective tissue production by cytokines released from IL-2 treated peripheral blood leukocytes: induction of PDGF and TGFβ gene expression. Submitted for publication.
2. Schmidt, JA, SB Mizel, D Cohen, and I Green. 1982. Interleukin-1, A potential regulation of fibroblast proliferation. J Immunol 128:2177.
3. Beutler, B, J Mahoney, N Le Trany, and A Cerami. 1985. A purification of cachectin, a lipoprotein lipase-suppressing hormone secreted by endotoxin induced RAW264.7 cells. J Exp Med 161:984.
4. Shimakado, K, EW Raines, DK Madtes, TB Barrett, EP Bendett, and R Ross. 1985. A significant part of macrophage-derived growth factor consists of at least two forms of PDGF. Cell 43:227.
5. Baird, A, P Mormede, and P Bohlen. 1985. Immunoreactive FGF in cells of peritoneal exudate. Biochem Biophys Res Commun 126:358.
6. Assoian, RK, BE Fleurdelys, HC Stevenson, PJ Miller, DK Madtes, EW Raines, R Ross, MB Sporn. 1987. Expression and secretion of type ß TGF by activated macrophages. Proc Natl Acad Sci 84:6020.

7. Kovacs, EJ. 1991. Fibrogenic cytokines: The role of TGFß and PDGF in the development of fibrosis. Immunology Today, in press.
8. Steis, RG, WJ Urba, LA VanderMolen, MA Brookman, JW Smith, JW Clark, RL Miller, ED Crum, SK Beckner, JE McKnight, RF Ozols, HC Stevenson, RC Young and DL Longo. Intraperitoneal lymphokine activated killer cell and interleukin-2 therapy of malignancies limited to the peritoneal cavity: Results of a phase I/II study. Submitted for publication.
9. Kovacs, EJ, B Brock, IE Silber, and JE Neuman. 1990. LAK cell expression of PDGF and TGF-ß mRNAs. (eds, MC Podwanda, JJ Oppenheim, M Kluger, and CA Dinarello), Molecular and Cellular Biology of Cytokines, New York, Alan Liss, p 407.
10. Kovacs, EJ, B Brock, L Varesio, and HA Young. 1998. IL-2 induction of IL-1ß mRNA expression in monocytes. J Immunol 143:3532.
11. Kovacs, EJ, JJ Oppenheim, and HA Young. 1986. Induction of c-fos and c-myc expression in T lymphocytes following treatment with IL-1α. J Immunol 137:3649.
12. Kovacs, EJ, SK Beckner, DL Longo, L Varesio, and HA Young. 1989. Cytokine gene expression during the generation of human lymphokine activated killer cells: Induction of IL-1ß by IL-2. Cancer Res 49:940.
13. Grotendorst, GR, HE Seppa, HK Kleinman, and GM Martin. 1981. Attachment of smooth muscle cells to collagen and migration towards PDGF. Proc Natl Acad Sci 78:3669.
14. Cormack, DT, MB Sporn, AB Roberts, MJ Merino, LL Dart, and JA Norton. 1987. Transforming growth factor-ß levels in rat wound chambers. J Surg Res 42:622.
15. Lynch, SE, JC Nixon, RB Colvin, and HN Antoniades. 1987. PDGF in wound healing. Proc Natl Acad Sci 84:7696.
16. Hoyt, DG and JS Lazo. 1988. Alterations in pulmonary mRNA encoding procollagens, fibronectin and transforming growth factor-ß precede bleomycin-induced pulmonary fibrosis in mice. J Pharmacol Exp Ther 1988; 246:765.

Cellular and Cytokine Networks in Tissue Immunity, pages 313-318

RETROVIRUS-TRANSFORMED MACROPHAGES: TOOLS TO INVESTIGATE LINEAGE HETEROGENEITY.

Marica Sassano, Laura Pirami, Brigitta Stockinger, Paola Ricciardi-Castagnoli and Marco Righi.

CNR - Center of Cytopharmacology and Università degli studi di Milano (M.S., L.P., P.R.-C., M.R.), 20129 Milano, Italy and Basel Institute for Immunology (B.S.), Basel, Switzerland.

INTRODUCTION

Cells of the monocyte-macrophage lineage derive from a common stem cell and seed multiple tissues of the organism where they display a large spectrum of functions (Walker and Hester, 1983). In spite of this common origin, differentiated macrophages show heterogeneity in functions, morphology and phenotypic markers (Gordon et al., 1988). Analysis of these differences have raised the question whether macrophage subsets exist. Alternatively, it can be conceived that mononuclear phagocytes can perform different immunological functions according to the stage of activation, or maturation, in which they are induced by extrinsic factors (Gordon et al., 1988). Therefore it results very important to analyze macrophage heterogeneity at a clonal level and in controlled conditions. In order to approach this issue, Leenen et al. (1990) have recently generated and used somatic cell hybrids obtained through the fusion of macrophage precursors with a transformed myeloid partner. This approach, however, suffers from a major disadvantage: it is difficult to demonstrate which genotype dictates the differentiated features observed, since it cannot be ruled out that the tumor associated phenotype is dominating the hybrid phenotype. An alternative approach to address this issue is the immortalization (i.e. promotion of indefinite growth) of normal macrophages by stimulating a quiescent proliferative mechanism. If the reproducibility of the experiment can be assured, the analysis of a large number of clones would reduce the risk of alterations introduced by the immortalizing procedure. In this respect oncogenic retroviruses can be very useful as immortalizing agents since they can transduce and express oncogenes inducing the proliferation of the infected cell. By choosing an appropriate oncogene combination it has indeed been possible to achieve immortalization of specific cells without affecting their functional characteristics (Anderson et al., 1985).

RESULTS AND DISCUSSION

With the aim of generating permanent macrophage cell lines, we have recently described the production of a complex of oncogenic retroviruses (Righi et al., 1989a) which was able to immortalize microglial cells (brain macrophages) from mouse embryos (Righi et al., 1989b). Southern and Northern analysis of two microglial clones, N-11 and N-13, demonstrated the presence in these cells of a wild-type AKR virus together with an AKR-derived recombinant retrovirus transducing a viral v-*myc* oncogene (Righi et al., 1991). As a consequence these clones produce infective oncogenic viral particles and can be used as source of immortalizing agents. In this respect we have tested the transforming potential of filtered N-11 and N-13 supernatants on primary cultures of adult mouse tissues.

Table 1. Surface markers and functions of immortalized clones.

Cell lines	MS-1	MT-2	M-1	M-2/1	M-2/9	M-2/13
Strain	C57	BL/c	B10/o	B10/n	B10/n	B10/n
Tissue	Sp	Th	Th	Th	Th	Th
F4/80	++	++	++	++	++	++
Mac 1	++	++	++	++	++	++
Fc receptors	+	+	++	+	+	++
SRBC * Phagocyt.	70%	60%	80%	50%	40%	80%

C57-C57Bl/6; BL/c-BALB/c; B10/o - B10D2/o; B10/n - B10D2/n
Sp - Spleen; Th - Thymus; SRBC - Sheep Red Blood Cells
* Percentage of cells having ingested at least 5 SRBC in 1 hour.

Experiments were performed on primary cultures of thymus or spleen obtained from BALB/c, C57Bl/6, B10D2/o and B10D2/n mice. In all the cases we obtained proliferation only in the infected cultures. The proliferating cells could be cloned by limiting dilution and 6 clones were characterized in detail. The cell lines obtained were analyzed by immune cytofluorimetry and found positive for the specific macrophage markers F4/80, Mac 1 and Fc receptors (Table 1). Phagocytic activity of opsonized sheep red blood cells could also be observed. These findings suggest that the infecting viruses show a tropism for cells of the monocyte-macrophage lineage. In addition, the process of immortalization seems to be independent from the age of the animal or the origin of the infected tissue.

The use of immortal cells cultured in vitro is based on the assumption that no major alterations are introduced during the immortalization procedure. In this respect it is important to know if the proliferative mechanism induced by the VN-11 or VN-13 oncogenic retroviruses is similar to that controlling macrophage proliferation in physiological conditions. For this purpose we carried out a detailed characterization of the oncogenic retrovirus harboured in clone N-11, and henceforward called VN-11, through the molecular cloning of its proviral form. As shown in Figure 1, a v-*myc* oncogene of avian origin but no other cell derived sequences can be located in the VN-11

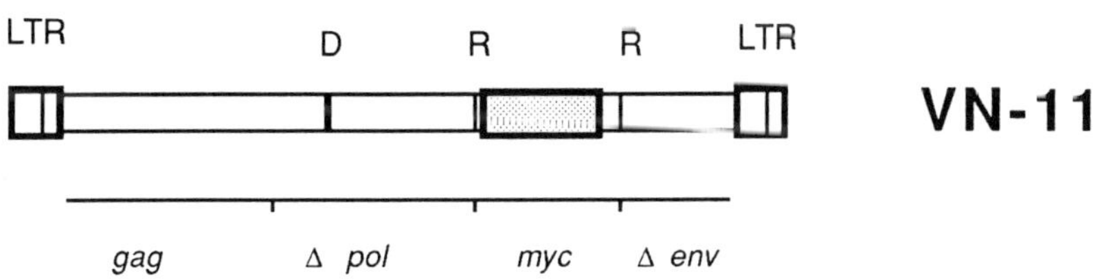

Figure 1. Genetic map of the VN-11 provirus. D indicates the site of the deletion in the *pol* gene. R map the sites of recombination. The dotted box maps v-*myc* sequences.

genome. Apart from this oncogene, VN-11 carries a deletion of about 1 kbp at the 5' portion of the *pol* gene. Otherwise, the map of VN-11 is colinear with that of the AKR retrovirus down to the beginning of the *env* gene where recombination with v-*myc* takes place. The last portion of

VN-11 is again colinear with AKR. A deregulated expression of the v- or c-*myc* oncogene is known to be necessary in macrophage immortalization (Vennström et al., 1984). However, the results reported in the literature point out that a second transforming event is necessary to induce indefinite growth of these cells (Baumbach et al., 1986). This event can be the expression of a second oncogene (e.g. *mil/raf*) or the estabilishment of an autocrine loop (Blasi et al., 1985; Baumbach et al., 1988). According to Southern or Northern blot analysis the *mil/raf* oncogene was not activated in our cell lines, therefore we analyzed the expression of myeloid growth factors. Whereas GM-CSF or

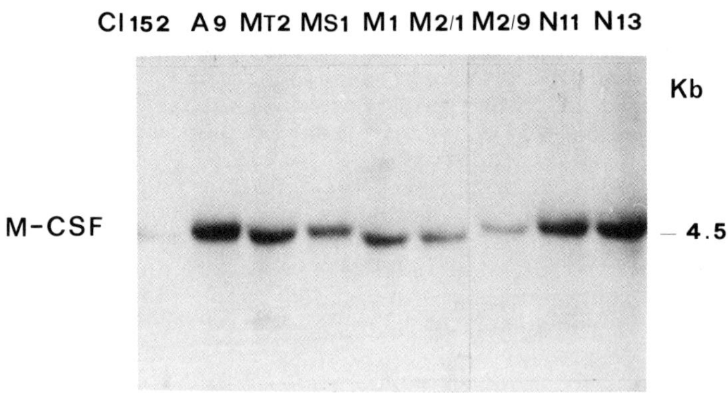

Figure 2. Expression of M-CSF transcripts in immortalized macrophages. Total RNA from the cell lines listed across the top of the figure where hybridized with a M-CSF probe. A-9 is a fibroblastic cell line expressing M-CSF. MSN-4 Cl 152 is a M-CSF dependent macrophage clone (Green et al., 1989) used as negative control.

Interleukin-3 were not expressed we observed in our cell lines the increased transcription of the M-CSF gene (Figure 2) in respect to a M-CSF dependent macrophage cell line (MSN-4 Cl 152: Green et al., 1989). The production of the M-CSF growth factor was confirmed by immunofluorescence with antibodies directed against the growth factor itself (data not shown). In addition to these results we observed that some of the cell lines under analysis were able to secrete M-CSF-like activity as detected by ^{3}H-Thymidine incorporation in the M-CSF dependent MSN-4 Cl 152 cell line (Table 2).

Table 2. ^{3}H-TdR incorporation stimulated in MSN-4 Cl 152 cells by the supernatant of different cell lines.

Cells	Medium	A-9	N-11	N-13	MS-1	MT-2
c.p.m.	10869	41647	23106	14317	25172	38934
± S.D.	±4133	±12133	±5484	±2246	±825	±7017

A9 - Fibroblastic cell line secreting M-CSF.

Since the M-CSF receptor is expressed constitutively in the cell lines tested, the production of the M-CSF growth factor and the resulting autocrine loop could be the synergistic event needed, in addition to v-*myc* expression, to induce macrophage proliferation . Although reported in the immortalization of fetal liver macrophages the activation of the M-CSF gene is not normally observed in cells carrying an activated *myc* oncogene (Birchenall-Roberts et al., 1989). In addition the analysis of the M-CSF locus performed on microglial cell lines allowed us to demonstrate the absence of retroviral integrations in the locus itself. Thus it remains unclear how the M-CSF gene can be activated by the infecting retroviruses.

It is well known that macrophages can be induced to proliferate for a short period of time by addition of the M CSF myeloid growth factor. When the cells proliferate, they express the normal c-*myc* proto-oncogene. Thus, in our system, the immortalizing viruses induce proliferative stimuli similar to those occourring in physiological conditions. In addition, we have demonstrated the possibility to obtain macrophage cell lines from different districts of the adult mouse. These results open the way to the estabilishment of large numbers of clonal cell lines derived from different organs and may be useful to test the existence of different macrophage subpopulations.

REFERENCES

Anderson SM, Klinken SP, Hankins WD (1985). A murine recombinant retrovirus containing the *src* oncogene transforms erythroid precursor cells in vitro. Mol Cell Biol 5: 3369-3375.

Baumbach WR, Keath EJ, Cole MD (1986). A mouse c-*myc* retrovirus transforms estabilished fibroblast lines in vitro and induces monocyte macrophage tumors in vivo. J Virol 59: 276-283.

Baumbach WR, Colston EM, Cole MD (1988) Integration of the BALB/c ecotropic provirus into the colony-stimulating factor-1 growth factor locus in a *myc* retrovirus-induced murine monocytic tumor. J Virol 62: 3151-3155.

Birchenall-Roberts MC, Engelmann GL, Keller JR, Lohrey N, Ruscetti FW (1989). Retroviral v-*myc* infection of primary fetal liver cells: transformation of monocytes in vitro. Oncogene 4: 731-735.

Blasi E, Mathieson B, Varesio L, Cleveland JL, Borchert PA, Rapp UR (1985). Selective immortalization of murine macrophages from fresh bone marrow by a *raf/myc* recombinant murine retrovirus. Nature 318: 667-670.

Gordon S, Keshav S, Chung LP (1988). Mononuclear phagocytes: tissue distribution and functional heterogeneity. Curr Opin Immunol 1: 26-34.

Green SM, Lowe AD, Parrington J, Karn J (1989). Transformation of growth factor dependent myeloid stem cells with retroviral vectors carrying c-*myc*. Oncogene 4: 737-751.

Leenen PJM, Slieker WAT, Melis M, Van Ewijk W (1990). Murine macrophage precursor characterization. I. Production, phenotype and differentiation of macrophage precursor hybrids. Europ J Immunol 20: 15-25.

Righi M, Pierani A, Boglia A, De Libero G, Mori L, Marini V, Ricciardi-Castagnoli P (1989a). Generation of new oncogenic murine retroviruses by cotransfection of cloned AKR and MH2 proviruses. Oncogene 4: 223-230.

Righi M, Mori L, De Libero G, Sironi M, Biondi A, Mantovani A, Denis-Donini S, Ricciardi-Castagnoli P (1989b). Monokine production by microglial cell clones. Europ J Immunol 19: 1443-1448.

Righi M, Sassano M, Valsasnini P, Shammah S, Ricciardi-Castagnoli P (1991). Activation of the M-CSF gene in mouse macrophages carrying a v-*myc* oncogene. Oncogene, in press.

Vennström B, Kahn P, Adkins B, Enrietto P, Hayman MJ, Graf T, Luciw P (1984). Transformation of mammalian fibroblasts and macrophages in vitro by a murine retrovirus encoding an avian v-*myc* oncogene. EMBO J 3: 3223-3229.

Walker WS and Hester RB (1983). In: Bellanti JA, Herscowitz HB (eds.), "The Reticuloendothelial System vol.6" New York: Plenum Press, pp 27-52.

Cellular and Cytokine Networks in
Tissue Immunity, pages 319-324

CAP37: A monocyte-specific chemotaxin released from the azurophilic granules of polymorphonuclear leukocytes

James W. Larrick[1], H. Anne Pereira[2], John K. Spitznagel[2], Teresa Sukiennieckl[1], John G. Morgan[1]

[1]Genelabs Inc., 505 Penobscot Drive, Redwood City, CA 94063.
[2]Dept. Micro. & Imm., Emory U. School of Med., Atlanta GA 30322.

INTRODUCTION

Inflammation is orchestrated by the sequential release of specific molecules that mediate the activation and chemotaxis of various cell types (1)[see figure 1]. Early inflammatory lesions are comprised primarily of polymorphonuclear leukocytes (PMN) followed by infiltration of mononuclear phagocytes. Evidence suggests that one or more factors derived from the PMN may modulate the subsequent chemotaxis of monocytes (2,3). In fact an early study described the absolute requirement of PMNs for the subsequent infiltration of mononuclear phagocytes (4).

Figure 1: Kinetics of inflammatory cell chemotaxis.

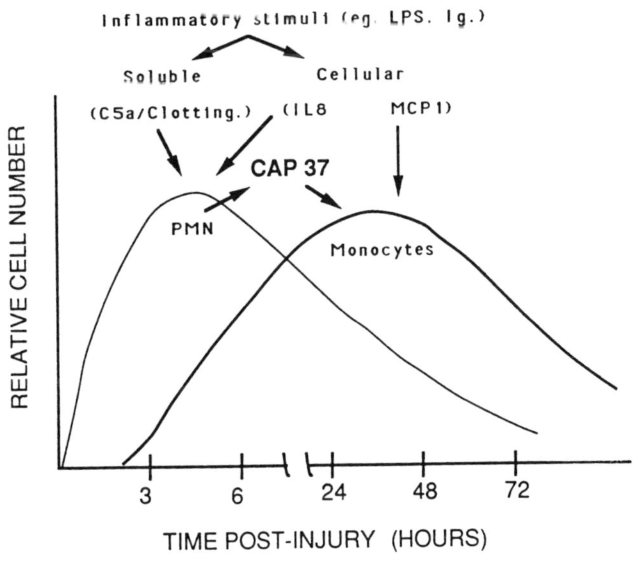

Previous work from this laboratory demonstrated the antimicrobial activity of a major PMN granule protein CAP 37 [designated Cationic Antimicrobial Protein of Mr = 37,000] (5,6). This protein is a potent mediator of monocyte specific chemotaxis and may act as a mediator of the second wave of inflammatory cell migration (7)[see figures 2 and 3]. Stimulation of PMN with opsonized Staphylococcus aureus resulted in a rapid release of approximately 89% of CAP37 into the extracellular milieu. This finding is important since, if a substance is to act as a chemotactic factor in vivo it must released extracellularly to effect its function. Immunocytochemical studies performed on peripheral blood cells indicated that CAP37 was present in PMN alone (7). Mononuclear cells, eosinophils, and red blood cells failed to stain positive with the monospecific mouse antibody to CAP37 used in these studies. Recently, we determined the N-terminal sequence of CAP37 (8).

Figure 2: CAP37 is a macrophage specific chemotaxin.

In vitro studies using a modified Boyden chamber demonstrated that purified CAP37 (but not elastase) was specifically chemotactic for human monocytes. Significant chemotaxis was apparent at 100 pM concentration. Details of these studies have been presented (7).

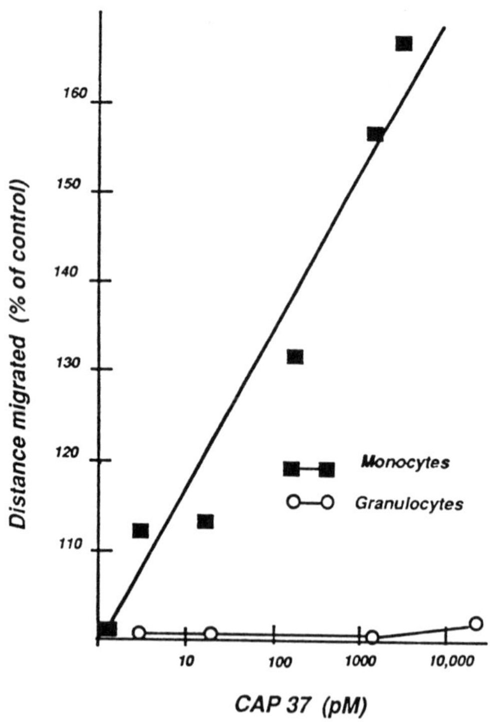

Figure 3: Specific chemotaxis of monocytes into peritoneal cavity of mice injected with purified CAP37 (1 ug). CAP37 is a potent chemotaxin in vivo. When purified CAP37 was injected IP into mice a significant emigration of monocytes was found versus saline control.

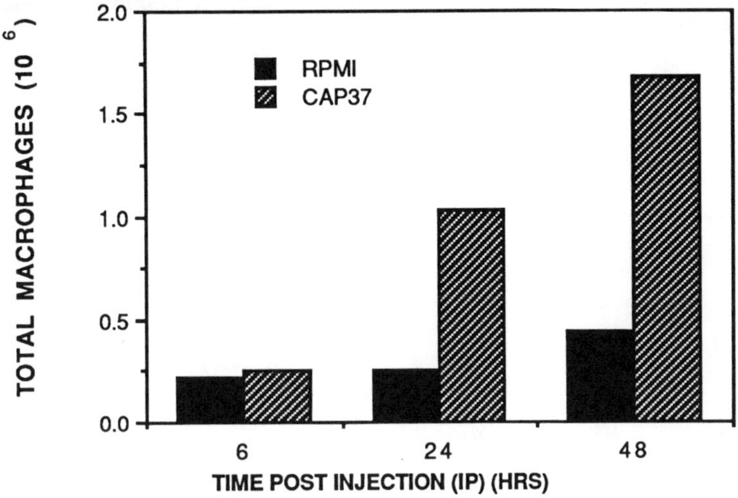

RESULTS AND DISCUSSION

Because immunohistochemistry demonstrated that the human promyelocytic cell line HL-60 contained CAP37 protein (7), a HL-60 cDNA library was constructed in lambda gt10. A CAP37 cDNA clone of 899 bp was isolated from an HL-60 cDNA library using degenerate oligonucleotide probes based on the N-terminal sequence of the CAP37 protein. Details of these studies will be published elsewhere (Morgan et al, submitted) and are summarized below. The sequence predicts an open reading frame of 753 bp encoding a protein of 251 amino acids. A 26-residue eukaryotic signal peptide and a potential 7 amino acid pro-peptide are present at the N-terminus of the protein. The cDNA sequence also predicts 3 N-linked glycosylation attachment sites and 8 intramolecular cysteines. The deduced amino acid sequence of CAP37 shows 44% and 32% homology at the amino acid level to neutrophil elastase and cathepsin G respectively, suggesting that CAP37 is member of the serine protease gene family. Figure 4 shows the hydropathic plots of CAP37 compared to elastase. CAP37 does not possess serine protease activity (8) probably due to mutations in two of three residues in the catalytic triad of the 'charge relay system' (see figure 5).

The mRNA for CAP37 is approximately 1.0 kb in size. Expression of CAP37 appears to be differentially regulated in myeloid cells. Whereas PMA-treated HL-60 cells undergoing monocytic differentiation turn off CAP37 mRNA, DMSO-treated HL-60 cells undergoing granulocytic differentiation express increased levels of CAP37 mRNA.

Figure 4. Comparison of hydropathicity plots for CAP37 and Elastase proteins.

Positive values on the y-axis indicate hydrophobic regions while negative values indicate hydrophilic regions. The x-axis refers to amino acid residue number in the mature protein sequence (9).

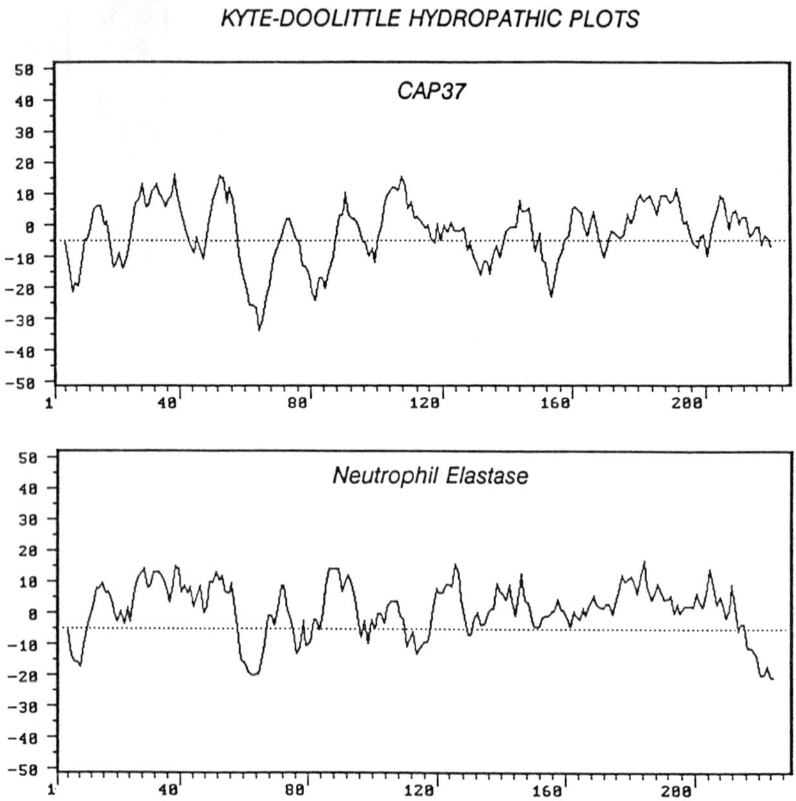

Figure 5. Mutations in the serine protease catalytic triad.

	Enzymatic Activity	Substitutions
ELASTASE:	Active	His^{41} — Asp^{88} — Ser^{173}
CAP37:	Inactive	Ser^{41} — Asp^{89} — Gly^{175}

The amino acid sequence of CAP37 shares strong homology to the serine proteinases. These endopeptidases are the largest class of mammalian proteinases. The strongest homology observed is to human neutrophil elastase/medullasin protein. Neutrophil elastase (PMN elastase) is a ppoteolytic enzyme with broad substrate specificity that resides in the azurophilic granules of PMNs and monocytes (10-12). It is a 28 kd protein which can degrade a wide range of substrates such as cartilage proteoglycan (13), elastin (14), fibronectin, laminin (15) and type I, type II and type IV collagens (16). Cathepsin G, also present in the azurophilic granules, is structurally and catalytically related to the pancreatic chymotrypsins and to the chymases of mast cell granules (17). A common feature of serine proteases is their conserved disulfide bonds. The positions of all 8 cysteines are conserved between CAP37 and elastase. In addition to the conserved disulfide bonds, another feature of the serine proteases is the residues forming the 'charge relay system' of the active catalytic site (18) which occur at his^{-57}, asp^{-102} and ser^{-195} (chymotrypsin numbering). The protein sequence (7) and cDNA sequence of CAP37 demonstrate that the conserved histidine (his^{-41}) is replaced by a serine residue, the aspartic acid (asp^{-89}) is conserved and the serine (ser^{-175}) is replaced by a glycine (Fig. 5). With such crucial mutations at these sites it is unlikely that CAP37 has serine proteinase activity and indeed recent studies have demonstrated that CAP37 does not cleave a number of substrates of elastase and cathepsin G (7). Comparison of the hydropathic plots of both CAP37 and elastase show very similar profiles particularly over the first 80 residues.

Expression of the recombinant protein will help define the role of CAP37 in homeostasis and inflammation. Important questions regarding the antimicrobial action can be investigated. It will be particularly interesting to examine cells exhibiting CAP37 receptors. At the present time it is not known if protease inhibitors block the chemotactic response of monocytes or whether conversion of the catalytic residues to those present in elastase restore proteolytic activity. Recombinant CAP37 may find uses in wound healing or cancer therapy.

REFERENCES

1. Wilkinson, P.C. 1982. Chemotaxis and Inflammation. 2nd Ed. Edinburgh: Churchill Livingstone, pp. 119.
2. Ward, P.A. 1968. Chemotaxis of mononuclear cells. J.Exp.Med. **128**, 1201.
3. Gallin, J.I. 1985. Neutrophil-specific granule deficiency. Ann.Rev.Med. **36**,

263.
4. Page, A.R. and Good, R.A. 1958. A clinical and experimental study of the function of neutrophils in the inflammatory response. Amer.J.Pathol. **34**, 645.
5. Shafer, W.M., Martin, L.E., and Spitznagel, J.K. 1984. Cationic antimicrobial proteins isolated from human neutrophil granulocytes in the presence of diisopropyl fluorophosphate. Infect.Immun. **45**, 29.
6. Shafer, W.M., Martin, L.E., and Spitznagel, J.K. 1986. Late intraphagosomal hydrogen ion concentration favours the in vitro antimicrobial capacity of a 37 kd cationic granule protein of human neutrophil granules. Infect.Immun.**53**, 651.
7. Pereira, H.A., Shafer, W.M., Pohl, L., Martin, L.E., & Spitznagel, J.K. 1990. CAP37, a Novel Monocyte-specific Chemotactic Factor. J. Clin.Invest. **85**, 1468.
8. Pereira, H.A., Spitznagel, J.K., Pohl, J., Wilson, D.E., Morgan, J., Palings, I. and Larrick, J.W. 1990. CAP37, a 37 kD human neutrophil granule cationic protein shares homology with inflammatory proteinases. Life Sci. **46**, 189.
9. Kyte, J., and Doolittle, R.F. 1982. A simple method for displaying the hydropathic character of a protein. J. Mol. Biol. **157**, 105-132.
10. Sinha, W., Watorek. W., Karr, S., Giles, J., Bode, W., and Travis, J. 1987. Primary structure of human neutrophil elastase. Proc.Natl.Acad.Sci. U.S.A. **84**, 2228.
11. Okano, K., Aoki, Y., Sakurai, T., Kajitani, M., Kanai, S., Shimazu, T., Shimizu, H., and Naruto, M.1987. Molecular cloning of complementary DNA for human medullasin: an inflammatory serine protease in bone marrow cells. J.Biol.Chem. **102**, 13.
12. Farley, D., Salvesen, G., and Travis, J. 1988. Molecular cloning of human neutrophil elastase. Bio. Chem. Hoppe. Seyler. **369**,(suppl.) 3.
13. Keiser, H., Greenwald, R.A., Feinstein, G., and Janoff, A. 1976. Degradation of cartilage proteoglycan by human leukocyte granule neutral proteases--a model of joint injury. II. Degradation of isolated bovine nasal cartilage proteoglycan. J.Clin. Invest. **57**, 625.
14. Barrett, A.J., 1981. Leukocyte elastase. Methods Enzymol. **80**, 581.
15. Campbell, E.J., Senior,R.M., McDonald, J.A., and Cox, D.L. 1982. Proteolysis by neutrophils. Relative importance of cell-substrate contact and oxidative inactivation of proteinase inhibitors in vitro. J.Clin.Invest. **70**, 845.
16. Pipoly, D.J. and Crouch, E.C. 1987. Degradation of Native Type IV Procollagen by Human Neutrophil Elastase. Implications for Leukocyte-Mediated Degradation of Basement Membranes. Biochem. **26**, 5748.
17. Roughley, P.J., and Barrett, A.J. 1977. The degradation of cartilage proteoglycans by tissue proteinases. Proteoglycan structure and its susceptibility to proteolysis. Biochem.J. **167**, 629.
18. Neurath, H. 1984. Evolution of proteolytic enzymes. Science **224**, 350.

Cellular and Cytokine Networks in Tissue Immunity, pages 325-330

TWO HUMAN TNF RECEPTORS: BIOCHEMICAL CHARACTERIZATION AND MOLECULAR CLONING

Werner Lesslauer, Manfred Brockhaus, Yu-Ching E. Pan, Hans-Werner Lahm, Ueli Gubler, Zlatko Dembic, Reiner Gentz, Hisahiro Tabuchi and Hansruedi Loetscher

Central Research Units, F. Hoffmann-LaRoche LTD, 4002 Basel, Switzerland, and Roche Research Center, Hoffmann-LaRoche Inc., Nutley, New Jersey 07110, USA (Y.C.E.P.and U.G.)

INTRODUCTION

Tumor necrosis factor (TNF) originally discovered as a serum component of BCG-primed mice which causes hemorrhagic necrosis of certain transplantable murine tumors (Old, 1985) comprises two related cytokines, TNFα and TNFβ, which have about 30% sequence homology (Pennica et al., 1984). A wide variety of pleiotropic activities of TNF *in vitro* and *in vivo* have been reported (for reviews see Beutler and Cerami, 1988; Beutler and Cerami, 1989; Tracey et al., 1989). A crucial role of TNF appears to be as a mediator in immune and inflammatory reactions. Studies of signal transduction pathways have shown that TNF induces NF-κB and thus takes part in the control of NF-kB inducible genes (Hohmann et al., 1990; Osborn et al., 1989).

Several groups have reported studies on TNF receptors from a variety of different cells and cell lines (for references see Loetscher, 1991). In most cases a single class of TNF binding sites with a K_d value in the pM range was found. Various TNFα- and TNFβ-reactive bands with molecular masses ranging from about 50 kDa to 138 kDa were detected in crosslinking experiments.

Here we present the molecular cloning of two human TNF receptors; in the past few month, independent groups have also isolated cDNA's coding for one or the other receptor (for review and references see Loetscher et al., 1990a).

RESULTS

1. Identification of Two TNF-Receptors

A thorough biochemical characterization of crosslinked TNFα-receptor complexes from various cells has indicated the existence of at least two distinct TNF receptor molecules which differ not only in molecular weight but also in ligand binding affinity, glycosylation, immunoreactivity and proteolytic fingerprints (Hohmann et al., 1989). Monoclonal antibodies raised against a partially purified TNF receptor preparation confirmed the distinct nature of the two receptors; no crossreactivity between the two classes of antibodies (htr and utr) was observed (Brockhaus et al., 1990). The two TNF receptors were purified from HL60 cells to apparent homogeneity (Loetscher et al., 1990c). SDS-PAGE analysis revealed for one receptor a double band at 55 and 51 kDa and for the other a major band at 75 kDa and a minor band at 65 kDa. Partial amino acid sequences were determined for both TNF receptors. In view of their different apparent molecular masses the two receptors will be called TNFRα (75 kDa) and TNFRβ (55 kDa).

2. Molecular Cloning and Expression of TNFRβ

The cDNA encoding human TNFRβ has been isolated using partial amino acid sequence information and a combination of polymerase chain reaction (PCR) and conventional cloning techniques (Loetscher et al., 1990b). Short fully degenerate sense and antisense oligonucleotide primers encoding the N- and C- terminal ends of the 22 amino acid residue N-terminal peptide sequence were used to amplify a 66 bp cDNA fragment from HL60 RNA by reverse transcriptase - polymerase chain reaction. This cDNA fragment as a probe identified several overlapping clones in a human placenta cDNA library. A restriction map of the TNFRβ cDNA is shown in Figure 1. The open reading frame of the cDNA predicts a protein with 455 amino acid residues. The single transmembrane region with 21 residues separates the extracellular N-terminal domain of 182 residues including 24 cysteines and the C-terminal domain of 223 residues. Three potential N-linked glycosylation sites are contained in the extracellular domain. A 29 amino acid leader sequence precedes the leucine (Leu^1) identified by protein sequencing as NH_2-terminus of the isolated mature protein. The mature human TNFRβ therefore comprises 426 amino acids with a theoretical molecular weight of 47.5 kDa. Posttranslational modifications, i.e. glycosylation probably account for the difference to the apparent molecular weight estimated from SDS-PAGE.

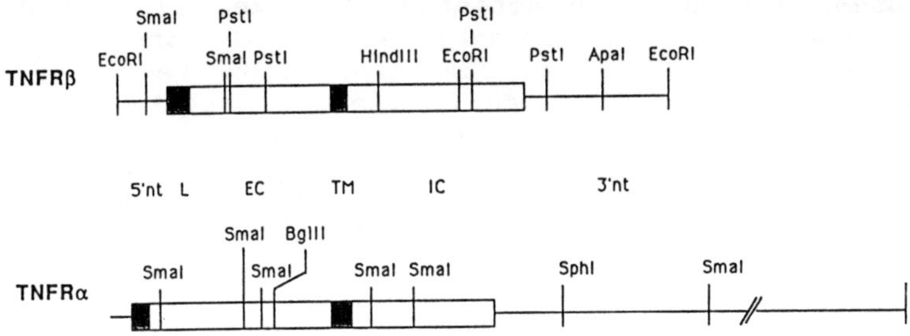

Figure 1. *Restriction Maps of the TNFRα and TNFRβ cDNA's.* The coding regions of the cDNA's are boxed and the putative leader (L), extracellular (EC), transmembrane (TM), intracellular (IC), and nontranslated (5' nt, 3' nt) regions are indicated.

The TNF binding activity of the protein encoded by this cDNA has been confirmed in two different expression systems. First, the 1.3 kb EcoRI-EcoRI fragment (see Fig.1) of the TNFRβ cDNA was cloned into a modified pXF3/ori vector which contains the human CMV immediate-early promoter and SV40 ori. This construct when tested in transient transfection in COS-1 cells resulted in the expression of a single class of high affinity ^{125}I-TNFα binding sites (K_d = 0.51 nM). Second, the 1.3 kb EcoRI-EcoRI fragment was recloned into a modified pVL941 plasmid under the control of the polyhedrin promoter, introduced into the AcNP virus by homologous recombination, and expressed in the baculovirus system. Virus-infected Sf9 cells displayed on their surface a highly significant and specific ^{125}I-TNFα binding similar to the binding observed on COS-1 cells after transfection with the pXF3/ori construct.

3.Molecular Cloning and Expression of TNFRα

A short cDNA fragment coding for a 17 amino acid tryptic peptide of human TNFRα was amplified from human genomic DNA by polymerase chain reaction (Dembic et al., 1990). A synthetic oligonucleotide derived from this cDNA was used as a probe to isolate the cDNA from human placenta and HL60 cDNA libraries. The isolated cDNA revealed a large open reading frame encoding a typical transmembrane protein (Fig.1). The N-terminal end of the predicted amino acid sequence was found to overlap with the N-terminal sequence of the purified protein. Thus, the mature TNFRα comprises 439 amino acids with extracellular (235 residues), transmembrane (26 residues), and intracellular (178 residues) regions. Two potential N-linked glycosylation sites are present in the extracellular domain. The HL60 derived cDNA in the pLJ268 expression vector after transfection into COS-1 cells yielded recombinant cell surface-located TNFRα which bound ^{125}I-TNFα with a K_d of about 0.1 nM. The positive staining of TNFRα in COS-1 cell transfectants with monoclonal antibody utr-1 in the fluorescence microscope further confirmed the identity of the recombinant protein.

DISCUSSION

The comparison of the predicted amino acid sequences of TNFRα and TNFRβ reveals a highly significant similarity of the extracellular regions when analyzed with the Mutation Data Matrix (Dayhoff et al., 1979). Four conserved domains are clearly delineated by a repetitive pattern of cysteine residues (see Fig. 2). The first two domains of both receptors contain six cysteines with a consensus pattern of $CX_{10-15}CX_{0-2}CX_2CX_{5-11}CX_{3-8}C$. The third and fourth domain each containing six (TNFRβ) or four cysteines (TNFRα) are less well conserved between the two receptors, but the alignement still scores significantly above random

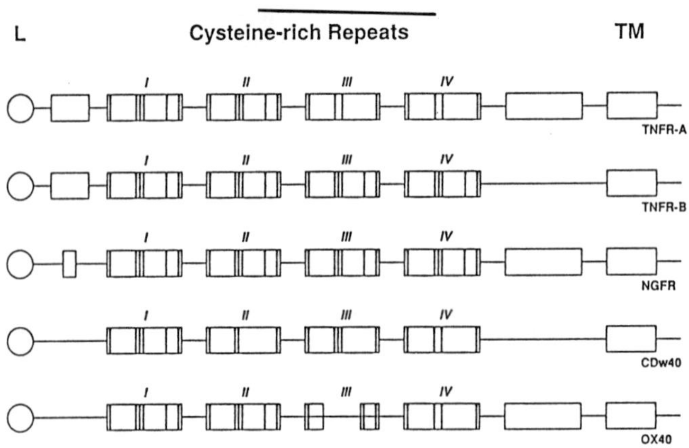

Figure 2. *Schematic Representation of the Domain Structure of the Extracellular Regions of the New Cytokine Receptor Gene Family.* The domains are boxed. Cysteine residues are represented by vertical lines. TNFR-A, TNFRα; TNFR-B, TNFRβ; NGFR, nerve growth factor receptor; CDw40, B cell surface antigen; OX40, surface antigen on activated CD4$^+$ rat T lymphocytes; L and TM, predicted leader and transmembrane regions, respectively.

score with the Mutation Data Matrix. A computer search in protein sequence databases reveals striking sequence similarities to five other known sequences : the human and rat nerve growth factor receptors, the B cell surface antigen CD40, the murine cDNA clone 4-1BB isolated from induced helper and cytolytic T cell clones, the transcriptionally active open reading frame T2 from the Shope fibroma virus, and the OX40 antigen present on activated CD4 positive rat T lymphocytes. However, the highly significant sequence similarity among the proteins mentioned above is restricted to the extracellular and therefore ligand binding regions of the known (TNFRα, TNFRβ, nerve growth factor receptor) and putative (CD40 and OX40) cytokine receptor molecule. It appears that the cysteine-rich extracellular domains of these receptors, presumably heavily disulfide-bonded, form a unique structural architecture defining a novel family of cell surface receptors. In sharp contrast to the high degree of similarity of the extracellular domains, the intracellular regions of the two TNF receptors do not display any obvious sequence similarity to each other nor to any other known mammalian sequence. In particular, similarities to catalytic domains of tyrosine or serine/threonine-specific protein kinases cannot be detected. An interesting feature of the cytoplasmic domain of both TNF receptors is the high content in serine, threonine, and proline. The presence of so-called PEST sequences (Rogers et al., 1986) in intracelluar portions of the TNF receptors might be indicative of rapid intracellular protein degradation leading to a high turnover rate.

REFERENCES

Beutler B, Cerami A (1988).Tumor necrosis, cachexia, shock, and inflammation: A common mediator. Ann Rev Biochem 57: 505 - 518.

Beutler B, Cerami A (1989).The biology of cachectin/TNF. A primary mediator of the host response. Ann Rev Immunol 7: 625 - 655.

Brockhaus M, Schoenfeld H-J, Schlaeger H-J, Hunziker W, Lesslauer W, Loetscher H (1990). Identification of two kinds of TNF receptors on human cell lines by monoclonal antibodies. Proc Natl Acad Sci USA 87: 3127 - 3131.

Dayhoff MO, Schwartz RM, Orcutt BC (1979). A model of evolutionary change in proteins. In: Dayhoff MO (ed.), "Atlas of protein sequence and structure", Vol.5 Suppl.3, Washington D.C: Natl Biomed Res Found, pp 345-362.

Dembic Z, Loetscher H, Gubler U, Pan YCE, Lahm HW, Gentz R, Brockhaus M, Lesslauer W (1990). Two human TNF receptors have similar extracellular, but distinct intracellular domain sequences. Cytokine 2: 231 - 237.

Hohmann H, Remy R, Brockhaus M, van Loon APGM (1989). Two different cell types have different major receptors for human tumor necrosis factor (TNF alpha). J Biol Chem 264: 14927 - 14934.

Hohmann HP, Remy R, Poeschl B, van Loon APGM (1990). TNFα and TNFβ bind to the same two types of TNF receptors and maximally activate the transcription factor NF-κB at low receptor occupancy and within minutes after receptor binding. J Biol Chem 265: 15183-15188.

Loetscher H, Brockhaus M, Dembic Z, Gentz R, Gubler U, Hohmann HP, Lahm HW, van Loon APGM, Pan YCE, Schlaeger EJ, Steinmetz M, Tabuchi H, Lesslauer W (1990a). Two distinct tumor necrosis factor receptors: Members of a new cytokine receptor gene family. In: Maclean N (ed.), "Oxford Surveys on Eukaryotic Genes" Vol.7, Oxford University Press. in the press.

Loetscher H, Pan Y-CE, Lahm H-W, Gentz R, Brockhaus M, Tabuchi H, Lesslauer W (1990b). Molecular Cloning and Expression of the Human 55 kDa TNF Receptor. Cell 61: 351 - 359.

Loetscher H, Schlaeger EJ, Lahm HW, Pan YCE, Lesslauer W, Brockhaus M (1990c). Purification and partial amino acid sequence analysis of two distinct tumor necrosis factor receptors from HL60 cells. J Biol Chem: in the press.

Loetscher H (1991). Purification and structural properties of two distinct TNF receptors on human cells. In: Aggarwal BB Vilcek J (eds.), "Tumor necrosis factors: Structure, function, and mechanisms of action", New York: marcel dekker, Inc. in the press.

Old LJ (1985). Tumor necrosis factor (TNF). Science 230: 630 - 632.

Osborn L, Kunkel S, Nabel GJ (1989). Tumor necrosis factor alpha and interleukin 1 stimulate the human immunodeficiency virus enhancer by activation of the nuclear factor κB. Proc Natl Acad Sci USA 86: 2336-2340.

Pennica D, Nedwin GE, Hayflick JS, Seeburg PH, Derynck R, Palladino MA, Kohr WJ, Aggarwal BB, Goeddel DV (1984). Human tumour necrosis factor:precursor structure, expression and homology to lymphotoxin. Nature 312: 724-729.

Rogers S, Wells R, Rechsteiner M (1986). Amino acid sequences common to rapidly degraded proteins : the PEST hypothesis. Science 234: 364 - 368.

Tracey KJ, Vlassara H, Cerami A (1989). Cachectin/tumor necrosis factor. Lancet I: 1122 - 1125.

Cellular and Cytokine Networks in Tissue Immunity, pages 331-336

INTERLEUKIN 10: A NOVEL T CELL GROWTH COFACTOR

Ian A. MacNeil, Takashi Suda, Kevin W. Moore, Timothy R. Mosmann, Maureen Howard, LuAnn Thompson-Snipes and Albert Zlotnik. DNAX Research Institute, 901 California Ave., Palo Alto, CA 94304.

Within the past few years, a greater understanding has emerged concerning the events which occur as cells differentiate and mature in the thymus. Many studies have focused on the alpha/beta T cell receptor and its interaction with thymic MHC molecules that results in the selection of the T cell repertoire. Less is understood concerning the role of both known and novel cytokines and their effect on T cell maturation.

We recently described a novel activity in the supernatants of several B cell lymphomas (CH12) which enhances the proliferative response of adult and fetal thymocytes to IL2, IL4 and IL7(1, 2). This factor, originally designated B-TCGF(B cell derived T cell growth factor), was shown to be distinct from other known cytokines. Fiorentino et al.(3) have also described a novel activity produced by a Type 2 helper T cell clone (D10-G4.1) that inhibits IFNγ production from Type 1 helper T cell clones and activated spleen cells.They called this activity cytokine synthesis inhibitory factor (CSIF).The presence of CSIF in supernatants from CH12 and the observation that partially purified CSIF has activity in the B-TCGF assay, suggested that the two factors were related. Mosmann et al.(4) have developed a series of neutralizing monoclonal anti-CSIF antibodies. These antibodies were shown to inhibit the thymocyte proliferation-inducing activity of B-TCGF derived from CH12LX.4866 (Figure 1A).

Moore et al. have isolated and expressed complementary DNA clones encoding CSIF and have assigned the designation Interleukin 10 (IL10,(5). Recombinant IL10 (rIL10) is also inhibited by anti-CSIF antibodies (not shown) and has activity in the B-TCGF assay (Figure 1B). Thus, we conclude that the IL10 in CH12 supernatants is responsible for the B-TCGF activity found in the supernatants.

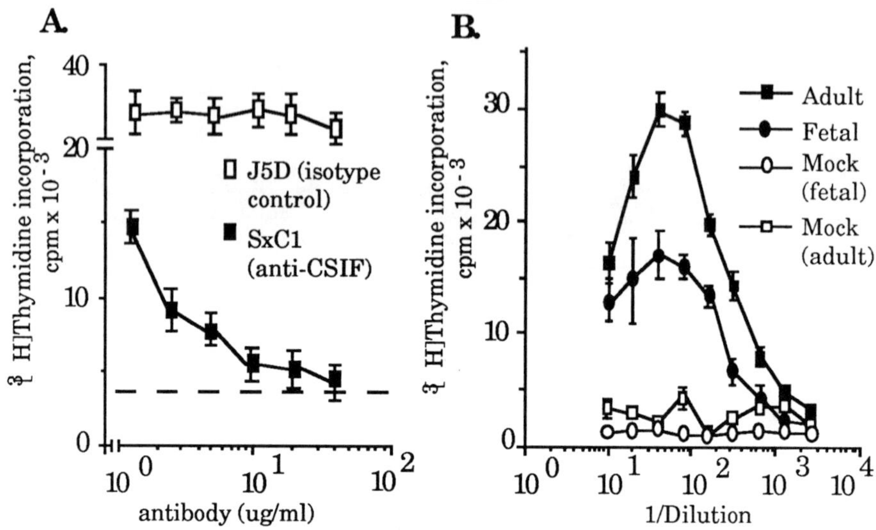

(Source: MacNeil, et al. J. Immunol.)

Figure 1A. Anti-CSIF antibodies inhibit B-TCGF activity. Adult thymocytes were incubated at $5x10^5$/ml with 500 U/ml IL2, 250 U/ml IL4 and B-TCGF (CH12.4866 supernatant diluted 1/6). Anti-CSIF antibody(SXC1, closed squares) or J5D, an unrelated mouse IgM (open squares) was added at the beginning of the culture. Figure 1B. IL10 enhances IL2/IL4 driven proliferation of adult and fetal thymocytes. Adult (squares) and day 15 fetal thymocytes (circles) were incubated as in 1A. Supernatants from IL10 cDNA transfected COS7 cells (closed symbols) or Mock transfected COS7 cells (open symbols) were added at various dilutions. Proliferation was assessed at day 4 by uptake of ^{3}H-Thymidine.

IL10 was also assayed for its ability to induce the proliferation of various thymic subsets. Adult thymocytes and splenocytes were sorted on the basis of CD4 and CD8 surface expression and tested for their response to IL10. As shown in Figure 2A, adult CD4-8-, CD4+8-, and CD4-8+ thymocytes proliferate in response to IL10 in the presence of IL2 and IL4. Adult CD4+8+ thymocytes did not proliferate in response to this combination of cytokines. Fetal thymocytes also exhibited an enhanced response to IL2/IL4 driven proliferation. The response of adult peripheral lymphocytes (lymph node and spleen) was also enhanced by the addition of IL10 although to a lesser degree. Splenic T cells appeared to be responsible for at least part of this response since the proliferation of sorted CD4 and CD8 spleen cells was enhanced by IL10. IL10 alone had no effect on any of the populations tested (not shown).

While the proliferative responses induced by IL10 in various thymocyte populations (especially the immature phenotypes) suggest a role for IL10 in T cell ontogeny, it is also important to demonstrate that this cytokine could be produced by cells present at this stage of development. We were able to detect IL10 in supernatants of thymocytes (including fetal thymocytes) or splenocytes stimulated with either calcium ionophore and phorbol ester, mitogens, or anti-CD3 monoclonal antibodies(1). In contrast, we failed to detect IL10 in supernatants of various cloned stromal cells (derived from either fetal or adult thymus) before or after stimulation with a variety of stimuli. Our inability to detect IL10 production from resting thymocytes suggests that the amounts of IL10 produced in vivo are below the level of detection in our assays; more sensitive methods are currently being tried.

As reported by Moore et al.(5) and Viera et al.(6), mouse and human IL10 are strongly homologous to the EBV open reading frame BCRFI (greater than 70% at the nucleic acid and 85% at the amino acid level for human IL10 and BCRFI). Since both IL10(5,6) and vIL10(BCRFI,7) inhibit IFN g synthesis we tested whether reombinant vIL10 also enhanced thymocyte proliferation. As shown in Figure 2B, recombinant vIL10 was unable to enhance the proliferation of adult murine thymocytes to IL2 and IL4, however human IL10 was active. Addition of vIL10 to cultures containing IL2+IL4+IL10 also had no effect on proliferation (data not shown). This inability of vIL10 to act as a growth stimulus is paralleled in other systems where IL10 is active such as B cell class II induction (8) and mast cell growth co-stimulation(6,9).

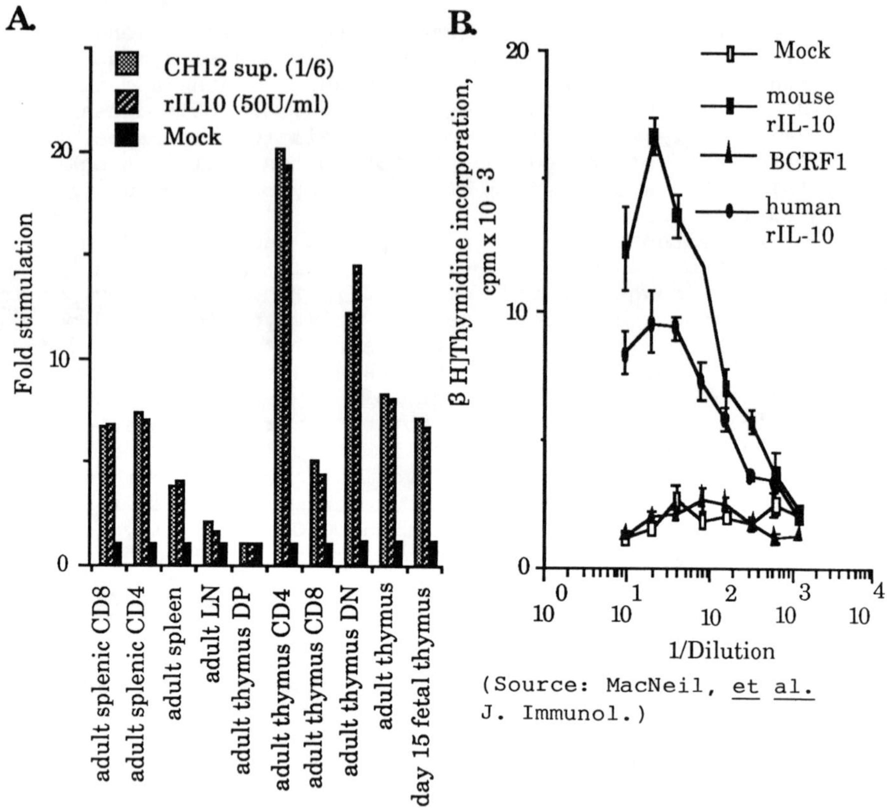

(Source: MacNeil, _et_ _al._ J. Immunol.)

Figure 2A. IL10 enhances IL2/IL4 driven proliferation of various adult and fetal T cell subsets. Cells were sorted on a Becton Dickinson FACSTAR-Plus as previously described (1). Supernatants from CH12, IL10 cDNA transfected COS7 cells (50 U/ml) or Mock transfected COS7 cells were added. Proliferation was expressed as fold stimulation over IL2 and IL4 alone. Figure 2B. Human IL10 but not vIL10 enhances the IL2/IL4 driven proliferation of murine adult thymocytes. mIL10 (closed squares), vIL10 (closed triangle), human IL10 (closed circle) or supernatant from Mock transfected COS7 cells (open squares) were added at various dilutions. Proliferation was assessed at day 4 via uptake of ^{3}H-Thymidine.

The pleiotropic nature of IL10 (Table 1) and its similarity to a viral product suggest that vIL10 may represent a captured cellular IL10 gene which has lost the ability to stimulate the immune system but retains the ability to inhibit IFNγ synthesis and potentially promote survival of the virus.

Table 1. Functional Relationship between IL10 and vIL10

Property	IL10	vIL10
1. CSIF activity	+	+
2. thymocyte co-stimulation	+	–
3. B cell class II induction	+	–
4. B cell viability enhancement	+	+
5. mast cell co-stimulation	+	–

These observations also suggest that IL10 may play a role in T cell ontogeny in the thymus. However, its effects on T cell growth are not restricted to thymocytes. IL10 can also enhance the proliferation of peripheral lymphocytes(1). While IL10 was originally described as a cytokine that inhibits IFNγ production by type 1 T helper cell clones and was therefore thought of as a cytokine capable of inhibiting certain T cell responses, its effects on T cell growth imply a second potential role in the expansion and/or activation of T cells during immune responses. Moreover, evidence presented by Fiorentino et al. (3) suggests that IL10 acts indirectly, via antigen presenting cells, to inhibit cytokine synthesis. However, since for many experiments we used sorted thymocytes and splenic lymphocytes, our data indicate that IL10 can act directly on T cells to stimulate a proliferative response. Future experiments will aim at clarifying the role of IL10 in T cell ontogeny and in the regulation of immune responses.

REFERENCES

1. MacNeil IA, Suda T, Moore KW, Mosmann TR, Zlotnik A (1990). Interleukin 10: A novel growth cofactor for mature and immature T cells. J.Immunol. In Press.
2. Suda T, O'Garra A, MacNeil I, Fischer M, Bond M, Zlotnik A (1990). Identification of a novel thymocyte growth promoting factor derived from B cell lymphomas. Cell. Immunol. 129:228-240.
3. Fiorentino D, Bond M, Mosmann T (1989). Two types of mouse helper T cells. IV. Th2 clones secrete a factor that inhibits cytokine production by Th1 clones. J. Exp. Med. 170:2081-2095.
4. Mosmann TR, Schumacher JH, Fiorentino DF, Leverah J, Moore KW, Bond MW (1990). Production of Mabs specific for a novel cytokine, Cytokine Synthesis Inhibition Factor (CSIF), as well as IL-4, IL-5, and IL-6, using a solid phase radioimmunosorbant assay: Isolation of blocking and nonblocking anti-CSIF Mabs. J. Immunol. 145:2938-2945.
5. Moore K, Vieira P, Fiorentino D, Trounstine M, Khan T, Mossmann T (1990). Homology of Cytokine Synthesis Inhibition Factor (IL-10) to Epstein-Barr Virus gene BCRFI. Science 248:1230-1234.
6. Vieira P, deWaal-Malefyt R, Dang M-N, Johnson KE, Kastelein R, Fiorentino DF, deVries JE, Roncorola M-G, Mosmann TR, Moore KW (1991). Isolation and expression of human cytokine synthesis inhibitory factor (CSIF/IL10) cDNA clones: homology to Epstein-Barr virus open reading frame BCRFI. Proc. Natl. Acad. Sci. USA In Press.
7. Hsu D, Malefyt R, Fiorentino D, Dang M, Vieira P, deVries J, Spits H, Mosmann T, Moore K (1990). Expression of IL10 activity by Epstein-Barr virus protein BCRFI. Science In Press.
8. Go N, Castle B, Barrett R, Kastelein R, Dang W, Mosmann T, Moore KW, Howard M (1990). Interleukin 10 (IL10), A Novel B cell stimulatory Factor: Unresponsiveness of "XID" B cells. J. Exp. Med. In Press.
9. Thompson-Snipes L, Dhar V, Bond MW, Mosmann TR, Moore KW, Rennick D (1990). Interleukin 10, A novel stimulatory factor for mast cells and their progenitors. Submitted for publication.

Cellular and Cytokine Networks in Tissue Immunity, pages 337-344

MOLECULAR ANALYSIS OF THE STRUCTURE AND FUNCTION OF THE HUMAN INTERFERON-GAMMA RECEPTOR

Robert D. Schreiber, Michael A. Farrar, Jose Fernandez-Luna, Gurjit Khurana Hershey, and Patrick W. Gray.

Department of Pathology, Washington University School of Medicine, St. Louis, MO 63105 and Genentech Inc, South San Francisco, CA 94080.

INTRODUCTION

It is now well established that IFNγ exerts its pleotropic effects on cells by interacting with a specific receptor expressed at the target cell surface. During the past 5 years, several laboratories have focused their efforts on studying IFNγ receptors on both human and murine cells (1-3). This work has provided a great deal of information concerning the structure and function of these proteins. Today we know that IFNγ receptors are 85-95 kDa single chained glycoproteins that are heavily glycosylated with N- and possibly O-linked oligosaccharides. Immunochemical analyses indicate that there is only one type of IFNγ receptor although receptors from different cells display modest (5-10 kDa) molecular weight heterogeneity due to cell-specific differences in N-linked glycosylation. IFNγ receptors are expressed at modest levels (1000-25,000 sites/cell) on nearly all cell types, with erythrocytes being the only normal cell found thus far that is devoid of receptor. IFNγ receptors bind ligand with high affinity in a totally species specific manner, i.e. human IFNγ binds only to the human IFNγ receptor and not to the murine IFNγ receptor, while murine IFNγ binds only to the murine receptor and not the human receptor. At physiologic temperatures, the receptor-ligand complex is internalized and traffics into an intracellular compartment where ligand dissociates and eventually is processed and degraded (1). Free receptors enter an intracellular pool and eventually recycle back to the cell surface.

Recently the complete primary structure of the human IFNγ receptor was elucidated following the purification of the protein and the cloning of its cDNA (4-7). The human IFNγ receptor is encoded by a 2.3 kb cDNA that gives rise to a 484 amino acid polypeptide containing a 17 amino acid signal sequence. The mature 472 amino acid polypeptide contains glutamic acid at its N-terminus and has a predicted Mr of 52.5 kDa. The molecule is symmetrically orientated around a single 21 amino acid transmembrane domain. The extracellular domain contains 229 amino acids including 10 cysteine residues. There are 5 N-linked glycosylation sites in this portion of the molecule and N-linked sugars contribute approximately 25 kDa to the apparent molecular weight of the fully mature receptor. In addition, there are 2 serine/threonine rich regions in the extracellular domain, one near the N-terminus and one near the membrane, that may serve as attachment sites for 0-linked oligosaccharides. The protein has a large, intracellular domain which consists of 220 amino acids. Interestingly, the intracellular domain of the human IFNγ receptor contains a high percentage (24%) of serine and threonine residues, and some of these residues are phosphorylated following interaction of the receptor with IFNγ in intact cells (8).

The availability of the human IFNγ receptor cDNA allowed several groups to examine whether this single polypeptide was both necessary and sufficient to generate a functional receptor system in the context of a heterologous cell. In the current paper, we review recent data that demonstrate the need for a second human component to form a functionally active human IFNγ receptor.

RESULTS

Demonstration that the IFNγ Receptor Polypeptide Is Not Sufficient to Form a Functionally Active Receptor in Heterologous Cells.

In order to assess the capacity of the human IFNγ receptor to induce biologic responses in cells we took advantage of the species specificity that human and murine IFNγ show in their interaction with their appropriate receptors and their ability to stimulate functional responses in human and murine cells. Murine L cells were stably transfected with an expression vector that contained the human IFNγ receptor cDNA, selected by G418 resistance, and then analyzed for receptor expression by FACS using one of our monoclonal antibodies specific for the extracellular domain of the human IFNγ receptor. Approximately 25% of the selected transfected cells stained modestly but specifically for the expression of the human IFNγ receptor. After repeated cycles of sorting and expansion, a homogeneous cell population was obtained that by Scatchard analysis using radiolabeled human or murine IFNγ expressed approximately 3500 natural murine IFNγ receptors and 22,500 recombinant human IFNγ receptors per cell. No binding of either human IFNγ nor the human IFNγ receptor specific antibody was detectable on nontransfected cells. Yet despite the expression of human IFNγ receptors in murine cells, the transfected fibroblasts remained responsive to murine IFNγ and not to human IFNγ as detected by monitoring IFNγ-dependent upregulation of MHC Class I antigen expression by flow cytometry. As expected the transfected murine L cells expressed MHC Class I antigen constitutively. However, although Class I expression was significantly augmented following incubation of the cells for 72 hr with homologous murine IFNγ, no upregulation of Class I was seen when transfected cells were incubated with human IFNγ. Thus, although expression of the human IFNγ receptor polypeptide was necessary to confer human IFNγ binding activity to murine cells, it was not sufficient to promote responsiveness to human IFNγ.

We therefore considered two possibilities that might explain this result: (1) that unresponsiveness was due to limiting expression of the human IFNγ receptor in murine cells, or (2) that formation of a functionally active human IFNγ receptor in the context of a murine cell required at least one additional human cellular component. The latter possibility had already been suggested by Jung et. al. (9) in 1987 based on cell fusion experiments. In these earlier studies, these investigators noted that when murine and human fibroblasts were fused, the resulting hybrids expressed a full complement of murine chromosomes but only some human chromosomes. All cells expressing human chromosome 6 bound human IFNγ suggesting that the IFNγ receptor gene was located on human chromosome 6. (This hypothesis was eventually confirmed by Merlin et. al. (10) who showed using *in situ* hybridization techniques that the receptor gene is located at 6q23.) However, hybrids that responded to human IFNγ showed an obligatory requirement for an additional human chromosome: chromosome 21. Based on these results these investigators concluded that formation of a functionally active human IFNγ receptor in the context of rodent cells required at least two human components: the receptor itself and a second accessory molecule.

Cloning and Expression of the Murine IFNγ Receptor cDNA.

We decided to analyze the most straightforward possibility first and determine whether the lack of responsiveness in the transfected murine cells was caused by the limited expression of the recombinant human IFNγ receptor. We approached this issue by cloning the cDNA for the murine IFNγ receptor and determining whether we could obtain high level expression of the murine protein in human cells (7). Using probes derived from the 3' and 5' ends of the human IFNγ receptor cDNA, we isolated and sequenced a 2.3 kb murine cDNA clone derived from a murine T cell hybridoma cDNA library that encoded the full length murine IFNγ receptor. A comparison of the predicted structures of the human and murine IFNγ receptors revealed that the two proteins were of similar size and had a similar molecular organization. They both consisted of nearly equivalent sized extracellular and intracellular domains that were separated by a single transmembrane domain of 21-23 amino acids. The extracellular domains of each protein contained the same number of N-linked glycosylation sites and the same two serine/threonine rich regions that could act as potential acceptor sites for 0-linked sugar addition. The intracellular domains of both proteins were extremely rich in serine/threonine residues and both proteins were phosphorylated following interaction with ligand in cells that express active IFNγ receptors. Yet despite the overall homology of protein structure, the two proteins displayed only modest (52%) homology at the amino acid sequence level. We found it particularly interesting that the relatively low level of sequence homology extended along the entire length of the two proteins and especially throughout the receptors' intracellular domains. This observation raised the possibility that the intracellular domains of the receptors were also involved in some form of species-specific interaction.

As we had hoped, the murine IFNγ receptor could be expressed at high levels in heterologous cells (7). Radioligand binding analyses performed on human 293 fibroblasts stably transfected with the murine IFNγ receptor cDNA showed that the transfected cells expressed 570,000 murine IFNγ receptors/cell and bound ligand with an affinity (1×10^9 M^{-1}) that was indistinguishable from the natural murine IFNγ receptor in the context of authentic murine cells. Biosynthetic labeling analysis of the expressed murine protein confirmed that it displayed the appropriate molecular weight. Finally, the recombinant murine receptor directed the internalization and degradation of murine IFNγ in a normal manner. Thus, based on these criteria, the recombinant murine IFNγ receptor appeared to be indistinguishable from its normal murine counterpart in authentic murine cells.

Since we had now been able to achieve the high level expression of murine IFNγ receptors in human cells, we returned to the issue of functional activity of recombinant receptors in heterologous cells and asked whether the deficiency could be overcome in cells that expressed high levels of receptor (7). For these experiments we monitored the ability of human or murine IFNγ to enhance MHC Class I antigen expression on the transfected human 293 cells. As expected, the human cells responded normally to their homologous human ligand and displayed a dose and time dependent increase in MHC Class I expression. In most experiments, human IFNγ (at concentrations of 100-1000 units/ml) produced nearly a doubling of HLA-A,B,C antigen expression. In contrast, the cells did not respond to any dose of murine IFNγ for any stimulation time tested despite the fact that these cells expressed 150 times more murine IFNγ receptor than human receptor. Similar results were obtained when we monitored induction of IFNγ-dependent anti-viral activity in these cells, i.e. the cells responded only to the homologous human ligand and not to murine IFNγ. Moreover, identical results were also obtained using a different transfected human cell line (Colo-205) that expressed more physiologic levels of the recombinant murine IFNγ receptor. Finally, similar observations were made simultaneously by three other groups working independently (11-13). Thus based on these experiments, we were able to rule out the possibility that the unresponsiveness of recombinant IFNγ receptors in heterologous cells was due to inadequate levels of receptor expression.

Demonstration that a Second Human Protein Was Required to Form A Functionally Active Human IFNγ Receptor in Murine Cells.

Based on the aforementioned data we considered the alternative possibility that an additional receptor component was needed to form a functionally active IFNγ receptor and that this component had to be species matched to the ligand binding protein. Based on the work of Jung et. al. (9) described above, we decided to examine whether a functionally active human IFNγ receptor could be constructed by transfecting the human receptor cDNA into a murine L cell that contained a single copy of human chromosome 21 (14). This cell line, denoted SCC16-5, was first characterized before transfection. As expected, SCC16-5 expressed murine IFNγ receptors and not human IFNγ receptors and responded (enhanced MHC Class I expression) only to murine IFNγ and not human IFNγ. Thus, by these criteria, SCC16-5 are identical with their normal murine L cell counterparts. To test for the expression of human chromosome 21 in SCC16-5, we took advantage of the fact that the gene for the human IFN–alpha receptor is also located on human chromosome 21 and we therefore determined whether SCC16-5 responded to a subclass of human IFNα, that was totally species specific. In fact, SCC16-5 responded (enhanced MHC Class I expression) to both species specific and non-species specific forms of IFN-alpha thereby demonstrating the presence of chromosome 21 in the cell line. The specificity of the induction was confirmed since normal L cells did not respond to the species specific form of IFNα.

SCC16-5 and normal L cells were then stably transfected with the human IFNγ receptor cDNA and receptor expression confirmed on both cell lines by FACS-, Scatchard- and surface labeling-analyses. As discussed above, expression of the human IFNγ receptor in normal murine L cells resulted in the generation of a receptor that, although it could bind and internalize human IFNγ, was unable to induce a cellular response (enhanced MHC Class I expression) to it. In contrast, a functionally active human IFNγ receptor was formed when the human IFNγ receptor cDNA was stably expressed in SCC16-5. Transfected SCC16-5 incubated with human IFNγ for 72 hr showed a 43 channel increase in MHC Class I staining as compared to cells incubated for the same time period in medium alone. Significantly, the response of the transfected SCC16-5 cell line to *human* IFNγ was indistinguishable from the response of the cells to their homologous *murine* ligand (48 channel shift). Thus, formation of a functionally active human IFNγ receptor in murine cells requires the presence of an accessory molecule, encoded by a gene on human chromosome 21, that collaborates with the IFNγ receptor polypeptide in a species specific manner.

SUMMARY

The results presented herein show that human and murine IFNγ receptors are 85-95 kDa, single chain glycoproteins that contain a single transmembrane domain located in the approximate middle of the molecule. The cDNAs for both proteins have been cloned, sequenced, and expressed. The IFNγ receptor polypeptide is required for ligand binding by cells. However, formation of a functionally active human IFNγ receptor in murine cells requires the additional presence of a gene product encoded on human chromosome 21. We are currently attempting to characterize the accessory molecule at the molecular level and determine the structure-function relationships that exist with the intracellular and extracellular domains of the IFNγ receptor.

REFERENCES

1. Celada A, Allen R, Esparza I, Gray PW, Schreiber RD (1985). Demonstration and partial characterization of the interferon-gamma receptor on human mononuclear phagocytes. J Clin Invest 76:2196-2205.
2. Rubinstein M, Novick D, Fischer DG (1987). The human interferon-gamma receptor system. Immunol Rev 97:29-50.
3. Langer JA, Pestka S (1988). Interferon Receptors. Immunol Today 9:393-400.
4. Aguet M, Merlin G (1987) Purification of human γ interferon receptors by sequential affinity chromatography on immobilized monoclonal

antireceptor antibodies and human γ interferon. J Exp Med 165:988-999.

5. Calderon J, Sheehan KCF, Chance C, Thomas ML, and Schreiber RD (1988). Purification and characterization of the human interferon-gamma receptor from placenta. Proc Natl Acad Sci (USA) 85:4837-4841.

6. Aguet M, Dembic Z, Merlin G (1988). Molecular cloning and expression of the human interferon-γ receptor. Cell 55:273-280.

7. Gray PW, Leong S, Fennie EH, Farrar MA, Pingel JT, Fernandez-Luna J, Schreiber RD (1989). Cloning and expression of the cDNA for the murine interferon γ receptor. Proc Natl Acad Sci (USA) 86:8597-8501.

8. Khurana Hershey GK, McCourt DW, Schreiber RD (1990). Ligand-induced phosphorylation of the human interferon-γ receptor: dependence on the presence of a functionally active receptor. J Biol Chem 265:17868-17875.

9. Jung V, Rashidbaigi A, Jones C, Tischfeld JA, Shows TB, Pestka S (1987). Human chromosomes 6 and 21 are required for sensitivity to human interferon γ. Proc Natl Acad Sci (USA) 84:4151-4155.

10. Merlin G, Van der Leede B-J, Aguet M, Dembic Z (1989). The human interferon gamma receptor gene. J Interferon Res 9:S89.

11. Kumar CS, Muthukumaran G, Frost LJ, Noe M, Ahn YH, Mariano TM, Pestka S (1989). Molecular characterization of the murine interferon γ receptor cDNA. J Biol Chem 264:17939-17946.

12. Munro S, Maniatis T (1989) Expression cloning of the murine interferon γ receptor cDNA. Proc Natl Acad Sci (USA) 86:9248-9252.

13. Hemmi S, Peghini P, Metzler M, Merlin G, Dembic Z, Aguet M (1989). Cloning of murine interferon γ receptor cDNA: Expression in human cells mediates high-affinity binding but is not sufficient to confer sensitivity to murine interferon γ. Proc Natl Acad Sci (USA) 86:9901-9905.

14. Farrar MA, Fernandez-Luna J, Schreiber RD (1990). A molecular analysis of the structure and function of the human interferon gamma receptor. J Interferon Res 10:S171.

Index